Medicines Management for Clinical Nurses

Edited by

Karen A. Luker
*Professor of Nursing, School of Nursing, Midwifery and Health Visiting,
University of Manchester*

David J. Wolfson
*Director, Mersey Academic Pharmacy Practice Unit,
Liverpool John Moores University*

**Blackwell
Science**

615. 14 MED

© 1999 by
Blackwell Science Ltd
Editorial Offices:
Osney Mead, Oxford OX2 0EL
25 John Street, London WC1N 2BL
23 Ainslie Place, Edinburgh EH3 6AJ
350 Main Street, Malden
    MA 02148 5018, USA
54 University Street, Carlton
    Victoria 3053, Australia
10, rue Casimir Delavigne
    75006 Paris, France

Other Editorial Offices:

Blackwell Wissenschafts-Verlag GmbH
Kurfürstendamm 57
10707 Berlin, Germany

Blackwell Science KK
MG Kodenmacho Building
7–10 Kodenmacho Nihombashi
Chuo-ku, Tokyo 104, Japan

The right of the Author to be identified as the
Author of this Work has been asserted in
accordance with the Copyright, Designs and
Patents Act 1988

First published 1999

Set in 10/12.5 pt Palatino
by DP Photosetting, Aylesbury, Bucks
Printed and bound in Great Britain by
The University Press, Cambridge

The Blackwell Science logo is a trade mark of
Blackwell Science Ltd, registered at the United
Kingdom Trade Marks Registry

DISTRIBUTORS

  Marston Book Services Ltd
  PO Box 269
  Abingdon
  Oxon OX14 4YN
  (Orders: Tel: 01235 465500
                  Fax: 01235 465555)

USA
  Blackwell Science, Inc.
  Commerce Place
  350 Main Street
  Malden, MA 02148 5018
  (Orders: Tel: 800 759 6102
                        781 388 8250
              Fax: 781 388 8255)

Canada
  Login Brothers Book Company
  324 Saulteaux Crescent
  Winnipeg, Manitoba R3J 3T2
  (Orders: Tel: 204 837 2987
                  Fax: 204 837 3116)

Australia
  Blackwell Science Pty Ltd
  54 University Street
  Carlton, Victoria 3053
  (Orders: Tel: 03 9347 0300
                  Fax: 03 9347 5001)

A catalogue record for this title
is available from the British Library

ISBN 0-632-04247-8

Library of Congress
Cataloging-in-Publication Data
Medicines management for clinical nurses/
    edited by Karen A. Luker and David J.
    Wolfson
        p. cm.
    Includes bibliographical references and
    index.
    ISBN 0-632-04247-8 (pbk.)
    1. Drugs – Administration.   2. Nursing.
    I. Luker, Karen A.
    II. Wolfson, David J.
    [DNLM: 1. Pharmacology nurses'
instruction.   2. Drug Therapy – nursing.
3. Prescriptions, Drug nurses' instruction.
4. Nurse Clinicians.   QV 4M489 1998]
615'.1'024613 – dc21
DNLM/DLC
for Library of Congress   98-35983
                                                          CIP

For further information on Blackwell Science,
visit our website: www.blackwell-science.com

This book is intended to help nurses understand drug protocols and the management of
patients under given drug regimes. This book should not be used as a prime source of
prescribing and dispensing drugs. The Editors, Contributors and Publishers have
undertaken reasonable endeavours to check medicines information and nursing content
for accuracy. Because the science of clinical pharmacology is continually advancing, our
knowledge base continues to expand. Therefore, the reader should always check the
manufacturer's product information before administering any medication.

Contents

List of Contributors

Lynn Austin RGN, MSc   Research Fellow, School of Nursing, Midwifery and Health Visiting, University of Manchester.

Christopher C. Braidwood BSc, MRPharmS   Chief Pharmacist, Whiston Hospital, St Helens and Knowsley Hospitals Trust, and Honorary Senior Teaching Fellow, School of Continuing Education, University of Leeds.

Adrian Brown BPharm, MSc, MRPharmS, MCPP   Chief Pharmacist, Pharmacy Department, Southport and Formby NHS Trust.

Neil A. Caldwell BSc(Hons), MSc, MRPharmS   Principal Pharmacist/ Lecturer, School of Pharmacy and Chemistry, Liverpool John Moores University, and Department of Pharmacy, Wirral Hospital NHS Trust.

Barbara Dicks BA, MBA, RGN, RM   Director, Mild May UK.

Simon Gelder BSc(Hons), MRPharmS   Deputy Chief Pharmacist and Drug Information Procurement Pharmacist, Whiston Hospital, St Helens and Knowsley Hospitals Trust.

Chris Green BSc(Hons), MRPharmS, DipClinPharm   Research Pharmacist, School of Pharmacy and Chemistry, Liverpool John Moores University.

Ross Lynton Groves BSc(Hons), MRPharmS   Community Pharmacist and Facilitator in Continuing Education, North-west England.

Nicholas W. Hough BPharm, MSc, MRPharmS   International Promotional Affairs Manager, Zeneca Pharmaceuticals. Formerly Director of MeReC (Medicines Resource Centre), Liverpool.

Michael P. Jackson MPSNI   Clinical Pharmacist, Belfast City Hospital.

Margaret Ling BA(Hons), MA   Lecturer in Medical Sociology, Department of Primary Care, University of Liverpool.

Karen A. Luker BNurs, PhD   Professor of Nursing, School of Nursing, Midwifery and Health Visiting, University of Manchester.

Mark Pilling BPharm, MPhil   Kirkby Locality Pharmaceutical Advisor, St Helens and Knowsley Health Authority.

Christine R. Proudlove BPharm, MSc, MRPharmS, MCPP, DipPressSci
Senior Information Pharmacist, The Infirmary, Liverpool.

John A. Sexton BPharm(Hons), MRPharmS, DipClinPharm, MSc, MCPP
Senior Pharmacist Lecturer-Practitioner, Royal Liverpool University Hospital,
and School of Pharmacy, Liverpool John Moores University.

Katrina Simister BPharm, MRPharmS   Principal Pharmacist, Drug
Information, The Infirmary, Liverpool.

Tracey Thornton BSc(Hons), MSc, MRPharmS   Senior Pharmacist – Clinical
Services, Whiston Hospital, St Helens and Knowsley Hospitals Trust.

David J. Wolfson BSc, PhD, FRPharmS, MIPharmM   Director, Mersey
Academic Pharmacy Practice Unit, Liverpool John Moores University.

Introduction

During this decade, as a consequence of the National Health Service (NHS) and Community Care Act 1990, there have been unprecedented changes in the way health care is organised and delivered. The most significant change in the modernisation of the health service has been the introduction of a market economy with health care purchasers and providers. The introduction of fund holding general practitioners, with a budget to purchase health care for their patients from provider units in hospitals, introduced an inequitable, and some would say a two-tier, system of health care into the NHS.

The structural changes in the NHS, introduced within a quasi-market ideology, have highlighted the centrality of the service user and the need for health care professionals to be more aware of the cost of health care and the need for cost containment through investment in cost effective practices. Nowhere is cost effectiveness more important than in prescribing and administration of medicines; containing the national drugs bill has been one of the biggest challenges for the government for a number of years.

In addition to structural changes, the traditional boundaries between the work of doctors, nurses and other health care workers have been reconfigured. These boundary changes have been driven by technological advances in the field of medicine, the need to achieve value for money for service users, and the aspirations of nursing and allied health professionals to extend their sphere of influence. The phasing-in of a shorter working week for junior doctors has provided additional impetus for nurses to extend their sphere of work into the domain previously considered to be the prerogative of doctors (Greenhalgh & Co. Ltd, 1994). The amendment to the Medicines Act in 1994 to enable community nurses with the relevant training to prescribe a range of products detailed in the *Nurse Prescribers' Formulary*, an appendix to the *British National Formulary* (reproduced in Appendix 1), is a clear indication of extending boundaries. In addition the Department of Health, through the appointment of a National Director of Research and Development, has moved the NHS towards the goal of evidence-based practice. In nursing, this has meant that the knowledge base of practice has come under scrutiny and has provided an impetus for nurses to study at higher degree level.

The United Kingdom Central Council (UKCC, 1992), in its documents on the scope of professional practice, endorsed the expanding role of the nurse but placed a clear emphasis on education for practice, in terms of appropriate skills and knowledge, to undertake new clinical activities. This document, along with the other developments detailed above, has acted as a catalyst to a proliferation of courses to prepare nurses to work at a more advanced level. Clearly, what can be achieved at an advanced level is constrained by the knowledge base of initial nurse preparation. The nursing profession cannot reach a consensus on an all graduate entry; hence the vast majority of nurses are only educated to diploma level. Provision of courses for advanced practice roles such as Nurse Practitioner is variable, and a review of the literature indicates a number of weaknesses, for example a lack of depth in the study of biological sciences including anatomy, physiology and pathology (Department of Health, 1989). There is also an inadequate amount of pharmacology in basic nurse training, and nurses often exhibit a low level of knowledge in drug therapy (Hampson, 1986).

The idea for this text arose because of a course innovation at the University of Liverpool where the first MSc designed to prepare Nurse Practitioners was introduced. The curriculum related to this programme is detailed elsewhere (see Gibbon & Luker, 1995). Suffice it to say here that one of the core modules for the course was pharmacology. In addition to providing the knowledge and skills necessary for limited prescribing and wide administration of drugs, the module aimed to place pharmacology in its political, social, regulatory and practical framework, and it soon became apparent that there was no single textbook suited to this purpose. Many of the authors of the chapters in this book were contributors to the original pharmacology module.

Medicines Management for Clinical Nurses is not a traditional pharmacology book. However, the traditional topics of pharmacology teaching are presented; for example, pharmacodynamics and pharmacokinetics. The emphasis in these chapters is on the responsibility of the nurse in the safe handling and administration of medicines. We use the term 'medicines' to reflect the fact that chemicals are formulated into medicines and due attention must be paid to the impact that different formulations have on individual patients. Whilst the book was written with advanced level practice in mind it will also be relevant to student nurses who want to know more about safe and effective medicines administration. All nurses are responsible for making sure that patients understand what medicines they are taking and why, including the likely side effects. According to Courtenay and Butler (1997), nurses need a thorough understanding of pharmacology including pharmacodynamics and pharma-cokinetics.

The increasing complexity of prescribing means that medicines adminis-tration is no longer a mechanistic response to the doctor's prescription; rather it requires thought and the exercise of professional judgement. Notwithstanding initial prescribing and protocol prescribing, it is also the case that nurses have an important role to play in educating patients and monitoring them for adverse drug reactions.

The book is loosely arranged into themes. The first part of the book examines the medicines' environment and it begins with the structures required to facilitate effective prescribing. It encompasses issues such as value for money, drug budgets, formularies and prescribing initiatives. This section introduces the NHS and some of the reference sources that are available to underpin safe prescribing and administration of medicines. Case management and high technology treatments are introduced. Chapter 2 entitled Policies and Practice, introduces a critical appraisal of advisory sources and their limitations.

The second theme deals with patients' considerations. Chapter 3 describes the absorption, distribution, metabolism and elimination of drugs in the body. A discussion of patient compliance serves to emphasise the importance of human behaviour in the success of the chemical process. That theme is taken further in Chapter 4, which examines the impact of age, pregnancy, disease and food on drug action. The functions of the liver and kidneys, introduced in the previous chapter, are described in more detail. The impact of tobacco smoking and alcohol is also described in Chapter 4. Those topics remind us that the social needs of the individual play a clear role in his or her behaviour related to medicines, and that theme is dealt with in depth in Chapter 5, the Patient's role in Optimising Treatment. It begins with the concept of self-medication and examines autonomy, normality, medication as food, compliance and patients' beliefs.

The third theme is that of medicines' prescribing. The factors influencing prescribing are described in Chapter 6. Beginning with the skills used in prescribing, the chapter introduces the roles of expert advisers, drug marketing, drug promotion, drug samples and the media. Clinical examination, drug history and clinical trials are described. Placebos, consent and ethics committees are introduced.

Those medicines obtained without the need for a prescription are the subject of Chapter 7, which introduces the legal framework. No analysis of bought medication would be complete without comments on drug abuse and drug misuse. Major categories of self-administered medicines, including analgesics, antacids, laxatives, antidiarrhoeals, 'cold' remedies, antitussives, antihistamines, topical products, hypnotics and vitamins, are described.

Chapter 8, entitled The Nurse's Role in Prescribing, presents the background to the nurse's role in prescribing and the legislative and administrative changes which have enabled community nurses to prescribe. The items included in the *Nurse Prescribers' Formulary* are described in detail, with some indications for use and side effects. In addition, protocol prescribing by nurses in the hospital setting is explored in terms of its legal framework and its potential for enhancing patient care.

Chapters 9 and 10 complete the prescribing scenario. Chapter 9 looks at prescribed medicines in primary care (general practice). Three specific but controversial therapeutic areas have been chosen to highlight the difficulties that GPs have in deciding which medicines to prescribe, namely acid suppressants, hypertension and non-steroidal anti-inflammatory drugs. Repeat prescribing, bulk prescriptions and prescribing for addicts are subjects on which some people require guidance, and are therefore included in this chapter.

Chapter 10 looks at prescribed medicines in secondary care. The emphasis is on general principles and practical elements of hospital prescribing with reference to five therapeutic areas led by, or mainly carried out in, hospital. The areas covered are anti-infective agents, anti-cancer drugs, cardiovascular agents, respiratory conditions and gastro-intestinal agents.

The fourth theme deals with medicines administration. Chapter 11 examines the legal and procedural framework within which nurses administer medicines. Among the topics described are the Medicines Act, the Misuse of Drugs Act, the Poisons Act, the Health and Safety at Work Act, the NHS and Community Care Act, the Aitken Report, the Gillie Report, the Roxburgh Report, the Duthie Report and the Breckenridge Report. Prescription forms, patients' own medicines and the regulatory framework surrounding the storage, handling and administration of medicines are described, and the background to unlicensed medicines and in-patient self-medication schemes are given.

Chapter 12 continues the topic of the nurse's role in medicines administration with an examination of the operational and practical factors. Topics covered include sources of administration error, names of medicines, strengths, forms, routes, rates and times. Parenteral therapy, fluid, electrolyte and cytotoxic administration, syringe drivers, topical and inhaled medication are included.

The patient's response is the fifth theme and is dealt with in Chapters 13 and 14. Chapter 13 is on the subject of adverse drug reactions (ADRs). No drug is free of side effects and the nurse can play a significant role in ADR monitoring. Nurses monitor patients at risk of ADRs; they monitor drugs with known toxic effects and newly marketed medicines. The chapter describes pharmacovigilance, post-marketing surveillance and the yellow card scheme. The impact of the patient's age, concurrent disease state, gender, race and genetic factors are examined.

Drug interactions is the topic of Chapter 14. An interaction occurs when the effects of one drug are changed by the presence of another drug, chemical, environmental agent or food. Since interactions may be harmful, the clinical nurse can play a pivotal role in minimising potential toxicity and optimising outcomes. The topics covered in this chapter should equip readers to play an important role in improving patient treatment.

The text is completed by inclusion of two appendices. The first is the Nurse Prescribers' Formulary. The second is Adverse Drug Reactions arranged according to body system.

As clinical care becomes more evidence based and medicines management comes under closer scrutiny, this book will become an essential text for the clinical nurse. In the context of community nursing, the white paper, *The New NHS* (SOSH, 1997), clearly indicates that the boundaries between medicine and nursing will continue to overlap and be reconfigured. General practitioners will no longer enjoy a non-cash limited prescribing budget. Nurse prescribing in the community will roll out on a larger scale during 1998 and cost effective prescribing will be the cornerstone of practice. In addition, it is anticipated that initial prescribing may be extended to other groups of nurses who undertake the relevant training. It is hoped that this textbook will become an important source of reference for nurses in any sphere of practice.

Karen A. Luker and David J. Wolfson

References

Courtenay, M. & Butler, M. (1997) Nurse prescribing – the knowledge base. *Nursing Times* **94** (1), 40–1.

Department of Health (1989) *Report of the Advisory Group on Nurse Prescribing*. HMSO, London.

Gibbon, B. & Luker, K. (1995) Uncharted territory: masters preparation as a foundation for nurse clinicians. *Nurse Education Today* **15**, 164–9.

Greenhalgh and Company Limited (1994) *The Interface between Junior Doctors and Nurses: a research study for the Department of Health*. HMSO, London.

Hampson, J. (1986) Prescribing by nurse practitioners. *The Lancet* **1** (8496), 1502.

Secretary of State for Health (1997) *The New NHS: modern, dependable*. HMSO, London.

United Kingdom Central Council (1992) *Scope of Professional Practice*. UKCC, London.

Chapter 1
Structures to Facilitate Effective Prescribing

Nicholas W. Hough and Mark Pilling

Introduction

In a book about medicines management, a good starting point is to describe the structures and mechanisms which are in place to facilitate effective prescribing. These have been established with the aim of ensuring, as far as is possible, value for money from the NHS drugs' budget. It is worth noting that the content of this chapter would have been very different before 1990, a year in which a wide range of new initiatives, both national and local, was introduced in the specific area of general practitioner (GP) prescribing. The use of medicines in primary care has since been subject to unprecedented attention in order to gain a clearer understanding of how best to encourage more rational and cost-effective prescribing.

It is also relevant in this opening chapter to consider the financial aspects of prescribing, both its impact on the total cost of the health service, and the means by which the costs and supply of medicines are regulated. This chapter therefore covers some of the important background information which will provide a basis for a better understanding of medicines management in the NHS.

The NHS drugs bill and the cost of medicines

Facts and figures about NHS prescribing

Most health care workers are probably unaware of the proportion of the total costs of the health service accounted for by medicines. The drugs' bill is actually the second largest single 'item' of expenditure after staffing costs, accounting for around 11% of NHS expenditure (Association of the British Pharmaceutical Industry, 1997). Primary health-care medicines expenditure is about four times that in the hospital sector (Audit Commission, 1994). In 1995, the figure for the Family Health Services Authorities (FHSAs) in England was £3681 million (net ingredient cost), an increase of 8.1% on 1994. Between 1985, when the FHSA drugs bill was £1333 million, and 1995 the average annual increase was around 10%.

When measuring the 'volume' of prescribing, that is how many prescriptions are written by GPs every year, it is important to differentiate between prescription items, which is the correct figure to quote, and the number of prescription forms (FP10s), because more than one item may be written on a single form. The number of prescription items dispensed in England in 1995 was 473 million, an increase of 3.8% over 1994. The number of items actually prescribed is always higher, because not all prescriptions are presented for dispensing. This happens for a variety of reasons and, for some patients, may represent a form of non-compliance.

From the cost and 'volume' figures it is possible to calculate the average net ingredient cost per prescription item; this was £7.78 in England in 1995, an increase of 4.2% over the previous year. The number of prescriptions received per head of the population for the same period was 9.7, an increase of 3.4% on the previous year.

The above figures exclude hospital prescribing which accounts for approximately 20% of the total NHS drugs bill per annum. Thus the main focus on managing prescribing costs has been in primary care, where 80% of the drugs bill is spent, although increasing attention is being paid to the effects of hospital-led prescribing on GPs. The creation of unified Health Authorities (HAs) in England and Wales in 1996 brought the two prescribing budgets closer together in the same management structure, and a future prospect may be a single drugs budget for hospitals and GPs. Similarly, in Scotland, health boards have similar functions to HAs in England and Wales, while these functions are the responsibility of health and social services boards in Northern Ireland.

It is not surprising, given the above figures, that the Department of Health (DH), and the Welsh, Scottish and Northern Ireland Offices, pay close attention to the size of the NHS drugs bill, and the most significant cost-containment measures were introduced as part of the wider NHS reforms in the early 1990s (Audit Commission, 1994).

The cost of medicines in hospitals

One of the main points to appreciate is that NHS hospitals have to work within fixed drugs budgets. However, hospital pharmacies can tender, either directly with manufacturers or wholesalers, for the best possible prices on the pharmaceuticals they purchase. Furthermore, bulk purchasing arrangements can be made, thus generating greater cost savings for a number of co-operating hospitals within a geographical area. All of this generally means that the same drugs cost less in the hospital service than in the community, i.e. those prescribed by GPs and dispensed in community ('high street') pharmacies.

Manufacturers are often willing to offer hospitals discounted prices in order to secure the use of their product(s) in place of therapeutically equivalent drugs made by their competitors. This opportunity arises because many hospitals operate 'formularies' which define the range of drugs which may be routinely prescribed. The criteria for inclusion usually include efficacy, safety, patient acceptability and cost. As there are generally several alternative drugs which fulfil the same therapeutic aim, a favourable cost will often be an important, though not overriding, factor in formulary decisions.

There is a secondary, perhaps more important, commercial benefit for companies whose products achieve formulary status within a hospital. This arises because treatments initiated in hospital, particularly drugs for chronic conditions, are often very likely to be continued after discharge. Understandably, GPs may be reluctant to interfere with a course of treatment recommended by a hospital specialist, and patients may become confused if their medicines are constantly changed every time they see a different doctor.

Consequently, some hospital formulary drugs become very widely used in general practice, and the manufacturer may soon recover any financial losses resulting from hospital discounting. Bearing in mind that approximately 80% of the NHS drugs bill is accounted for by GPs' prescribing, from a manufacturer's point of view there is much to be gained from the use of so called 'loss leaders' which are accepted onto the hospital formulary. There have been several examples of medicines being heavily discounted to hospitals which have then gone on to displace less expensive therapeutically equivalent drugs in general practice. In the future, however, it is expected that decisions on hospital prescribing policy should not be driven exclusively by hospital cost minimisation. The selection of medicines for formularies is described in Chapter 2.

The cost of medicines in primary care

For drugs prescribed by GPs, the vast majority of which are dispensed in community pharmacies, there are manufacturers' 'list prices' which represent the price the NHS pays through reimbursement of the pharmacist (or dispensing doctor) who supplies them. The 'list prices' of branded medicines can be found in the *Monthly Index of Medical Specialities* (MIMS), a commonly used reference source for GPs, or the *Chemist and Druggist Price List*, which is more commonly used by pharmacists.

Community pharmacists have to reclaim the costs of the medicines they dispense against GP prescriptions. On a monthly basis, all the prescription forms (FP10s) collected at the pharmacy are forwarded, in England, to the Prescription Pricing Authority (PPA) where they are processed and the amount owed to the pharmacy calculated. The pharmacy is then reimbursed by the local HA for the appropriate amount. This takes into account the fact that the pharmacy will have already collected a certain amount of money through the prescription charge system. This must be declared to the PPA, and it is then deducted from the reimbursement sum. The Scottish equivalent to the PPA is the Prescription Processing Division (PPD), the Welsh is the Prescription Information and Pricing Services and the Northern Ireland equivalent is the Central Services Agency for Health and Social Services.

Where various pack sizes exist, the pharmacist must annotate the prescription accordingly to show which one was used to make up the prescription. This is because larger pack sizes are usually less expensive per unit dose, and the PPA needs to be able to calculate the appropriate level of remuneration. The pharmacy does not receive 100% of the total 'list price' of the medicines dispensed each month, because there is a 'discount clawback' mechanism in place to account for the fact that pharmacies obtain varying levels of discount from wholesalers and manufacturers. This 'clawback', which is deducted from the monthly remuneration, encourages pharmacists to get the best deals they can on the medicines they purchase. The process of setting generic drug prices has a similar effect, and this is described below.

The cost of generic medicines

Generic medicines are those which are produced after patent expiry, usually by manufacturers other than the originator. Since less research and development costs are incurred in making 'copies' of original brands, their production costs and consequently their NHS prices are usually much lower. Hence generic medicines are much less expensive for the NHS compared to their branded counterparts, and with a few well known exceptions (see Chapters 3 and 12), they can be regarded as clinically equivalent. There has therefore been considerable effort on the part of the various national prescribing initiatives and also by HAs to encourage generic prescribing, and the rate has increased markedly from a national average of 35% to 60% over the last 5 years.

The costs of generic drugs to the NHS are listed in the *Drug Tariff*, a DH publication, for England and Wales and their equivalents in Scotland and Northern Ireland. These represent the basic costs against which the government reimburses community pharmacies for the generic drugs they dispense. There is an incentive for pharmacists to purchase at or below the *Drug Tariff* price, since a financial difference in their favour represents a legitimate source of profit. However, the 'discount clawback' mechanism also operates to compensate for this. The *Drug Tariff* price is kept up to date to reflect the prices being charged by a number of leading generic manufacturers (thus it follows rather than sets costs), so that any major differences between the actual purchase prices and the costs reimbursed to pharmacists are reconciled on a regular basis.

The pharmaceutical price regulation scheme

The costs of branded medicines to the NHS are subject to a voluntary agreement between manufacturers and the DH. This is known as the Pharmaceutical Price Regulation Scheme (PPRS). It is regularly reviewed by both parties to ensure that it achieves its dual purpose of ensuring reasonable prices for the NHS, whilst providing a secure environment for the pharmaceutical industry to make enough profit to invest in future developments. The way that the PPRS operates is unfamiliar to most health care professionals, and to those who do understand the basic principles, there is much which remains hidden as a result of confidential negotiations between individual companies and the DH.

One of the main principles of the PPRS is that it does not regulate the prices of individual medicines, but sets an upper allowable limit on the total profits, or return on capital employed, which individual companies may earn from sales of medicines to the NHS. There are a number of considerations which determine this limit, for example the level of investment in research and development. These factors work in favour of a company, thus helping it to achieve an allowance at the upper end of the permitted scale. The profit allowed is not guaranteed by the PPRS, so manufacturers still have to promote and sell their products as effectively as possible to achieve their maximum earnings potential. Companies can set the prices of individual medicines with some freedom, although they may have to repay the DH at the end of the financial year if they exceed their overall profit allowance.

The present agreement, which came into being in 1993, initially imposed a 2.5% overall price reduction across the whole industry. This was at a time when the drugs bill was rising very much faster than the rate of general inflation. Although unpopular with the industry, many companies felt that this move was better than some of the other measures the DH might have imposed. Since 1993 there has been some slowing down in the rate of rise of the drugs bill, which may in part be due to the effects of the present PPRS.

The selected list scheme

In 1984, the DH introduced prescribing restrictions on a range of drugs within seven particular therapeutic categories – an initiative known as the Selected List Scheme (SLS). The drugs affected could no longer be prescribed at NHS expense. Many well known branded medicines were involved, including some of the more popular benzodiazepine preparations, for example Valium, Mogadon and Librium. In many cases the same active ingredients remained available, providing they were prescribed generically.

The scheme had some teething troubles, with patient groups and the pharmaceutical industry arguing that many products were no longer available for which there was a genuine clinical need. Doctors and pharmacists also took time getting used to what they could prescribe and dispense, and there were many patients who needed convincing that the 'generic' they had been given to replace a 'banned' branded medicine was therapeutically equivalent. In some instances, patients requested private prescriptions, for which they had to pay, in order to stay on their preferred form of medication.

Some adjustments were made to the original list and a number of 'banned' medicines were subsequently added to the list of drugs that could be prescribed. The DH set up the NHS Advisory Committee on Drugs (ACD) to make recommendations on the range of drugs which were to constitute the 'blacklist', i.e. those which were banned. Their decisions were to be based on ensuring that medicines would remain available to meet all clinical needs at the lowest possible cost to the NHS. The more expensive therapeutically equivalent alternatives therefore became unavailable.

Some commentators saw the SLS as the beginnings of a restricted national formulary, covering all therapeutic areas. However, only a few additional categories of medicines have been added to the original seven since 1985. The last major announcements about the SLS were in 1992, when a further ten categories were proposed. These and the original seven categories are shown in Table 1.1.

Table 1.1 The selected list scheme.

Initial categories affected in 1984	New categories proposed in 1992
Cough and cold remedies	Appetite suppressants
Analgesics for mild to moderate pain	Anti-diarrhoeal drugs
Indigestion remedies	Drugs acting on the skin
Vitamins	Drugs acting on the ear and nose
Laxatives	Drugs for vaginal and vulval conditions
Bitters and tonics	Contraceptives
Benzodiazepines	Drugs for allergic disorders
	Topical antirheumatics
	Hypnotics and anxiolytics
	Drugs used in anaemia

Some of the newer proposals generated heated debate, particularly in the areas of contraceptives and dermatologicals. However, after the deliberations of the ACD, few major new restrictions were introduced. One category particularly affected, however, was topical non-steroidal anti-inflammatory drugs, and what eventually happened, in effect, was that a reference price was introduced. Above this, the preparation would not be available at NHS expense. Not surprisingly, there was then a round of price cuts by the manufacturers and the respective products remained prescribable on the NHS.

The new NHS structure and government prescribing initiatives

One of the key NHS reforms was the creation of purchasers and providers of health care. The former were mostly District Health Authorities (DHAs) and fundholding GPs, and the latter were usually hospital trusts. Some further changes to the NHS in England were introduced on 1 April 1996. These changes included the removal of two key elements which have existed in one form or another since 1948, namely the Regional Health Authority (RHA) and the Family Health Services Authority (FHSA), the latter formerly known as Family Practitioner Committees (FPCs). Similar changes to organisational structures and responsibilities have also taken place, or are likely to take place, in Wales, Scotland and Northern Ireland. On 1 May 1997, a new Labour Government came into office with a manifesto commitment to look at changes to the internal market arrangements within the NHS. While the Government is still to confirm its long-term plans for the NHS, one of their aims is to pilot different GP locality commissioning models as a more effective and efficient mechanism than fundholding for purchasing hospital and community services for patients (Secretary of State for Health, 1997).

The new Health Authorities

The new HAs became statutory bodies on 1 April 1996. There are just under 100 of these new HAs, and they replace the previously separate DHAs and FHSAs. It is important to realise that their function is quite different from the two previously separate types of health authority. Although the new HAs incorporate the functions of the former FHSAs (managing primary care contractors, e.g. GPs and community pharmacists) and also their existing responsibilities of negotiating, managing and monitoring contracts with NHS trusts, they were created primarily to lead on strategic developments. HAs are therefore responsible for planning and developing new patterns of service to effect health improvements for their populations.

The Department of Health and NHS Executive

The Secretary of State for Health is responsible to Parliament for the running of the NHS, and the DH (including the Scottish, Welsh and Northern Ireland Offices) advises him on policy matters. The NHS Executive (NHSE) manages the NHS directly through the new HAs, and is organised with a central unit and eight Regional Offices (ROs) to carry out its functions (Fig. 1.1). Unlike the former RHAs, the ROs are part of the DH and not part of the operational NHS, and their staff are civil servants, not NHS employees. ROs relate to services in their region only as part of a central monitoring function and do not have an operational management role.

Department of Health prescribing initiatives

Alongside the NHS 'structural' reforms, there have been specific changes taking place around prescribing. The definitive plans were published in May 1990 in *Improving Prescribing* (DH, 1990), which placed an emphasis on improving the quality of prescribing, with cost savings as a secondary benefit. On 1 April 1991, prescribing budgets were introduced for all GP practices

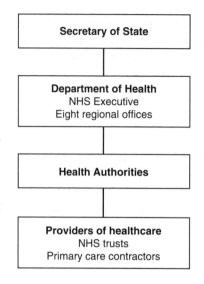

Fig. 1.1   The new NHS structure in England.

following their announcement in the White Paper *Working for Patients* (DH, 1989); further details were given in the working paper *Indicative Prescribing Budgets for General Medical Practitioners* (DH, 1991). This was significant because it represented the first suggestion of a move away from a non-cash limited drugs budget in primary care, and also introduced an element of accountability for the money spent on medicines. The White Paper *The New NHS* published in December 1997 (SOSH, 1997) confirmed a cash limited budget for primary care.

As previously mentioned, prescribing costs in the secondary care sector were already subject to strict budgetary control, with hospital pharmacy departments playing an important role in containing drug costs. However, whilst the primary care sector accounts for 80% of the prescribing market in cash terms, GPs had long enjoyed almost complete prescribing freedom, without any external monitoring procedures to ensure cost-effectiveness. In addition to the Indicative Prescribing Scheme (IPS), the DH expanded the range of educational and advisory initiatives and resources available to GPs and HAs in the area of prescribing and medicines usage. In addition to the appointment of HA prescribing advisers, both medical and pharmaceutical, there was also the establishment of the Medicines Resource Centre (MeReC), the National Medical Advisers Support Centre (MASC), and the development of Prescribing Analysis and Cost (PACT) data, including electronic PACT and the inclusion of therapeutic advice in the 'centre pages' of the 'paper copy' reports. Eventually, MeReC and MASC, which began work in 1990, merged in 1996 and became part of the National Prescribing Centre (NPC) in Liverpool, although their roles continue within the new structure. In common with MeReC, Scotland has the Scottish Medicines Resource Centre which is part of the Scottish Pharmacy Practice Centre, and in Wales there is the Welsh Medicines Resource Centre.

These units provide independent prescribing information in the form of bulletins to general practitioners, pharmacists and prescribing advisers in Scotland and Wales, respectively. In Northern Ireland, the Drug Utilization Research Unit (DURU) has provided a similar function. Scotland, Wales and Northern Ireland have no organisation, equivalent to what was MASC or the NPC, providing formal support to professional advisers.

The DH also began, in a more proactive manner, to encourage the development of local formularies, generic prescribing policies, and guidelines or protocols for the use of specific classes of medicines, for example antibiotics and benzodiazepines. More recently, some HAs have built upon this by establishing local area prescribing committees, which have joint representation from hospital and general practice, to tackle issues at what has become known as the 'prescribing interface'. Their role is described in more detail later.

The National Prescribing Centre (NPC)

Established in 1996, the purpose of the NPC is to promote high quality cost-effective prescribing through a co-ordinated programme of activities in support of HAs and GPs. As stated, some of its functions are a continuation of the activities of MASC and MeReC; the former's role was to provide educational support and training for HA prescribing advisers, and the latter's to produce a monthly advisory and information bulletin for GPs to assist them in prescribing.

The NPC continues to support prescribing advisers by providing them with education and training, usually through workshops and lectures, so that they are kept up to date with the latest evidence on the cost-effective use of medicines. Advisers are given regular overviews of all the main therapeutic areas, for example the drug treatment of cardiovascular, respiratory, gastro-intestinal and central nervous system disorders, so that they are better equipped to advise GPs. Any new information or evidence arising from the publication of major studies is discussed in detail, and the implications for prescribing in routine clinical practice evaluated.

The NPC is well placed to help advisers share best practice and avoid duplication of effort. Initiatives undertaken by individual HAs to improve prescribing can be brought to the attention of others responsible for managing HA drug budgets. Materials produced to support local campaigns around improving prescribing, for example prescribing newsletters or patient information leaflets, can be adapted for more widespread use. Advisers are able to meet colleagues from other HAs who face similar issues, and this also enables them to identify solutions together.

The provision of evaluated information and advice on new medicines launched by the pharmaceutical industry, both prior to and around the time of marketing, is likely to be an increasingly important aspect of the NPC's work. This is achieved partly through the advisers' workshops and through material published by, or commissioned on behalf of, the centre.

At the time of writing, the NPC has only been established for about 2 years and so its presence has not yet been fully appreciated, although the activities formerly undertaken by MASC and MeReC are still very much in evidence.

Information and advice about medicines and prescribing

Published information and advice on medicines and prescribing

There are two major sources of information on medicines and their use; one is the DH, through various publications and the NPC, and the other is the pharmaceutical industry. Depending on what type of information is required, either may be regarded as a useful source, although the 'official' independent publications are generally favoured by those whose responsibility it is to provide advice to GPs on the development of local formularies or treatment guidelines. These are described below. The role of the pharmaceutical industry is outside the scope of this chapter.

Drug and Therapeutics Bulletin (DTB)

This is probably the best known and most widely respected of the regular publications, and it has been in existence for over 30 years. It is published every month in an eight-page format by the Consumers' Association, and a subscription is paid by the DH on behalf of both GPs and hospital doctors in England. It covers a wide range of subjects, mainly, but not exclusively, around prescribing, and is known for its sometimes forthright opinions. Critical reviews of new and established pharmaceutical products, the treatment of specific conditions, and general articles on the regulation of medicines feature regularly in the *DTB*. Each article remains unsigned, having been subjected to a thorough editorial process which takes into account the recommendations of many different commentators.

Prescribers' Journal

This has also been circulated for over 30 years, and is owned and published by the DH under the direction of a management committee and advisory board comprising a number of experts. It is published four times a year in the form of a small booklet containing upwards of 60 pages. There are usually several different topics covered and each article is written by a named author. In contrast to the *DTB*, the articles provide a more personalised account, which is also peer-reviewed, of the treatment of a specific condition or an assessment of a particular type of drug or group of drugs. Occasionally, the whole of one issue is devoted to a special symposium edition featuring a range of articles on the same subject, for example paediatrics.

MeReC Bulletin

This is a specifically GP orientated publication which first appeared in 1990 and is now published by the NPC, the name *MeReC* being retained for reasons of familiarity. It began as an independent initiative, funded by the DH and managed through one of the former RHAs (Mersey RHA in Liverpool). It is a monthly four-page bulletin focusing on primary care prescribing. Topics include assessments of major new drugs recently marketed and targeted at GPs, comparative reviews of groups of drugs for the same condition, and the treatment of common conditions seen in general practice. The writing team are all pharmacists who work full time in the centre. It is distributed to all GPs and community pharmacies in England; similar bulletins are published in Scotland and Wales.

British National Formulary (BNF)

This is regarded as the official pocket reference book on medicines and prescribing. Updated every 6 months, it is published by the British Medical Association and the Royal Pharmaceutical Society of Great Britain, and paid for on behalf of all NHS doctors and pharmacists by the DH. It is a comprehensive guide to virtually all prescribed medicines, providing vital information on uses, dosages and any special prescribing considerations. The latter includes prescribing in, for example, pregnancy, hepatic and renal disease. The *BNF* contains a series of separate chapters on each of the main therapeutic categories of drugs, and there are prescribing guidance notes at the beginning of each section. These notes contain some very useful information on drug choice and highlight the main features of the products listed in each chapter. The *BNF* also contains advice on prescription writing, controlled drugs, drug interactions, intravenous additives, and ADR reporting. The *Nurse Prescribers' Formulary* is published in the *BNF*, and is reproduced in this book as Appendix 1.

Other publications

The above are the main published sources of prescribing information provided by the DH for doctors and pharmacists in the NHS. There are two others which should be mentioned for completeness. These are *Current Problems in Pharmacovigilance* and *PACT 'Centre Pages'*. The former is published as a four-page bulletin by the Committee on Safety of Medicines about three or four times a year, and provides the latest information on any safety issues with prescribed medicines, for example when major pharmaco-epidemiological studies identify new hazards. The latter are part of the PACT reports that GPs receive every quarter; they consist of the 'centre' four pages and feature reviews of different therapeutic drug groups or the management of a common medical condition. Some practice-specific prescribing feedback data are also provided along with comparisons against local HA and national averages. The topics are sometimes planned to complement subjects covered in the *MeReC Bulletin*. All of the above are intended to ensure that prescribers and those who advise them have access to independent evaluated information on medicines and prescribing. The range of publications available and their different formats help to ensure that most people should find something of interest which also enables them to keep more up to date. There are, of course, other published sources of information which are widely used by prescribers, two of which are the *Monthly Index of Medical Specialities* (MIMS) and the *Data Sheet Compendium*. *MIMS* only contains very brief details of different drugs, but it is very useful for checking up on the costs of branded medicines. The *Data Sheet Compendium* contains detailed technical information on the licensed indications of branded pharmaceutical products. For all new medicines, data sheets are now being replaced by Summaries of Product Characteristics.

Professional support for prescribing

All HAs are expected to have access to professional advice on prescribing matters. Medical advisers, usually GPs recruited from general practice, and pharmaceutical advisers, usually from a hospital or community pharmacy background, are employed in almost all new HAs. Most professional advisers at HAs see their role as promoting high quality prescribing and helping to reduce unnecessary or ineffective medicine use (Audit Commission, 1994).

While a system of providing some feedback to GPs on their prescribing costs already existed, the introduction in 1988 of PACT reports, described in detail later in this chapter, meant that all GPs began to receive regular feedback on their prescribing.

Monitoring prescribing and visiting practices to discuss prescribing is a large element of the work of most prescribing advisers. The information available in PACT reports is frequently shared with practices during visits, and facilitates exchange of information on local circumstances and ideas.

HA prescribing advisers are usually responsible for setting prescribing budgets for general practices. There are also many other areas of work in which advisers may become involved, for example, attending hospital drug and therapeutics committees and area prescribing committees, developing clinical guidelines and prescribing policies, producing prescribing bulletins and developing local strategies for the introduction of new drugs. Production of practice formularies is often facilitated by a prescribing adviser who is able to analyse current drug usage from PACT data and provide independent clinical evidence on the safety, efficacy and cost of available drugs in a particular treatment area. The development of practice formularies encourages and enables doctors in a practice to share their knowledge and clinical experience of drug usage. Chapter 2 gives more detailed information about drug formularies.

The role of pharmacists

Drug information pharmacists play an important role in answering drug related enquiries from health care professionals in hospital and community practice. They are usually based in large NHS hospital trusts or regional centres. Historically, their role has centred upon the production of drug information bulletins and the answering of drug related enquiries, for example, information about the administration, dosage and adverse effects of drugs which is not often found in standard reference sources available to doctors and pharmacists. Increasingly, drug information pharmacists are providing purchasers and HA advisers with advanced intelligence and objective information about forthcoming new drugs. This assists purchasers in managing the entry of new drugs into their HA, which is becoming increasingly important in the case of expensive biotechnology products. This development has resulted in several drug information centres appointing primary care liaison posts to provide dedicated support to purchasers in their district.

Recent initiatives have also sought to expand the role of the community pharmacist, and there are reports of increasing collaboration between them and GPs (Schneider & Barber, 1996; Pilling *et al.*, 1998). The DH is keen to examine the feasibility of more formal arrangements between community pharmacists and GPs in order to improve the pharmaceutical care of patients, the management of repeat prescribing and the overall quality and cost-effectiveness of prescribed medicines. Many HAs are already encouraging meetings between GPs and local community pharmacists as a valuable means of facilitating communication about prescribing and improving medicines management.

Prescribing costs and budgets

Drug expenditure in the UK is funded almost exclusively by central government. Estimates of the amount of money likely to be required for the drug bill in the forthcoming year are agreed during the Public Expenditure Survey discussions held between the Treasury and the DH. Drugs budgets allocated to the new HAs are based on historical spending patterns and expected population changes, but may also give some allowance for demographic factors such as the age mix of patients, and for local morbidity which will influence the demand for health care. HA drugs budgets are not cash limited. However, any overspend in the national total for the current financial year is carried forward, requiring either reductions in the funding for other NHS services or further economies in prescribing. A contingency reserve is held at HA level to meet exceptional prescribing costs for which an individual practice could not reasonably plan; for example, a patient starting on a particularly expensive therapy. There is usually a formal mechanism within each HA for the funding of specific high-cost drugs from these contingency reserves.

Each year the NHS Executive issues guidance to HAs on the setting of practice budgets. While the method by which budgets are set is broadly the same for fundholding and non-fundholding practices, the prescribing alloca-tion to fundholders is 'real', in that it forms part of the total practice fund. Unlike non-fundholding GPs, who prescribe within a non-cash limited budget, an overspend by a GP fundholder has to be taken from other parts of the practice budget, i.e. either their staffing or their hospital and community health-care budget.

Fundholders therefore have a clear incentive to contain their prescribing costs, while any savings made must be used for the benefit of patients. Non-fundholding practices are now given a target prescribing budget that is in fact a range of expenditure within which it is reasonable to expect the practice to meet the needs of patients by rational, cost-effective prescribing. Formal incentive schemes for non-fundholding practices were first established in 1991. These practices can be given a portion of any savings they make in defined areas, provided they do not exceed their overall target budget. Target ranges tend to be more challenging for high prescribing practices. These targets should not be purely financial, but may include, for example, levels of generic prescribing and participation in a practice audit of repeat prescribing (NHSE, 1995a).

Capitation-based funding

Since the introduction of drugs budgets, a great deal of work has been carried out to improve the methods used in allocating drugs budgets to general practices. Progress is being made towards a more equitable and needs-based system, away from using historical spending patterns to determine future requirements (Majeed *et al.*, 1996). It has also been recognised that dividing up and distributing the NHS drugs budget to practices solely on the basis of list sizes (i.e. the total number of registered patients), would fail to take account of several other factors which are well known to affect GPs' prescribing costs. Budgets may therefore be set partly according to the size and age/sex dis-tribution of the population, but can also take into account the standardised mortality ratio (SMR), which is used as a crude indicator of morbidity for the local population (Sleator, 1993). This is a reasonable approach at HA level, but is more difficult to achieve at practice level, where individual patients needing expensive drugs may drastically distort a practice budget calculated using these factors alone.

The most frequently used baseline figure to estimate a practice's prescribing costs is the net ingredient cost (NIC) per prescribing unit (PU). The PU is the factor used to provide the comparative data included in PACT reports: each patient under 65 years of age represents one PU and each patient 65 years of age and over represents three PUs. More recently, the ASTRO-PU (Age, Sex and Temporary Resident Originated Prescribing Unit) has been developed to help allow total costs to be assessed in a way which is more sensitive to the popu-lation characteristics of individual practices (Roberts & Harris, 1993). Pre-scribing budgets may then be set by multiplying the HA average cost per

ASTRO-PU by the number of ASTRO-PUs in each practice to produce an outline practice budget. This is then adjusted by considering local morbidity and the number of patients requiring particularly expensive treatments.

While budget setting will take into account historic prescribing costs of each practice, HA advisers will make judgements about where potential savings or increased costs may be expected. For many practices, potential savings may be achieved, for example, through more rational use of ulcer healing drugs and antibiotics, while practices developing more preventive care for asthma patients are likely to have increased costs. In general, the budget set will tend to reflect the quality and cost-effectiveness of the prescribing of each practice.

Prescribing analysis and cost (PACT) information

Prescribing analysis and cost (PACT) information was introduced in 1988 as a tool to enable GPs to monitor change in drug usage and prescribing costs, and to assist prescribing audit. Analysis and action on the basis of PACT data can enable improvements in patient care. PACT reports are produced by the PPA and provide information on all items prescribed and dispensed on FP10 prescriptions by GPs and their trainees. This is possible because every FP10 that is written and handed in at a pharmacy or dispensed in the surgery is forwarded to the PPA, and the details are entered onto a very large computer database. Data equivalent to PACT are produced in Scotland (Scottish Prescribing Analysis data, (SPA data)) and also in Wales and Northern Ireland, where equivalent prescribing and cost information is made available to prescribers and prescribing advisers.

In 1994, the format of PACT reports was changed to include extra information presented in a more accessible way. There are now two levels of report, the Standard Report, which is sent to every GP each quarter, and the Prescribing Catalogue which is available only on request. The Standard Report is eight pages long and is arranged to provide an increasing level of detail. It compares the practice's prescribing costs and volume (number of items prescribed) with local and national averages, and includes the practice's top 20 drugs, the proportion of new drugs prescribed, and the percentage of drugs prescribed generically. The Standard Report also contains a four page pull-out section which gives prescribing advice and comparative data in a specific therapeutic area. The Prescribing Catalogue provides details of every item prescribed and dispensed by the practice or individual GP (with the quantity prescribed and the associated costs) over a specific period of time.

Health Authorities also have access to electronic prescribing data which allow advisers to examine trends and patterns of prescribing in considerable detail. There are two such prescribing programs, PACTline, which provides comparative data at *BNF* chapter and section level, and the more detailed HAePACT, which provides more information about an individual practice's drug usage.

PACT data can be very helpful to doctors who want to examine their pre-scribing in detail. For example, it can be used to audit a practice's prescribing for asthma, and may indicate whether too many patients are relying on bronchodilators alone, rather than receiving preventive inhaled corticosteroids. PACT data can also be used to compare the rates of growth of new versus 'older' drugs prescribed. For example, the proportion of newer antidepressants used, such as paroxetine, can be compared with the proportion of traditional antidepressants used, such as amitriptyline. This information can then be used by the practice when discussing safety, effectiveness, and cost-effectiveness of their prescribing for depression.

Quality prescribing indicators

Increasingly, reference is being made to indicators of prescribing quality. These indicators usually refer to what is regarded by 'an expert panel' as markers of appropriate prescribing in a given disease or therapeutic area on what is considered to be best practice. These indicators are often specified as a ratio. For example, it is suggested that, for individual general practices, the ratio of prescribed corticosteroid to bronchodilator prescribed for asthma should approach 0.5. But, as with any statistical information, indicators have their limitations and potential pitfalls. In particular, GPs and HA advisers need to be aware of local and practice-specific demographic factors when comparing a practice's prescribing with local and national averages. This should help them to avoid using the data inappropriately and drawing the wrong conclusions.

Prescribing: the primary and secondary care interface

Key decisions about hospital drug usage are usually agreed at hospital drug and therapeutics committees (Leach & Leach, 1994). Before the introduction of GP drugs budgets, the majority of the membership of these committees con-sisted of hospital consultants from each of the main clinical directorates, senior hospital pharmacists and representatives from the finance directorate of the trust. More recently, however, there has been greater representation from primary care, and these committees now include one or two local GPs, and prescribing advisers from local HAs. Committees with a wider representation can be a useful way of ensuring that community interests are represented in hospital decisions; for example, decisions about the inclusion of new drugs in formularies or about where clinical responsibility lies for the prescribing of drugs that need specialist monitoring.

Guidance from the DH in 1994 indicated that HAs should ensure that hos-pital initiated prescribing is appropriate in relation to general practice, and stressed the importance of addressing issues surrounding the introduction of new drug products which could have a considerable impact on GP prescribing costs and budgets (NHSE, 1994a). This guidance also highlighted the need for purchasers to closely involve clinicians and other key professionals including GPs, chiefly through the establishment of area prescribing committees (APCs). APCs, sometimes referred to as primary care drug and therapeutics committees, tend to have more flexible membership arrangements, with the majority of representatives from primary care including a number of GPs and medical and pharmaceutical advisers from HAs, together with clinical directors from local hospital trusts. APCs are accountable to the HA; their aim is centred on the need for the development of a strategic approach from HA purchasers to prescribing in both primary and secondary care. The aims of such committees may include some or all of the following:

- To derive a common and considered approach with hospital consultants to the adoption of new drug products
- To advise local HAs on appropriate and cost effective drug therapy, and to inform the contracting process
- To work with hospital consultants and GPs in the development of shared care guidelines
- To liaise with the local hospital drug and therapeutics committees.

Shared care arrangements

It is becoming increasingly common for hospital consultants to seek the agreement of the patient's GP to share the subsequent care of patients needing long-term drug treatments that require special monitoring (Crump *et al.*, 1995). These types of drug treatment tend to be unfamiliar to most GPs, and are usually initiated by hospital specialists; for example, growth hormone and the immunosuppressant drug cyclosporin. GPs would not generally be expected to prescribe in the absence of their agreement to a *shared care arrangement*. When there is a transfer of prescribing responsibility, the patient's GP will need to receive from the hospital consultant all the necessary information, in order to be in a position to monitor treatment and adjust the dose if necessary. In addition, when a treatment is not licensed for a particular indication, then full justification for its use should usually be given by the consultant to the GP. It is important to recognise that whichever clinician signs the prescription, he/she accepts clinical responsibility for the treatment and its outcomes, and in cases where there is doubt or dispute about where clinical responsibility rests, it will normally be considered to lie in secondary care if the patient is still under the care of the consultant.

High-tech healthcare for patients at home

Recent NHS reforms have resulted in an increasing trend towards transferring care into the community. Expensive, high-technology treatments such as total parenteral nutrition and intravenous antibiotics may increasingly be provided to chronically sick patients at home. Other examples of 'high-tech homecare' include continuous ambulatory peritoneal dialysis (CAPD) and home intravenous chemotherapy, and these are usually provided as a 'package of care'. These typically include the delivery of everything required for the patient to manage their treatment at home effectively.

Until April 1995, these specially formulated treatments and the necessary equipment were prescribed by the patient's GP, usually at the request of a hospital clinician, and were funded by the NHS prescribing budget. The NHS Executive Letter EL(95)5 issued in January 1995, Purchasing High-Tech Healthcare for Patients at Home, required HA purchasers to place contracts for effective high-tech homecare services (NHSE, 1995b). This change prevented the need for GPs to accept clinical and financial responsibility for these unfamiliar treatments and placed the responsibility for decisions about funding new patients and high-tech treatments with HAs.

Case management

Case management originated from the USA and is the process by which all those responsible for prevention, diagnosis and treatment of a disease agree to the standards, personnel and cost of the care to be provided. Managed care, a closely related term, is the process that delivers and finances health-care services. Therefore the concept of case management is a change of emphasis from control of individual costs (e.g. for drugs) to the total cost of management, thereby enabling a case to be managed as a coherent package of activities rather than as a series of separate interventions (Panton *et al.*, 1995).

Particular interest in this area has been generated by the desire for joint disease management ventures between the NHS and private sector companies, including pharmaceutical companies. The NHS Executive issued guidance, in the form of an Executive Letter EL(94)94 in December 1994, on commercial approaches to the NHS regarding disease management packages (NHSE, 1994b). This preliminary advice forbids NHS purchasers, including fundholding GPs, from making commitments to purchase drugs which exclusively link prescribing to a particular company's products.

Case management may prove to be attractive to HAs because it establishes clinical pathways of care, and states the quality standards within the service to be provided. HAs can also ensure that clinical pathways and guidelines are based on evidence of clinical effectiveness, are set to agreed standards, and that monitoring systems and clinical audit are included within contracts for disease management. While a structure is in place, the ability of HAs to develop managed care is limited in current legislation and is limited because of the likely inadequacy of current patient information systems. Nevertheless, the potential to reallocate resources to managed care exists, and change will also be promoted by a need for improved patient care, measurable outcomes in health gain, and cost-containment.

Summary

Recent NHS reforms and pressure to contain GP prescribing costs have resulted in many and varied initiatives and mechanisms to facilitate medicines management and to promote cost-effective prescribing. There is an increased emphasis placed on understanding medicines management in the NHS, and initiatives to regulate the financial aspects of the cost and supply of medicines within the NHS, such as the Selected List and the Pharmaceutical Price Regulation Scheme, have achieved moderate success.

There is increasing support in the NHS, in many HAs and among GPs, for the developing role of pharmacists as prescribing advisers. Prescribing advisers are supported by the National Prescribing Centre which is instrumental in providing educational support and training for this group. Published information and advice on medicines and prescribing, such as the *MeReC Bulletin* and *Drug and Therapeutics Bulletin* containing the latest evidence on the cost-effective use of medicines, are regularly received by GPs and welcomed by prescribing advisers. The introduction of Prescribing Analysis and CosT (PACT) data, GP prescribing budgets and prescribing indicators have further enabled prescribing advisers to promote better quality and more cost-effective prescribing.

The role of HAs and their medical and pharmaceutical advisers, is also important in influencing both hospital and community prescribing policies, including the development of shared care policies and agreements on repeat prescribing policies. In the future, changes in legislation and improved collection and use of health data may facilitate the development of disease management and integrated care, which may lead to improved patient care and measurable outcomes in health gain and cost-containment.

References

Association of the British Pharmaceutical Industry (1997) PHARMA *Facts and Figures*, ABPI, London.

Audit Commission (1994) *A Prescription For Improvement. Towards more rational prescribing in general practice*. HMSO, London.

Crump, B.J., Panton, R., Drummond, M.F., Marchment, M. & Hawkes, R.A. (1995) Transferring the costs of expensive treatments from secondary to primary care. *Br. Med. J.* **310**, 509–12.

Department of Health (1989) *Working for Patients*. HMSO, London.

Department of Health (1990) *Improving Prescribing*. HMSO, London.

Department of Health (1991) Indicative prescribing budgets for general medical practitioners. *Working Paper 4*, HMSO, London.

Leach, R.H. & Leach, S.J. (1994) Drug and therapeutics committees in the UK in 1992. *Pharm. J.* **253**, 61–3.

Majeed, A., Cook, D. & Evans, N. (1996) Variations in general practice prescribing costs – implications for setting and monitoring prescribing budgets. *Health Trends* **28**, 52–5.

NHS Executive (1994a) *Purchasing and Prescribing* (EL(94)72). NHS Executive, Leeds.

NHS Executive (1994b) *Commercial Approaches to the NHS Regarding Disease Management Packages* (EL(94)94). NHS Executive, Leeds.

NHS Executive (1995a) *Prescribing Expenditure: Guidance on Allocations and Budget Setting 1996/97* (EL (95)128). NHS Executive, Leeds.

NHS Executive (1995b) *Purchasing High-tech Healthcare for Patients at Home* (EL (95)5). NHS Executive, Leeds.

Panton, R.S., Cox, I.G. & Norwood, J. (1995) The development of managed care in the United Kingdom. *Pharm. J.* **255**, 781–2.

Pilling, M., Geoghegan, M., Wolfson, D.J. & Holden, J.D. (1998) The St Helens and Knowsley Prescribing Inititative: a model for pharmacist-led meetings with GPs. *Pharm. J.* **260**, 100–102.

Roberts, S.J. & Harris, C.M. (1993) Age, sex and temporary resident originated prescribing units (ASTRO-PUs): new weightings for analysing prescribing of general practices in England. *Br. Med. J.* **307**, 485–8.

Schneider, J.S. & Barber, N.D. (1996) Community pharmacist and general practitioner collaboration in England and Wales. *Pharm. J.* **256**, 524 –5.

Secretary of State for Health (1997) *The New NHS: modern, dependable.* HMSO, London.

Sleator, D.J.D. (1993) Towards accurate prescribing analysis in general practice: accounting for the effects of practice demography. *Br. J. Gen. Pract.* **43**, 102–6.

Chapter 2
Policies and Practice

Katrina Simister

Introduction

Health care systems in developed countries are under pressure currently to provide services within limited budgets. An increase in the number of elderly people, the development of new therapies which enable prescribers to offer treatments to the chronically sick and the rapid growth in medical knowledge mean that society must address the issue of appropriate funding for future health services.

The members of all health care professions will become increasingly involved in the delivery of evidence-based health care and in evaluating the cost-effectiveness of the various treatments and procedures with which they are involved. Nurse prescribing will further extend the role of the nursing profession and its need for reliable information. More of the current prescription medicines are likely to be transferred to over-the-counter prescribing, hence expanding the role of the community pharmacist. Current drug treatments are extremely potent and their pharmacology is often complex. It is therefore of vital importance that all clinical staff involved in the prescribing or administration of such drugs should have access to accurate information and know how to obtain it when required. Links are developing between community and hospital pharmacists, which will enable access by the former of therapeutic information previously used by hospital pharmacists. Pharmacists are working with doctors and nurses in both primary and secondary care to facilitate cost-effective prescribing. Multi-disciplinary working is an essential component for patient care in the future.

This chapter discusses different sources of information, their relative advantages and disadvantages.

Advisory sources and their limitations

There is a wide variety of advisory sources available. These include textbooks, journals, and CD-ROM databases, on-line computer sources and specialist centres. They are divided into primary, secondary and tertiary sources of information.

Primary information sources

Scientific journals

The publication of scientific trials in medical journals allows a critical evaluation of methodology, results and conclusions, which is not possible with any other information sources. However, journals are of variable quality. Those with high standards, e.g. *British Medical Journal* and the *New England Journal of Medicine*, usually insist that the editorial process for articles submitted for publication includes peer review by independent referees. When reading articles published by these reputable journals, it is important to remember that no clinical paper will be perfect and to assess it critically.

Other journals publish data which may be subject to less critical review, and even the best scientific journals contain material in the form of letters and short reports which have not been refereed, although they may be subject to editorial control. All material requires critical appraisal before use (Greenhalgh, 1997).

Secondary information sources

Abstracting and alerting systems

The publishers of alerting systems provide a means of current awareness by scanning selected journals as soon as they are published, writing brief but informative abstracts and mailing them direct to the customer. Thus a superficial knowledge of new developments, published in a large number of journals, can be maintained.

Systems that rely on abstracts must be used with care: while it may be reasonably accurate, an abstract can only give a brief résumé of the particular paper concerned. The restrictions on space mean that important data may be omitted; a misleading bias may be imposed on the data; there is normally no criticism of procedures, results or conclusions. Abstracting systems must therefore be used as means of selection and access to relevant journals.

Examples of some abstracting systems on drug therapy used in the UK are given below.

Pharmline. This is a computer-based system of abstracts produced by the UK regional drug information centres which scan over ninety journals for articles of pharmaceutical interest. The system is also available in a CD-ROM version. Experienced NHS drug information pharmacists prepare the abstracts.

International Pharmaceutical Abstracts. This database is published fortnightly by the American Society of Health-Systems Pharmacists, covering over seven hundred journals. Subjects include pharmaceutics, adverse reactions, toxicology and many others from pharmacy practice to pharmacy history.

Review journals and books

Several journals predominantly publish reviews of pharmacology and therapeutics. The most notable of these is *Drugs,* which is published monthly. The most useful reviews are those that consider drugs in depth and do not usually appear until 1–2 years after a drug has been marketed. The reviews present evaluated data and opinion, and are particularly valuable in summarising large volumes of literature published worldwide. They are well referenced and may be considered as a route to primary information sources.

Computerised secondary sources

Using a computer is essential when searching a database of any size (and therefore usefulness), is contemplated. Keywords can often be selected from a thesaurus before starting a search. This is a useful discipline to adopt in order to plan a search strategy. These keywords can then be linked using the Boolean (logical) operators AND, NOT and OR. For example, two sets of citations A and B may be manipulated as shown in Fig. 2.1.

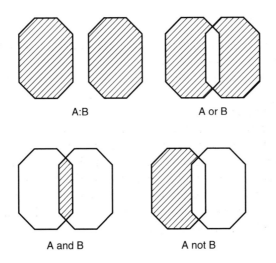

Fig. 2.1 Method of manipulating two sets of citations.

Databases that have controlled vocabularies are quicker and more economical to search, since they do away with the need to think of, and ask the computer to search for, synonyms. While computerised databases can still be searched directly 'on-line', the majority of libraries now purchase CD-ROM versions and the use of this route will increase in the future.

The Internet is becoming an increasingly popular route for the transmission of information and will continue to be so. However, there is now considerable debate concerning the quality of the material available via this route, and recently various American medical and pharmaceutical journals have expressed concern over this issue. A means of guaranteeing quality is required, and at present a large quantity of the information available should be treated with caution (Jadad & Gagliardi, 1998; Silberg *et al.*, 1997; Wyatt, 1997; D'Emanuele, 1998).

Examples of various electronic databases are given below.

Medline. This is an electronic version of the familiar *Index Medicus*. It is produced in the USA by the National Library of Medicine using over 3200 journals published in 70 countries and contains approximately 3 500 000 citations. Like *Index Medicus* it is a means of locating primary references, although 40% of more recent records also contain an author's abstract.

The use of Boolean operators makes possible within minutes an exhaustive literature search which produces a number of references specifically dealing with the subject in question. However, there are some disadvantages. The time lag for abstracts to appear may be 4–6 weeks for major journals, and several months for others. The vocabulary used in indexing articles is strictly limited to highly structured terms specified in the medical subject headings (MeSH) and a familiarity with the vocabulary is essential to get the best from the database.

Excerpta Medica. This is another large database, produced from 3500 journals and, as it has a wider coverage of European journals than *Medline*, it only overlaps with some 60% of the latter. It is a useful additional resource, but its lack of an easily used vocabulary and relatively high on-line charges make searches expensive. The lag time is also greater than with *Medline*.

Tertiary information sources

These comprise reference books, which present a distillation of information from the primary sources in the context of therapeutic practice and opinion. Topics are covered very broadly and therefore may be poorly referenced. The interpretation of the data is subject to the opinion, comment, evaluation and bias of the author.

The time constraints involved in the editing and publishing of textbooks usually mean that they are already out of date in rapidly developing areas by the time that they are published, and long delays between revised editions mean that a book's usefulness declines as current thinking changes. Textbooks are, however, useful as a means of obtaining background information.

Martindale – The Extra Pharmacopoeia

This is a widely used and well-respected source of information on drugs, a new edition of which is published every 5 years; computerised on-line and CD-ROM versions are also available. Information is provided on over 5000 drugs; therefore such detail is highly selective and brief. However, the drug monographs provide general background on pharmacology, therapeutics, adverse effects and formulations plus the relevant references (Reynolds, 1996).

Meyler's Side Effects of Drugs

This is the standard reference on adverse effects. A new issue is produced every 4 or 5 years, with annuals published as an updating exercise during the intervening years. The series presents monographs on major drugs and their pharmacological groups. The international list of authors provides comment and evaluation. The field of adverse reactions is fast changing, and this text should be used in conjunction with the annuals. Much of the material published in the annuals has been published in the preceding 2 years. However, the books are useful in providing a broad and fairly current view of the subject, and are sufficiently well referenced to allow important primary sources to accessed (Dukes, 1996).

Data Sheet/Summary of Product Characteristics Compendium

This is produced by the Association of the British Pharmaceutical Industry (ABPI) and is a collection of manufacturers' data sheets arranged in alphabetical order of manufacturers. Information to be included in a data sheet is specified by the Medicines (Data Sheet) Regulations 1972. Data appear under standardised headings, although manufacturers select what information goes under which headings, so this may vary from one data sheet to another. However, from January 1998 all new drugs introduced to the market are subject to the European licensing system and have a Summary of Product Characteristics (SPC) monograph rather than a data sheet. The two documents are similar, but as the SPC must be approved by all member states of the European Union (EU), phrasing is much broader and reflects clinical practice throughout the EU. It does, however, include more detail on certain aspects of drug therapy, such as use in pregnancy (Anon., 1996a).

Data sheets/SPCs are contributed by individual manufacturers:

(1) Only if companies are members of ABPI
(2) The compendium contains the data sheets of products the company has selected, usually those which are being actively promoted. It is not comprehensive for all drugs on the market, particularly generics.

The British National Formulary (BNF)

This is produced jointly by the British Medical Association (BMA) and the Royal Pharmaceutical Society of Great Britain (RPSGB). It is available in hard copy and an electronic version. A joint formulary committee of doctors and pharmacists determines the content. The *BNF*'s content has been presented in Chapter 1. Some professionals have been critical of the style adopted in the *BNF*. Doctors are asked to contribute to the chapters relevant to their speciality, and their comments may reflect their personal experience, although the editorial staff write the basic monographs. The introductory chapters and appendices give some prescribing guidelines and information on intravenous additives, drugs in pregnancy, drugs in breast milk and interactions. The presentation is sometimes confusing and dosage data need to be checked. Not all of the chapters are updated in each new edition. This is done only when it is thought necessary (Mehta, 1997).

Manufacturers' promotional material

Information from the manufacturer of a medicine or dressing may be valuable, particularly if it contains data not published elsewhere, termed data on file (Anon., 1996a,b). However, it should be assessed objectively to ensure that it is not following a particular promotional line. Many companies will supply, on request, copies of internal reports if they have been referenced in promotional material.

Other information sources

Should the sources outlined above provide insufficient information, the following may be useful.

The United Kingdom Drug Information Pharmacists' Network

Established over 25 years ago this is a co-ordinated network of over 200 centres throughout the UK. Usually based in a major teaching hospital or district general hospital, the drug information pharmacist is available to answer queries and provide independent, evaluated advice on all matters pertaining to drug therapy. The majority of drug information pharmacists are also involved with ward commitments, lecturing and the production of formularies.

The Poisons Information Service

This is organised on two levels. On one level it is a national service, recognised by the Department of Health which receives details of products and their ingredients from major industrial companies. This information is confidential and used to answer specific questions. Additionally, three centres offer advice on poisoning, but do not receive national funding. The telephone numbers for individual centres can be found in the BNF (Mehta, 1997).

Malaria Reference Centres

Advice on prophylaxis of malaria for people travelling abroad can be obtained by contacting one of the centres that are listed in the BNF. The service is available to both the general public and health professionals.

Formularies

Hospitals have had formularies for many years, the aim being to encourage rational, safe, cost-effective prescribing by the provision of independent, evaluated information (Anon., 1994a,b).

The selection of drugs for a formulary is commonly overseen by the hospital drug and therapeutics committee (DTC). Membership of the committee usually comprises medical representatives from clinical directorates, pharmacists, medical and pharmaceutical advisers of health authorities (HAs) and GPs. In a few cases community pharmacists may also be included.

Background work and comparative data on various treatments will have been produced by either the drug information or formulary pharmacist. The committee will then discuss those drugs to be included in different therapeutic sections of the formulary. While some formularies may be a list of drugs that can be prescribed within the hospital, others will contain more background information on the drugs; however, all will reflect local policies.

A major criterion to be considered when producing a formulary is the introduction of new drugs. Such a request is usually dealt with by the DTC, and decisions taken after a case has been made by the head of the appropriate clinical directorate. Factors such as cost-effectiveness and the therapeutic importance of the product are taken into account.

The impact of new drugs on NHS budgets is now of major importance due to the introduction of products produced via high-technology or biotechnology techniques. Inevitably these agents are expensive, and, as the frontiers of our knowledge are pushed back, many more patients can be treated. These include those patients with chronic illnesses who previously had no or limited choice of drug treatment. Costs are therefore increased and discussions occur concerning equity of treatment, for example the treatment of multiple sclerosis patients.

While much debate has taken place concerning the introduction of a limited national formulary or national guidelines, it is more likely that decision taking will remain at local level.

Protocols and guidelines

An increasing role for DTC is in the production of shared care protocols and treatment guidelines. The increasing emphasis on primary care has led to a sharing of responsibility for a patient's treatment between the individual's hospital doctor and GP. This transfer of care, particularly when expensive and costly drug treatments are involved, has led to the production of shared care protocols incorporating the views of both primary and secondary care staff.

Local guidelines, sometimes based on national guidelines, are often produced for diseases such as asthma, and for the use of expensive new drugs such as interferon-beta for multiple sclerosis.

In 1994 an NHS Executive Letter was published on aspects of prescribing (EL(94)72). This identified a development agenda for HAs and GPs, particularly in improving the management of new drugs into the NHS. As a result of this paper many HAs have now established area prescribing committees (APCs) comprising representatives of both the medical and pharmaceutical professions.

Evidence-based practice

There is a move within the NHS to obtain evidence concerning the effectiveness of drug treatments and other technologies (Sackett *et al.*, 1997; Muir Gray, 1997). It is hoped that this information will help in making decisions about resource allocations. Various initiatives have been put in place, as part of the NHS Research and Development (R&D) Strategy, to provide evidence concerning many of the procedures that are provided currently. The roles of the Cochrane Centre and the NHS Centre for Reviews and Dissemination are discussed below.

The Cochrane Centre. This was established in Oxford in 1992 to facilitate and co-ordinate the preparation and the maintenance of systematic reviews of research on the effects of health care. The main output of the centre is the Cochrane Library. The Cochrane Collaboration is an international network of individuals who prepare, maintain and disseminate systematic reviews of research on the effects of health care.

The Cochrane Library is available electronically and is updated four times a year. It contains four related databases and other information relevant to evidence-based practice. The four main databases are:

- The Cochrane Database of Systematic Reviews (CDSR)
- The Database of Abstracts of Reviews of Effectiveness (DARE)
- The Cochrane Controlled Trials Register (CCTR)
- The Cochrane Review Methodology Database (CRMD)

The subjects covered in the databases include surgical, diagnostic and drug therapy interventions. The reviews are concentrated mainly in the areas of pregnancy and childbirth, sub-fertility and stroke. However, there are newer reviews covering musculo-skeletal disease, schizophrenia, acute respiratory infections, diabetes and peripheral vascular disease.

The NHS Centre for Reviews and Dissemination (CRD). This unit was established in January 1994 in the University of York, and it publishes reviews of health-care procedures in two bulletins entitled *Effective Healthcare Bulletins* and *Effectiveness Matters*. The CRD works closely with the Cochrane Centre and produces the DARE database, which can be accessed as part of the Cochrane Library.

Summary

The drive for cost-effective health care has focused the minds of many health-care providers. On the evidence available to guide practice, pharmaceutical interventions are costly to the NHS and many drug treatments involve complicated regimens. It is therefore important that clinical staff have access to the best and most up to date information in order to evaluate treatment potential and provide a safe service. This chapter explores a wide range of information sources and attempts to highlight their strengths and weaknesses. The coverage includes textbooks, journals, CD-ROM databases, on line computer sources and specialist centres. The chapter does not claim to be exhaustive of all relevant sources, but provides a useful starting point for the thoughtful practitioner.

References

Anon. (1994a) *Paediatric Formulary*, 3rd edn. Guy's, Lewisham and St Thomas' Hospitals, London.

Anon. (1994b) *Alder Hey Book of Children's Doses*, 6th edn. Royal Liverpool Children's Hospital (Alder Hey), Liverpool.

Anon. (1996a) *ABPI Compendium of Data Sheets and Summaries of Product Characteristics 1996–1997*, Datapharm Publications, London.

Anon. (1996b) *ABPI Compendium of Patient Information Leaflets 1996–1997*. Datapharm Publications, London.

D'Emanuele, A. (1998) The Internet. *Pharm. J.* **260**, 26–8.

Dukes, M.N.G. (1996) *Meyler's Side Effects of Drugs*, 13th edn. Elsevier, Amsterdam.

Greenhalgh, T. (1997) *How to Read a Paper. The Basics of Evidence Based Medicine.* BMJ Publishing Group, London.

Jadad, A.R. & Gagliardi, A. (1998) Rating health information on the Internet. Navigating to knowledge or to Babel? *J. Am. Med. Assoc.* **279**, 611–4.

Mehta, D.K. (1997) *British National Formulary No. 34*, British Medical Association and Royal Pharmaceutical Society of Great Britain, London.

Muir Gray, J.A. (1997) *Evidence Based Health Care.* Churchill Livingstone, Edinburgh.

NHS Executive (1994) *Purchasing and Prescribing* (EL(94)72). NHS Executive, Leeds.

Reynolds, J.E.F. (1996) *Martindale. The Extra Pharmacopoeia*, 31st edn.

Royal Pharmaceutical Society of Great Britain, London.

Sackett, D.L., Richardson, W.S., Rosenberg, W. & Haynes, R.B. (1997) *Evidence-based Medicine. How to Practice and Teach EBM.* Churchill Livingstone, Edinburgh.

Silberg, W.M., Lundberg, G.D. & Musacchio, R.A. (1997) Assessing, controlling and assuring the quality of medical information on the Internet, *J. Am. Med. Assoc.* **277**, 1244–5.

Wyatt, J.C. (1997) Commentary: measuring quality and impact of the World Wide Web. *Br. Med. J.* **314**, 1879–81.

Further reading

Evans, D.M.D. (1989) *Special Tests. The procedure and Meaning of the Commoner Tests in Hospital*, 13th edn. Faber and Faber, London.

Salisbury, D.M. & Begg, N.T. (1996) *Department of Health. Immunisation Against Infectious Disease*. HMSO Publications, London.

Stockley, I.H. (1996) *Drug Interactions*, 4th edn. Pharmaceutical Press, London.

Walker, R. & Edwards, C. (1994) *Clinical Pharmacy and Therapeutics*. Churchill Livingstone, Edinburgh.

Chapter 3
Drug Absorption, Distribution, Metabolism and Elimination

Neil A. Caldwell

Introduction

Pharmacokinetics specifically addresses the processes and time course of drug absorption, distribution, metabolism and elimination. By applying pharmacokinetic principles we aim to achieve the desired therapeutic response in each and every individual. We do so by taking account of every individual's ability to clear drugs. An understanding and appreciation of the significance and influence of these four processes may improve, and indeed optimise, treatment outcome following drug therapy.

Many examples of applied pharmacokinetics can be drawn from clinical practice. In the case of an individual with staphylococcal septicaemia, vancomycin, becuase it is a very large molecule unable to cross the intestinal wall into the systematic circulation, is administered by pulsed intravenous infusion, rather than by the oral route. Oral vancomycin is, however, effective for localised gastro-intestinal colonisation, such as by *Clostridium difficile*, because it does not require absorption. Similarly, amphotericin in the treatment of fungal sepsis requires parenteral administration rather than lozenges which are commonly prescribed for topical effect in the management of oropharyngeal candidiasis.

Pharmacokinetic principles are used to describe and quantify the movement of drug from dosage form to the intended site of action, and its consequent elimination or excretion. Those principles have a strong influence on dose selection and frequency of dosing.

The primary focus of all activity under the clinical pharmacokinetic banner, however, must always be patient outcome (Fig. 3.1).

Absorption

For a drug to exert a clinical effect, it must move from the pharmaceutical dosage form (tablet or capsule, liquid, suppository, injection, or topical for-

CLINICAL PHARMACOKINETICS

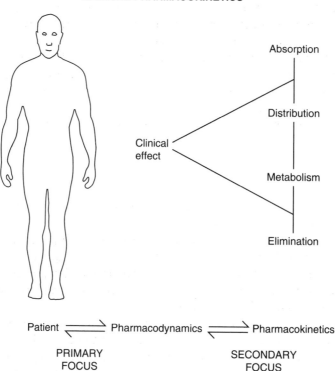

Patient ⇌ Pharmacodynamics ⇌ Pharmacokinetics

PRIMARY   SECONDARY
FOCUS   FOCUS

Fig. 3.1 The primary focus of all 'pharmacokinetic' activity must be the patient and clinical response.

mulation) to the intended site of action within the body. In addition to the oral route, absorption follows administration rectally (metronidazole suppositories in systemic anaerobic infection), intramuscularly (depot neuroleptics for schizophrenia), subcutaneously (insulin in diabetes mellitus), inhalation (anaesthetic gases), topically (anti-inflammatory corticosteroid creams in eczema) and by most other routes to varying degrees. It is now possible to achieve systemic clinical effect within the body by applying patches to the skin: specially formulated patches are available for analgesia, nausea, hormone replacement therapy and chest pain.

Bioavailability

The proportion of an administered dose of medicine, which is absorbed intact without undergoing hepatic breakdown and reaches the systemic circulation of the patient, is known as the bioavailability. (Hepatic breakdown is described below under Metabolism.) Assuming that 100% of a drug enters the circulation after intravenous injection, bioavailability is the relative proportion which enters the systemic circulation after administration by any other route.

The maximum value for bioavailability is unity, and if no drug is absorbed the bioavailability is zero. For most drugs and routes of administration the value is somewhere in between. Digoxin tablets, used in the management of atrial fibrillation, have a bioavailability of between 0.5 and 0.9. With iron salts normally around 10% of oral intake is absorbed; hence bioavailability is 0.1. This factor will increase in deficiency states and decrease in cases of iron overload. Vancomycin, which was mentioned previously, has an oral bioavailability of less than 0.05.

Bioavailability does not take into account the rate of drug absorption, it merely estimates the extent of absorption.

Rate of absorption

The rate of absorption is influenced by a number of factors including dosage form and gastro-intestinal transit time. Before absorption, tablets and capsules must disintegrate or dissolve in the intestine. Consequently liquid or soluble medicines are absorbed faster than tablets. For rapid symptom relief, such as for pain or heartburn, it therefore makes sense to dose with liquid preparations. Aluminium hydroxide liquid will therefore relieve the symptoms of indigestion much faster than calcium carbonate tablets.

Modified-release preparations are a poor choice for 'when needed' therapy, because once the patient complains of symptoms there will be a significant delay between dose administration, drug absorption and therapeutic response. In those with slow gastro-intestinal motility (e.g. as a side effect of opiate analgesics), absorption may be delayed somewhat because of the time the dosage form takes to reach the appropriate site within the gut. In patients with rapid transit, the drug may reach the site of absorption quickly, but it may also rapidly pass through the gastro-intestinal tract, and less of the drug may be absorbed. This can be a particular problem with modified release preparations of drugs such as theophylline, a bronchodilator, which require some time to leach out or release the drug within the gastro-intestinal tract. An example of such a preparation is Theo-Dur. Care must be taken to continue therapy with the patient's usual dosage form, because different formulations of the same drug may produce varying concentrations, and possibly a different clinical response, despite an equivalent dose (Fig. 3.2).

The brand name of a number of medicines should be specified on the prescription. Examples would include most modified-release preparations plus some calcium-channel blockers (e.g. nifedipine and diltiazem), lithium, theophylline and antiepileptics. For these particular medicines prescribing by generic name is not advisable (Mehta, 1997). Thus clinical economy must be forfeited in a small section of pharmacotherapeutics by implementing brand-name prescribing. Once the patient is stabilised on a particular brand, the preparation should not be altered unless recognition has been made of the different absorption properties and possible changes in clinical effect.

Certain modified-release preparations confer no added benefit over the non-

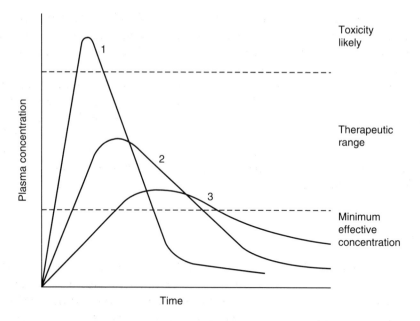

Theophylline concentration following the same oral dose but administered in different dosage forms:

(1) Theophylline liquid
(2) Theophylline tablet
(3) Theophylline sustained release tablet

Different modified release preparations will produce different concentration-time profiles, hence brands are not interchangeable.

Fig. 3.2   Concentration–time profile illustrating the influence of dosage form on absorption for theophylline following the same oral dose administered in different dosage forms.

branded equivalent. Formulations of sustained release iron are a case in point. These preparations are designed to slowly release the iron along the gastro-intestinal tract. It is suggested, however, that they carry the medicine past the initial part of the duodenum into an area of gut where iron absorption is less efficient. The fact that such preparations produce fewer side effects than conventional ferrous sulphate tablets may simply be a reflection of the inefficiency of the particular modified release dosage form. *The British National Formulary (BNF)* states that such preparations have no therapeutic advantage and should not be used.

Food may influence the rate and extent of absorption. A number of medicines form insoluble salts with calcium and iron, thus administration at the same time can severely compromise absorption. Cyclical therapy with bisphosphonates, such as etidronate disodium in the treatment of osteoporosis, requires patients to consume their tablets on an empty stomach and omit food for 2 hours afterwards. Pharmacists will advise that certain penicillins, such as flucloxacillin, be taken on an empty stomach, because gastric acid stimulated by food breaks down the drug before it can be absorbed. Ketoconazole, an antifungal medicine, on the other hand, actually requires an acid environment for absorption, and it must be consumed with meals to take advantage of the post-prandial acid environment.

It is important that instruction to take a medicine at a particular time-point in relation to meals or food is followed to optimise treatment and avoid therapeutic failure. Whilst the pharmacist may indicate when drugs should be taken, it is equally important that the nurse understands the underlying pharmacokinetic reasoning in order to explain the significance of the instruction to the patient. Guidance on the labelling of medicines in relation to food is listed in Appendix 10 of the *BNF*.

Distribution

Most drugs have their site of action beyond the bloodstream. To reach this site, drugs commonly have to enter a number of different organs. Distribution occurs when the drug is present in the blood and it penetrates different tissues or organs. It does not happen instantaneously but over a time period of minutes or hours. The extent to which the drug distributes out of the bloodstream depends on its physicochemical properties. Each drug in each individual patient displays a unique distribution volume, although the actual value may be similar among groups of patients.

Volume of distribution

The volume of distribution is a theoretical term describing the relationship between the quantity of drug absorbed and the plasma concentration of the drug. It reflects how widely the drug has distributed into the organs and tissues (Fig. 3.3). A drug with a large volume tends to be present in the blood in low concentration relative to the dose given. Digoxin has a large volume of distribution (around 400 litres) because it distributes out of the plasma into skeletal muscle. Hence the plasma concentration is low compared with the administered dose. A small volume of distribution suggests most of the absorbed or administered drug remains predominantly in the plasma. Warfarin has a small volume (around 10 litres) because it binds to plasma proteins and remains in the bloodstream. Its concentration in the blood, therefore, is relatively high compared with the administered dose.

A number of clinical conditions may alter the distribution volume of a drug. For drugs which distribute into body fluid, such as penicillins or aminoglycosides, conditions which affect fluid balance (oedema, pleural effusion, ascites, dehydration) will influence volume. With drugs which distribute into fatty tissue, such as benzodiazepines, certain conditions including obesity or malnutrition may alter volume. Patients in whom the volume of distribution has increased may require larger doses of medicine to achieve the same rise in

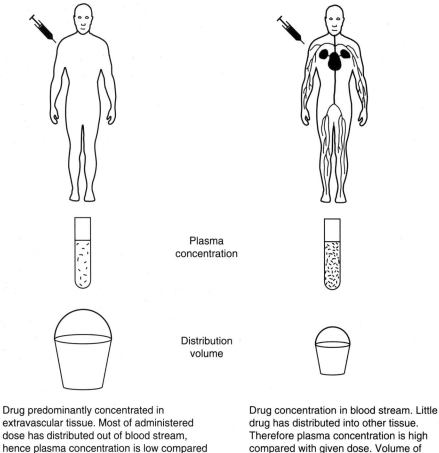

Plasma
concentration

Distribution
volume

Drug predominantly concentrated in
extravascular tissue. Most of administered
dose has distributed out of blood stream,
hence plasma concentration is low compared
with given dose. Volume of distribution is
thus large.

Drug concentration in blood stream. Little
drug has distributed into other tissue.
Therefore plasma concentration is high
compared with given dose. Volume of
distribution is thus small.

Fig. 3.3   Volume of distribution.

serum drug concentration. The converse may apply in those individuals in whom the volume of distribution has decreased.

If the volume of distribution of a drug is known, one can calculate the rise in concentration following an administered dose. The antibiotic gentamicin may have a volume of distribution of around 15 litres. It is water soluble and distributes predominantly into body fluids. We can thus estimate that if a dose of 160 mg were administered by intravenous bolus injection, the concentration would rise by around 10 mg/l. This figure is simply calculated by dividing the dose of drug which reaches the systemic circulation by the volume into which it distributes. This process is slightly more complicated with medicines given orally, because not all of an oral dose of medicine is absorbed; bioavailability is often less than unity. In addition, absorption is not instantaneous; there may be some delay. Once the drug has been absorbed it is subject to elimination processes and a fraction of the drug may be metabolised or excreted before the whole dose of medicine has been absorbed.

Distribution volume has a very strong influence on drug dose. It is, however, a theoretical term and does not necessarily equate with the fluid balance of the individual patient. If the volume changes dramatically, the effective dose of drug may require modification. Because the volume of distribution is often influenced by the patient's weight it is very important that weight is documented in medical or nursing notes, especially when dealing with infants and children.

Elimination

Drug elimination from the body can be very complex and is influenced by many factors. Elimination from the acutely ill individual can be complicated. However, in simple terms the liver and the kidneys are the two major organs in the body responsible for elimination of both waste product and drugs. The liver is principally responsible for metabolism. The kidneys are primarily responsible for elimination via the processes of glomerular filtration, tubular secretion and tubular reabsorption. Elimination also occurs via other body systems, but the relative contribution, compared with hepatic and renal routes, is slight.

There are notable exceptions to the monopoly held by the hepatic–renal waste disposal systems. Suxamethonium, a short-acting muscle relaxant, is inactivated by hydrolysis in the plasma. Rifampicin, used in tuberculosis, can appear in patients' sweat, tears and spit causing an orange-red discolouration: this may prove to be an alarming occurrence if the patient has not been well informed. A number of drugs are excreted in the bile as conjugated metabolites, which may be broken down by the action of gut bacteria and the active drug reabsorbed: examples include the antibiotic chloramphenicol and oestrogens in the oral contraceptive pill.

Metabolism

Following the administration of medicines, most drug metabolism (or biotransformation) occurs in the liver. The liver does not simply convert the pharmacologically active substance to the inactive form(s); it can also transform inactive to active, or change active chemicals to slightly different but equally active entities. For example, a proportion of carbamazepine, an anticonvulsant, is hepatically metabolised to carbamazepine epoxide which also acts to prevent epileptic seizures.

Metabolism changes the chemical structure of the drug in either of two phases:

(1) Phase 1 metabolism tends to involve the breaking of chemical bonds within the drug molecule by processes such as hydrolysis, oxidation or reduction. For example, ethanol is metabolised within the body via oxidation to acetaldehyde.

(2) Phase 2 metabolism commonly involves the addition of other chemical structures to the drug via conjugation reactions. Conjugation reactions generally increase the water solubility of the transformed product. Examples of conjugation reactions include glucuronidation, methylation, sulphation and acetylation. Oestrogens are conjugated within the liver via glucuronidation before their elimination through biliary secretion. Paracetamol is also eliminated from the body via a glucuronidation reaction.

A number of drugs undergo extensive first-pass hepatic metabolism. Following absorption from the small intestine a drug will enter the hepatic portal vein and flow to the liver. If a substantial proportion of the absorbed drug is metabolised, or broken down into inactive substances on first passage through the liver, the pharmacological or therapeutic response will be greatly reduced. Propranolol shows significant first-pass effect, undergoing a hydroxylation reaction to an inactive agent. Patients with hepatic cirrhosis have an impaired ability to remove propranolol on first-pass through the liver and consequently the doses used in such patients must be much smaller. If the usual daily dose of 80–160 mg of propranolol were administered to such patients they would demonstrate marked clinical signs of excessive doses of beta blockers.

Some drugs undergo such extensive removal on first-pass that an alternative route of administration must be implemented. Examples of such therapy include glyceryl trinitrate, used to relieve myocardial ischaemia, which is administered via the buccal cavity, sublingually, intravenously or transdermally; all these routes avoid high concentrations entering the hepatic vein and thus first-pass removal by hepatic metabolism. If patients experience side effects, such as a throbbing headache, with buccal or sublingual glyceryl trinitrate, instruction to swallow the tablet once the chest pain has resolved will greatly reduce the likelihood of dose related adverse effects.

A number of factors may influence hepatic drug metabolism including:

(1) *Liver disease.* The liver has great reserves, and hepatic damage must be quite severe before significant changes in drug metabolism are evident. Unfortunately routine liver function tests do not give a useful indication of the extent of hepatic impairment with regard to drug metabolism.

(2) *Concurrent drug therapy.* A wide range of drugs may induce and increase, or alternatively inhibit and decrease, the hepatic metabolism of other drugs (see Chapter 14). These changes in metabolism must be taken into account when commencing, or discontinuing, medicines.

(3) *Age.* Elderly people and the very young, in particular babies less than 6 months old, may show evidence of impaired metabolism of certain drugs.

Very young children may eliminate drugs by different metabolic pathways due to the relative immaturity of their evolving hepatic systems. In the neonate, theophylline (which may be used in the management of apnoea of prematurity) is metabolised to caffeine. This represents a very minor pathway in adults.

(4)   *Concurrent illness.* Conditions which alter hepatic blood flow or change the extent of hepatic oxygenation may also influence the metabolic process. Patients with acute or chronic respiratory illness, or those with severe congestive cardiac failure, will not metabolise drugs efficiently.

(5)   *Genetic influence.* Both acetylation and oxidation reactions may be, at least in part, determined by genetic factors. The process of acetylation (the addition of an acetyl grouping to the drug) is involved in the biotransformation of hydralazine, which produces arteriolar dilatation, and isoniazid, which is used to treat tuberculosis. Phenytoin, the antiepileptic drug, is broken down by oxidative metabolism, which is also subject to genetic influence (Reynolds, 1996).

In very simplistic terms, the end result of metabolism is the production of a more water soluble substance, which is less pharmacologically active than the initial compound, although this may involve transition through a range of intermediate pharmacologically active agents which can then be eliminated from the body, most commonly in the urine.

Elimination half-life

The elimination half-life of a drug describes the time taken for the plasma concentration of the drug to fall by 50% (Fig. 3.4). Half-life is influenced both by the distribution volume and clearance. Values for half-life vary enormously from minutes (soluble insulin, 6 minutes; benzylpenicillin, 40 minutes) to days (amiodarone (used in the management of cardiac arrhythmias) around 50 days, range 20–100 days). Values for drugs show inter-patient variation, and depend very much on how an individual handles the particular drug. The half-life of digoxin may be 30 hours in someone with normal renal function, but as long as 120 hours in a patient with both renal impairment and congestive cardiac failure.

A drug with a short half-life will be removed quickly from the body and often requires frequent dosing during the day. A drug with a long half-life will remain for a prolonged period and may require dosing on a daily basis or sometimes even less frequently. Following discontinuation, the elimination half-life indicates how long the drug will remain in the system. The clinical effect of a penicillin may last only a few hours, but amiodarone will remain in the body for many months. This can have a very important bearing on how long a patient should be monitored when a drug is discontinued following an adverse event. When commencing patients on angiotensin-converting enzyme (ACE) inhibitors it is common practice to give a test dose of captopril at night

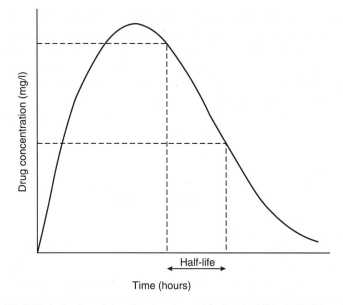

Fig. 3.4   Half-life is the time taken for drug concentration to fall to half of its original value, assuming no further dose of drug has been administered.

and monitor consequent blood pressure response. Captopril has a half-life of 1–2 hours and duration of clinical effect of about 6 hours. Enalapril has a half-life of 5–11 hours and lasts about 24 hours. If the patient was test dosed with enalapril and subsequently suffered first dose hypotension, the side effects would last considerably longer than they would after a dose of captopril.

The benzodiazepine, diazepam, will remain in the circulation for a long time after overdose because of its long elimination half-life and biotransformation to active metabolites. Heroin, on the other hand, has a short elimination half-life and will normally be removed from the bloodstream within hours.

In addition to describing elimination, the half-life of a drug will determine the time period over which accumulation occurs with repeated dosing, and thus the time to achieve steady state.

Creatinine clearance

Creatinine enjoys centre stage and headline billing in clinical practice as a reliable indicator of renal function and hydration status. The biochemical is produced following breakdown of muscle creatine. Production is thus related to lean body or muscle mass. Creatinine is eliminated from the body via the kidneys, mainly by glomerular filtration. When the patient has stable renal function the rate of creatinine production will equal the rate of elimination through the kidneys. The serum concentration of creatinine at this point will be relatively constant. If we assume that production of creatinine does not change significantly, when the serum concentration rises it must be because elimination has decreased and kidney function has fallen. Likewise, if the creatinine concentration decreases it may be explained by an increase or recovery of renal function. By measuring serum creatinine concentrations we may thus obtain some indicator of renal function. Quantification of renal function is important in clinical practice because it can greatly influence choice of therapy, as well as dosage and frequency of drug administration.

Creatinine clearance, a measure of kidney function, can be calculated using the method of Cockcroft and Gault (1976):

Creatinine clearance (ml/min) =
$$\frac{[140 - \text{Age (years)}] \times \text{weight (kg)} \times [1.04 \text{ (females) or } 1.23 \text{ (males)}]}{\text{Serum creatinine } (\mu\text{mol/l})}$$

A simple mnemonic to remember is that creatinine clearance is as simple as 123ABC. For male subjects creatinine clearance equals 1.23 multiplied by 140 minus A for age, multiplied by B for body weight, divided by C for serum creatinine. The multiplication factor for females is 1.04 to allow for their smaller muscle mass, which contains creatine, the precursor of serum creatinine.

Calculation of creatinine clearance using the above method is not possible for all individuals. A number of clinical and physiological conditions preclude the use of the Cockcroft and Gault method. Unstable or changing renal function, muscle wasting conditions or emaciated individuals, patients immediately post-surgery or following trauma, in pregnancy, those with severe liver disease or ascites, obese individuals, the critically ill, or infants and children, are all excluded from this particular method of creatinine clearance calculation. Obese individuals' renal function can be estimated if ideal body weight is substituted for actual weight.

As patients age, their renal function declines and their ability to handle drugs decreases. As a general rule we all lose around 10% of our kidney function for every 10 years over the age of 40 years. Thus an 80 year old man will have a maximal kidney function of only 60%. This is an important fact to remember when designing drug regimens for older people.

The *BNF* assigns renal impairment amongst adult individuals into one of three groups (mild, moderate or severe) based on a creatinine clearance (or glomerular filtration rate) of 20–50 ml/minute, 10–20 ml/minute, and less than 10 ml/minute, respectively. For those drugs, or drugs whose metabolites are, eliminated predominantly by the renal route, dosage adjustment is commonly required to minimise side effects and adverse events. Appendix 3 of the *BNF* provides a useful summary of dose adjustment in renal impairment.

Example

An 84 year old widow is admitted to hospital in an acute confusional state. She has no previous medical records as she stated, 'I've never been ill in my life.' She weighed only 42 kg. A biochemical screen reveals her serum creatinine to be 118 μmol/l (normal range 50–120 μmol/l). On first examination her serum creatinine is within normal limits but does this mean her renal function is normal? This is more readily answered if we calculate her creatinine clearance:

$$\text{Creatinine clearance} = 1.04 \times \frac{(140 - \text{Age}) \times \text{Body weight}}{\text{Serum creatinine}}$$

$$= 1.04 \times \frac{(140 - 84) \times 42}{118}$$

$$= 21 \text{ ml/minute}$$

So, in spite of a seemingly normal serum creatinine result, the patient has mild to moderate renal impairment. Such marked renal insufficiency may have a significant influence on both choice and dose of any subsequent drug therapy.

It is impossible to look at a serum creatinine result in isolation from the patient and quantify the extent of renal impairment. Creatinine clearance is influenced, amongst many other factors, by age, sex, weight and stable serum creatinine. All these parameters must be considered when quantifying the degree of renal impairment.

Therapeutic drug monitoring

Drugs within the body follow a general pattern: namely, in excess they will produce side effects or toxicity, whereas too little of a drug will induce therapeutic failure. Somewhere in between resides the correct dosing schedule which will effect a therapeutic or clinical response (Fig. 3.5). For many drugs this 'therapeutic window' is large and there is a wide margin between therapeutic failure and toxicity. Examples of such drugs include penicillins, vitamins and benzodiazepines. Other drugs have a very narrow window: the transition between toxicity and no response is a fine line. Therapeutic concentrations have been defined for a number of drugs. If exceeded there is an increased likelihood of toxicity, and if under-dosed the treatment will probably be ineffective. Concentrations within the target range are likely, but not guaranteed, to be effective. Therapeutic ranges can thus be viewed as a probability factor. Blood concentrations of a number of drugs are regularly measured in clinical practice to facilitate optimal patient outcome (Table 3.1).

Dosing regimes

There are two concentration–time profiles that we aim to achieve with drug administration (Fig. 3.6). We may wish to see high peak concentrations for clinical efficacy, and then allow drug elimination to occur down to a low trough before the next dose is given. Pulsed therapy, the intermittent administration of bolus doses, is often necessary with treatments such as antimicrobial and

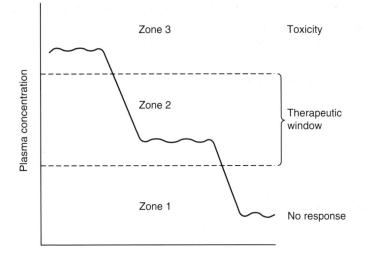

Fig. 3.5   The therapeutic window.

Table 3.1   Drugs that should have plasma concentrations measured to guide therapeutic management in certain clinical situations.

Drug	Therapeutic use
Aminoglycoside antibiotics	Infection
Caffeine	Neonatal apnoea
Carbamazepine	Anticonvulsant
Cyclosporin (Ciclosporin)	Immunosuppressant
Digoxin	Atrial fibrillation
Lithium	Mania
Phenobarbitone (Phenobarbital)	Anticonvulsant
Phenytoin	Anticonvulsant
Theophylline	Bronchodilator
Tricyclic antidepressants	Depression

cancer chemotherapy which cause dose-dependent side effects. With amino-glycoside antibiotics (Fig. 3.6a), high peak concentrations are necessary to penetrate the focus of infection and kill the micro-organisms responsible for the clinical symptoms of infection. However, if the plasma concentration remains high for a period of time, the patient may suffer kidney damage (nephro-toxicity) or hearing impairment (ototoxicity). Dosing in this manner relies on an estimation of the individual's volume of distribution and rate of clearance.

For other drugs we may wish to maintain the concentration at a steady level with few peak and trough values. A plateau concentration with little variation is most desirable for conditions which are present all the time with minimal circadian variation. To quantify dosing requirements in this instance we simply

(a)

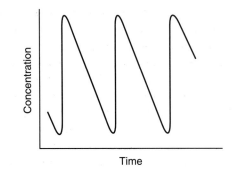

High peak concentrations and low trough concentrations
are desirable with aminoglycoside antibiotic therapy

(b)

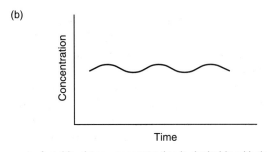

A stable plateau concentration is desirable with theophylline,
digoxin, antiepileptics

Fig. 3.6 Concentration–time profiles.

need an estimate of drug clearance. Examples of therapy requiring a flat concentration–time profile include anticonvulsants for managing epilepsy, digoxin in atrial fibrillation and lithium in the management of mania (Fig. 3.6b).

A simple approach to dosing regimes is to picture everyone as a leaking bucket. If we imagine all patients as a bucket of fluid with a known volume, every time we add a quantity of drug, defined by the product of dose administered and bioavailability, the concentration will rise. Over time the concentration will decline as the drug is cleared by elimination pathways. The rate of elimination can be quantified in terms of clearance. The resultant concentration at any point in time is thus dependent on the interplay between administered dose, dosing frequency, volume of distribution and clearance.

Steady state

When a new dose regimen is commenced the plasma concentration will rise with each subsequent dose until an equilibrium exists whereby the rate of administration equals the rate of elimination. This equilibrium is known as steady state. At least four or five elimination half-lives must pass before the patient is at steady state. At steady state the drug concentration will rise and fall by the same amount if both the dose and dosing frequency remain unchanged.

If blood samples are withdrawn before steady state, concentrations must be interpreted with great caution. Digoxin has a long elimination half-life, commonly around 2 days but varying with renal function. If plasma concentrations are reported before steady state has been achieved, perhaps after only 2 or 3 days' therapy, the result may appear within the target range. If the same dose is continued and the concentration measured after 2 weeks it may have increased further to a potentially toxic value. Care must therefore be taken to ensure blood samples for plasma drug concentration analysis are drawn at an appropriate time.

Loading dose

For drugs with a long elimination half-life it may be necessary to give a loading dose at the start of treatment to achieve 'therapeutic concentrations' sooner rather than later. The loading dose is simply an initial total dose which is required to readily achieve the desired plasma concentration. The decision to give such a dose would obviously be influenced by the clinical acuity of the condition under discussion. Loading doses of digoxin (half-life 2 days), amiodarone (half-life 54 days) and warfarin (exists in two different forms with half-lives of 32 and 54 hours, respectively) are commonly prescribed in clinical practice. If loading doses are not given, the plasma drug concentration will rise slowly over four or five half-lives (Fig. 3.7). A wait of 10 days to bring a life-threatening arrhythmia under control is obviously unacceptable. Clearly for

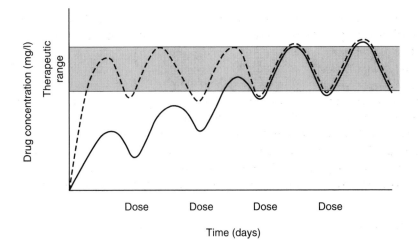

Fig. 3.7 To achieve therapeutic concentrations quickly a loading dose may be necessary. It takes four or five half-lives to achieve steady-state. If the drug has a short half-life, a loading dose may not be necessary: if the drug has a long half-life, a loading dose will help to attain therapeutic response sooner.

drugs with a short elimination half-life, the time delay in attaining steady state is much shorter, and the loading dose may be omitted.

Maintenance dose

The regular or maintenance dose describes the quantity of drug which we must administer to our patient to replace the amount of drug which has been lost from the body since the last dose was given. By replacing the drug lost through elimination the desired plasma concentration can be maintained.

The meaning of measured plasma drug concentrations

The interpretation of plasma drug concentrations is a complex process. Unfortunately, a simple comparison of the reported value with the target range gives no meaningful information unless all background data are taken into account.

Therapeutic concentrations, or target ranges, have been defined for a number of drugs (Table 3.2). The process of therapeutic drug monitoring is not simply a comparison of the reported drug concentration for each particular patient with the intended target result; it must be much more patient centred.

Table 3.2   Therapeutic concentrations for the most commonly measured drugs.

Drug	Therapeutic range
Carbamazepine	6–12 mg/l for monotherapy
	4–8 mg/l for multiple anticonvulsant therapy
Cyclosporin (Ciclosporin)	60–180 μ/l for renal transplant
Digoxin	1–2 μg/l sampled at least 6 hours after dose
Gentamicin	Trough less than 2mg/l
	Peak 4–12 mg/l drawn 60 minutes after intravenous bolus dose
Lithium	0.4–1.0 mmol/l sampled 12 hours after previous dose
Phenytoin	10–20 mg/l
Theophylline	10–20 mg/l

Adapted from Anon. (1998).

Patients and their clinical response must always be the primary focus of all therapeutic drug monitoring activity. Consider the case of an elderly female prescribed digoxin for atrial fibrillation. If the steady state concentration is less than the therapeutic range but the patient remains in controlled fibrillation, clearly the dose for that particular individual is, by definition, therapeutic. The oft quoted truism, worth stating once again, is that we should aim to treat the patient, not the level.

To interpret plasma drug concentrations, the blood sample is of paramount importance. If blood is drawn at an inappropriate time or from an inappropriate site the reported concentration may prove meaningless. It is impossible to detail the correct time to draw bloods for analysis because practice varies depending on the individual drug, what the result is being used for, and local practice. Some generalisations are, however, worth highlighting.

- If samples are drawn too soon after administration, a falsely elevated concentration may result. It takes time for a drug to distribute out of the blood into the various tissues and organs.

- Following ingestion of a digoxin tablet, blood samples should not be drawn for at least 6–8 hours to allow time for it to distribute out of the bloodstream into muscle.

- Aminoglycosides commonly take around 60 minutes to distribute. Hence peak concentrations measured before this time are often meaningless.

- If possible, plasma lithium concentrations should be measured 12 hours after the previous dose. For most drugs a sample drawn immediately before the next dose is a useful reference point, as it reflects the lowest point in the concentration–time profile.

When a patient is on long-term maintenance therapy, bloods drawn immediately before the next dose will contain the lowest concentration of drug. This is known as the trough concentration. The trough is fairly reproducible because it is not influenced by any absorption or distribution phenomena. Concentrations after ingestion of a medicine will obviously increase and be greater than the trough result. Trough results are often useful to monitor for patients on anticonvulsant therapies, such as phenytoin, carbamazepine and phenobarbitone (phenobarbital), or those prescribed modified release medicines, for example many branded theophylline preparations, which slowly release drug into the gastro-intestinal tract and may support absorption over a prolonged time period.

When serum drug concentrations are reported as unexpectedly high or low, a rational explanation may not be immediately obvious. If the patient shows clinical signs of neither toxicity nor of therapeutic failure, in spite of such biochemical indices, the easy solution is to blame the laboratories. 'Obviously they've done it wrong!' However, a thorough examination of the drug-use and blood sampling process will often prove very illuminating.

How compliant was the patient? Does the low drug concentration suggest low or non-compliance with prescribed medication? Was the drug dose actually administered or was it omitted because the patient was off the ward or there was no supply on the ward? Was the patient sick after the drug round? Witnessing patients placing tablets in their mouths is no guarantee that they actually swallow them. Occasionally, by measuring serum drug concentrations it is possible to uncover cases of non-compliance because the result is at great variance with previous reports, or it is physically impossible.

Does the low concentration indicate that the patient has not yet reached steady state because of a long elimination half-life? If blood was sampled some time later the serum drug concentration would be greater. Remember that it takes around four or five half-lives to achieve a new steady state concentration following a change in dosing regimen.

Does the low concentration suggest that blood was sampled before the full dose of drug actually entered the patient's bloodstream? For aminoglycoside antibiotics a peak concentration should be monitored 1 hour after administration of an intravenous bolus injection. If the drug is injected into a giving set through which a large volume infusion is running, such as sodium chloride 0.9% or glucose 5%, it may take some time for the aminoglycoside to actually reach the patient's bloodstream. If blood is sampled for concentration analysis 60 minutes after the drug is injected into the giving set, the result may be falsely low simply because it has not yet reached the systemic circulation. This often appears to be a problem in paediatrics because injections tend to be administered into burettes or giving sets rather than via venflons directly into the bloodstream.

High serum drug concentrations may also have a number of less obvious explanations. Once more, is patient compliance in question? Has the patient deliberately ingested more than the prescribed quantity of medicine? If one is prescribed theophylline tablets 'to help the breathing', does it not seem entirely reasonable for an individual with chronic obstructive airways disease to take a handful of the tablets when their chronic dyspnoea becomes a bit more debilitating? An elevated theophylline concentration in this case may not necessarily indicate that the patient has been prescribed an overdose, merely that through injudicious medication instruction the patient has misunderstood the therapeutic intention.

Immunosuppressed patients undergoing chemotherapy and/or radiotherapy are at risk of neutropenic septicaemia. In the event of systemic infection, various antibiotics including vancomycin may be administered into central venous lines, such as Hickmann catheters. If the line into which a drug is infused is not properly flushed with saline, results can be spuriously high when blood is subsequently withdrawn for concentration analysis, because the blood sample will have mixed with high concentrations of drug solution. The result does not reflect the drug concentration in the patient's bloodstream because it has been contaminated. Dose reduction in such cases of elevated serum antibiotic concentrations may result in therapeutic failure.

Similarly, it is not unheard of for the person sampling bloods for antibiotic concentrations to try and beat the patient's circulation. I have heard the story of the newly qualified doctors who, on giving a dose of gentamicin, suddenly realised they had not withdrawn bloods for measuring the pre-dose, trough concentration. On recognising their mistake they immediately ran round the bed and sampled blood from the opposite arm. Unfortunately, the patient's heart had beaten them for speed and the trough concentration was reported as unexpectedly toxic.

If blood is withdrawn before complete distribution of the drug, serum concentrations may be falsely elevated. Importantly, however, this is not an indication of imminent toxicity; it merely reflects the fact that the drug has not yet distributed out of the central blood pool. This is a common problem with digoxin which takes approximately 6 hours for distribution. Morning drug rounds within hospital often take place around 8 a.m. If the phlebotomist visits at 10 a.m., blood samples will be taken a mere 2 hours after digoxin ingestion and serum drug concentrations will be erroneously reported as potentially toxic. To circumvent this common event, within Wirral Hospitals NHS Trust, we now administer digoxin at 6 p.m. When the phlebotomist comes the following morning, it is at least 14 hours after ingestion of digoxin. Other hospitals operate an 'omit the morning dose until the patient is bled' policy. Both procedures, if adhered to, are satisfactory means of avoiding spuriously elevated distribution phase drug concentrations.

Nursing contribution

An accurate history of drug administration and sampling strategy must be available to the professional who interprets the serum drug concentration. As a bare minimum, the information required to make a meaningful interpretation of any measured drug concentration should include the following:

- Was there an accurate dosing history including dose and time?
- When was the last dose of drug given/taken?
- When was the blood sample drawn?
- From where was the blood sample drawn?
- Was there a reason for concentration analysis?
- Was there concurrent medication?

Clinical nurses are ideally positioned to ensure that the above information is both accurate and readily accessible. By so doing the success of any subsequent therapeutic drug monitoring event will be greatly enhanced, with resultant patient benefit. In the absence of such information serum drug concentration analysis will tell us very little.

Summary

The pharmacokinetic process, including drug absorption, volume or distribution, metabolism and elimination, is introduced and illustrated by clinical example. The four parameters inform optimal drug dosing, and a full understanding by clinical nurses will facilitate appropriate outcomes from drug therapy.

The chapter described the influence of age, concurrent illness and drug therapy on the elimination of medicines. Elimination half-life and its influence on drug accumulation and clearance is discussed. Calculation of creatinine clearance as an indicator of renal function, the major route of drug elimination, is described. Quantification of the degree of renal impairment has an important bearing on the appropriateness or otherwise of drug dosing. Therapeutic drug monitoring and the rationale for measuring serum drug concentrations of certain drugs in selected patients is explained. The concept of steady state and the difference between loading dose and maintenance dose is discussed. The interpretation of reported serum drug concentrations is reviewed. By concluding with a critique of why mistakes may be made, it is hoped that readers will be in a stronger position to influence the therapeutic drug monitoring process and achieve optimal outcomes in their future practice.

References

Anon. (1998) *Wirral Prescribers Guide*, 4th edn 1998/99. Wirral Hospitals NHS Trust, Upton.

Cockcroft D.W. & Gault, M.H. (1976) Prediction of creatinine clearance from serum creatinine. *Nephron* **16**, 31.

Mehta, D.K. (1997) *British National Formulary No. 34*, British Medical Association and Royal Pharmaceutical Society of Great Britian, London.

Reynolds, J.E.F. (1996) *Martindale. The Extra Pharmacopoeia*, 31st edn. Royal Pharmaceutical Society of Great Britain, London.

Further reading

Fitzpatrick, R. (1994) Practical pharmacokinetics. In: *Clinical Pharmacy and Therapeutics* (ed. R. Walker & C. Edwards). Churchill Livingstone, Edinburgh.

Grahame-Smith, D.G. & Aronson, J.K. (1992) *Oxford Textbook of Clinical Pharmacology and Drug Therapy*, 2nd edn. Oxford University Press, Oxford.

Chapter 4

Impact of Age, Pregnancy, Disease and Food on Drug Action

Michael Philip Jackson

Introduction

The development of a new drug takes several years, starting from its initial discovery to marketing the product for human use. This time is spent testing the drug in animal and human subjects in order to highlight any potential problems or side effects, and gauge the therapeutic and toxic concentrations. Trials carried out on healthy individuals may not reflect the population to which the drug might be given eventually. Trials carried out on children, the aged, pregnant women and those with hepatic and renal problems are unethical in most cases, and dose adjustments may need to be made by extrapolating data taken from healthy individuals. After the drug is launched, post-marketing surveillance is carried out by the Committee on Safety of Medicines (CSM). However, even this rigorous monitoring may not identify rare, potentially fatal, side effects of the drug.

If the same single dose of a drug was given to several individuals of different ages, variation would be observed in the final drug concentration in the blood. The concentration may be sub-therapeutic in some, but toxic in others. This is because the drug's characteristics (onset of action, duration and concentration) are influenced by the body's individual characteristics, which change with age. It is not just the physiology of ageing which affects drug concentration, but any factor which affects the absorption, distribution, metabolism and excretion of that drug.

This chapter is intended to apply what you have learned about these concepts in the previous chapter to people of different ages and disease states. It will look at how a drug's characteristics are altered in neonates, children, elderly people, pregnant women, and patients with liver, renal and other diseases. In addition, consideration will be given to the presence of food on drug metabolism.

Neonates

Much less is known about the way in which drugs are handled (pharmacokinetics) in neonates and children due to ethical constraints surrounding drug testing. The majority of the information collected about drugs in this age bracket comes from experience during the drugs' use by consultant paediatricians. In general, neonates and children require a lower dosage of drug than adults because of their relatively low body weight. However, they should not be classed as 'small adults'. When dealing with neonates and children, there are similarities and differences for altered drug pharmacokinetics, which will be explored in the next two sections. The definitions below are common terms used in paediatric medicine.

Pre-term baby	less than 38 weeks' gestation
Full term baby	38–42 weeks gestation
Neonate	up to 1 month
Child	1–12 years.

Drug absorption

Oral route

The oral route is probably the most practical in terms of drug administration. However, many different factors can affect the rate and extent of drug absorption via the oral route. The most influential is stomach acidity, which can affect the drug's solubility properties and therefore the total amount of drug that reaches the systemic circulation. A newborn baby's stomach is pH 7 (neutral) at birth. This is because of the presence of amniotic fluid which is swallowed during gestation. Within minutes acid production begins, the stomach reaching pH 1.5–3.0 after a few hours. There quickly follows a fall in acid production lasting 10 days, before acid production starts to climb again. Pre-term neonates may not follow this pattern, with an estimated 20% having a decreased capacity to secrete gastric acid. Consequently this leaves them with a gastric acid output referred to as 'achlorhydria'. An adult pH value is reached after 2 years.

Both gastric and duodenal pH affect drug ionisation and subsequently absorption. An ionised drug is usually the salt of a drug, e.g. phenytoin sodium, which is very water soluble but has low lipid solubility. Alternatively an unionised drug, e.g. phenytoin, has less water solubility but greater lipid solubility. An acidic environment (low pH), favours the absorption of acidic drugs (e.g. phenytoin), because these drugs will be less ionised and therefore more lipid soluble, enhancing movement of the drug through membranes. However, in neonates with achlorhydria these drugs will be ionised because of the higher pH in the stomach, and therefore they are not absorbed as well as in older children and in adults. Alternatively, basic drugs, such as penicillins and erythromycin, will be less ionised at a higher pH, and therefore they are absorbed to a greater extent in neonates with achlorhydria than in adults.

The rate at which the stomach empties can also influence drug absorption. Gastric emptying time is increased in the neonate, resulting in drugs remaining in the stomach much longer. Since the stomach has a less absorptive surface than the small intestine, this may prolong the time to reach peak drug concentration. Adult values are attained after 6–8 months.

Bile acids aid the absorption of fat-soluble drugs and vitamins (vitamin A, D, E and K). Neonates have a reduced bile output; therefore this is likely to alter the absorption of fat soluble drugs. Table 4.1 summarizes the factors affecting oral absorption.

Table 4.1 Factors affecting oral absorption.

Factor affecting absorption	Increased drug absorption	Decreased drug absorption
High pH of stomach	Basic drugs: penicillins, erythromycin	Acidic drugs: phenytoin, phenobarbitone (phenobarbital)
Gastric emptying time prolonged	Generally reduces rate of absorption	
Bile output reduced		Fat-soluble drugs

Intramuscular (IM) absorption

The rate and extent of drug that is absorbed via the IM route is dependent upon several factors that vary with age: the surface area of muscle in contact with the drug; the blood flow to that muscle; and the activity of that muscle. Muscle mass and subcutaneous tissue in the newborn are directly proportional to gestational age. During the first few days there is a reduced muscle blood flow which may be made worse by concomitant illnesses such as heart failure. A paralysed or severely ill neonate would have reduced movement, resulting in less muscle blood flow. Therefore in newborn babies, IM absorption is poor, and is less reliable as a route of administration.

Percutaneous absorption

Percutaneous absorption refers to the absorption of drugs from a reservoir (i.e. patch) when applied topically to the skin. The epidermis (top layer of skin) in the full term neonate is well developed and similar to that of an older child or adult (Choonara, 1994). The pre-term infant, however, has an immature epidermis with decreased thickness of the skin, increased skin hydration and increased ratio of surface area per kilogram body weight (approximately three times that of an adult), resulting in an increased percutaneous absorption of a topically applied drug. Drug toxicities have been reported for topical salicylic acid and corticosteroids, therefore caution is advised.

Drug distribution

Drug distribution is an active process involving drug partitioning into body compartments to form a constantly changing equilibrium. The relative distribution between compartments is dependent upon the drug's lipid/water solubility, protein binding, membrane permeability and blood flow to each compartment. Membrane permeability is generally greater in the neonate compared to the adult, and this is particularly true of the blood–brain barrier, allowing more drug to affect the brain.

Water-soluble drugs

Total body water content changes with increasing age as shown in Fig. 4.1. The higher percentage total body water content of the pre-term neonate increases the volume of distribution (V_d) for water soluble drugs (digoxin, warfarin, gentamicin, caffeine, and theophylline). Because distribution into water is increased, a greater dose (mg/kg) is required to achieve similar concentrations to those in the adult.

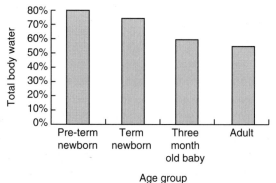

Fig. 4.1   Total body water in different age groups. (Data taken from Walker & Edwards (1994).)

Lipid-soluble drugs

In contrast to total body water content, the amount of adipose tissue is reduced in the pre-term neonate (1% of body weight in pre-term; 15% in full-term; 30% in adults), thereby reducing the V_d for lipid-soluble drugs, e.g. diazepam. A lower dose (mg/kg) is therefore required.

Drug–protein binding

Drug–protein binding refers to the temporary binding of a drug molecule to a protein (usually albumin) in the blood. The bound drug is not able to act on receptors in the body and is therefore inactive. However, when the concentration of free (unbound) drug in the blood starts to fall, the bound drug releases itself from the protein to become active. The degree of protein binding is different for every drug. The following shows that the binding of a drug with a protein in the blood is a two-way reaction:

Drug (unbound, active) + Protein ↔ Drug–protein complex (inactive drug)

Protein binding is reduced in the neonate compared with older children and adults. Possible reasons for this include the presence of competing endogenous substances (bilirubin, free fatty acids and steroids) which occupy the protein binding sites available for drug binding; a reduction in protein concentrations, and a lower affinity of the protein for drug binding. For drugs that are protein bound in the plasma, there will be a larger fraction of unbound drug in neonates than in adults. It is the unbound (free) drug that gives rise to the pharmacological and toxic actions of the drug, and in general lower plasma concentrations must be attained to take into account the increased free drug by a reduction in the administered dose. Drugs implicated include ampicillin, carbamazepine, diazepam, lignocaine (lidocaine), phenobarbitone (phenobarbital), phenytoin, propranolol, sulphonamides and theophylline.

Certain drugs (sulphonamides, ceftriaxone) can cause jaundice in neonates by displacing bilirubin from albumin binding sites, facilitating the deposition of unconjugated bilirubin in the brain which may produce neurological damage (kernicterus).

Metabolism

Liver metabolism is reduced in the neonate because of decreases in the following: hepatic blood flow, cellular uptake of drugs, liver enzyme capacity and biliary excretion. These result in a reduced clearance from the body for certain drugs (e.g. diazepam, phenobarbitone (phenobarbital), phenytoin, sodium valproate, theophylline, morphine, indomethacin (indometacin) and metronidazole). A dose reduction is therefore advised.

The influence of drugs that increase the metabolism of other drugs (enzyme-inducers) have a faster and greater response in neonates than adults. For example, phenobarbitone (phenobarbital) induces the enzymes responsible for the metabolism of phenytoin. Consequently, lower phenytoin levels are observed.

Renal elimination

Renal clearance for drugs and their metabolites is greatly reduced in the neonate. As a result maintenance doses of drugs that are eliminated renally (e.g.

digoxin, vancomycin, aminoglycosides) must be reduced. Benzylpenicillin is cleared from the premature neonate at about 30% of the rate seen in adults when adjusted for body weight.

In contrast, an increase in dosage (mg/kg) may be required for drugs that depend upon renal excretion to exert their effects, e.g. thiazide and loop diuretics.

Pharmacodynamics

Pharmacodynamics deals with alterations in the way a drug interacts with its receptor to produce an effect. Digoxin-binding receptors on cardiac tissue have been shown to be more numerous but less sensitive to digoxin in the neonate and children than in adults. This leads to a larger dose (mg/kg) being required in the neonate and child.

Children

As children grow, there are maturational changes in body composition and organ function that can affect drug pharmacokinetics. This leads to a large inter-patient and intra-patient variation in which drugs are handled by the body. Factors that should be taken into account when prescribing drugs are maturational changes in organ structure and function, enzyme activity and quantity, body composition, and concomitant disease states. Certain organs in the body will mature faster than others, some reaching adult values within months.

Various disease states (including renal and hepatic disease and cystic fibrosis) are known to significantly alter drug pharmacokinetics in paediatric patients (see later sections).

The following section will look at changes in drug pharmacokinetics in children up to the age of 12 years.

Drug absorption

The route of administration for a drug chosen by the clinician is influenced by age. Very small children may not be able to take drugs by the oral route and instead receive injections. Rectal administration is generally disliked by children, and the IM route is very painful. Children will usually be administered liquids instead of solid dosage forms. Liquids will increase the rate of absorption of the drug because the time for a tablet to disintegrate is eliminated.

Oral route

The rate and extent of gastro-intestinal absorption of a drug depends on many factors, including the gastric emptying time, the acidity of the stomach, the presence of food, metabolism during passage through the intestinal wall, the presence of bacteria in the gut (microflora) and the effect of disease. Between the neonatal period and maturity these factors change little, so with few exceptions gastro-intestinal absorption varies little.

Rectal route

Rectal absorption of drugs given to paediatric patients, in general, is poor and erratic. However, rectal absorption of certain drugs (diazepam) is adequate when given as a rectal enema rather than a suppository. Solutions and suspensions are the preferred dosage form for rectal drug administration in neonates and young children.

Drug distribution

The main factors that influence drug distribution are the same as in the neonate, total body water being the main factor. The adult value of 55–60% is reached by the age of 12 years. Therefore, up to the age of 12 years there is a gradual decrease in total body water and therefore a reducing V_d for water soluble drugs.

Total body fat also changes throughout childhood. In full-term neonates, fat constitutes 15% of the total body weight. This quickly reaches the female adult value of 30% by 9 months of age for both sexes. During puberty females retain the same percentage of fat while there is a reduction in fat seen in male subjects. The increase in fat by 9 months of age will increase the V_d for lipid-soluble drugs.

Protein binding

As with neonates, infants have a reduced amount of circulating plasma proteins that bind to drugs, and the plasma proteins that are available have a lower affinity to bind to drugs. This leads to an overall reduction in drug–protein binding. Drug–protein binding will usually reach adult values by 12 months of age. This is usually of little clinical significance, except when two drugs compete for the same protein binding site.

Cystic fibrosis

The apparent volume of distribution and renal clearance of drugs, especially broad-spectrum antibiotics, are increased in children with cystic fibrosis. The increased V_d is mainly from the increased amount of viscous sputum in the lungs and other organs. The effect of this is that larger doses of antibiotics (aminoglycosides, cephalosporins and penicillins) are required to saturate the increased volume. There have been reports of an increase in liver metabolism of drugs in patients with cystic fibrosis.

Metabolism

Young infants metabolise drugs more slowly than older children and adults. The 'grey baby' syndrome in infants receiving chloramphenicol is a good example of what can happen when a metabolic pathway is deficient in young children but present in older children, and the capacity to remove a potentially toxic drug is exceeded, leading to accumulation of the parent drug in the body.

Older infants and children can metabolise certain drugs (carbamazepine, phenytoin, quinidine, theophylline) faster than can adults; the clearance rates for these drugs decrease steadily throughout childhood to adult values. Dosages for these drugs are generally larger than those for adults on a mg/kg basis.

Renal elimination

As with neonates, renal function is reduced in young infants. The glomerular filtration rate (GFR), an indicator of renal function, reaches the adult value by about 12 months of age. Until this age a lower dose of renally excreted drug must be given to avoid drug toxicity. Conversely certain drugs such as digoxin have a greater renal clearance in children than adults.

Elderly people

It is now well recognised that individuals age at different rates, i.e. chronological age and biological age are not synonymous. Distinct separation of these interrelated factors is difficult, because both may contribute to variability in drug response. Drug trials using healthy elderly patients may not be relevant to the rest of the elderly population, who probably have other factors to be taken into account, such as disease, concomitant drug treatment, smoking, alcohol intake, diet and general physical status.

Cardiac output decreases by about 1% each year from the age of 20. This reduction is likely to affect most of the body's organs, especially those concerned with drug absorption and elimination. The frequency of drug–drug interactions and adverse reactions associated with unexpectedly high blood drug concentrations are increased in elderly people. However, anaphylactic reactions and allergic reactions appear not to increase in frequency with age. Therefore elderly people have an increase in adverse drug reactions at therapeutic as well as toxic levels.

Drug absorption

Physiological changes in elderly people likely to affect drug absorption are:

- Reduced gastric acid output
- Reduced production of saliva

- Blood flow to the gastro-intestinal tract (GIT) reduced
- The absorptive surface area of the GIT reduced (up to 20%)
- Gastric emptying time increased.

Reduced acid secretion

At least 25% of elderly people have little or no acid in their stomach (Saltzman *et al.*, 1994). An elevation in the pH of the stomach can affect drug ionisation, dissolution, degradation and gastric emptying time. A few drugs, including ketoconazole, ampicillin related drugs and iron compounds, require a low pH in the stomach to render them non-ionised so that they may be absorbed. Bacterial overgrowth is also more common when the ability to produce acid is lost. Bacterial overgrowth may contribute to gastro-intestinal symptoms of distention, gaseousness and looseness of the bowels, and make the threshold for common adverse drug effects much lower.

Reduction in saliva

Saliva production in elderly people is reduced, and patients may thus find it difficult to swallow large tablets and capsules. The dissolution of buccal and sublingual tablets, e.g. glyceryl trinitrate (GTN) tablets would be greatly affected by reduced saliva, and the patient would appear not to benefit from such treatment. The use of saliva stimulants (e.g. malic acid pastilles), artificial saliva (e.g. carmellose, Salivace®) or the frequent sipping of water would help remedy this problem. Dryness of the mouth will be made worse by drugs with antimuscarinic side effects, e.g. hyoscine, and some antidepressants, e.g. amitriptyline.

First-pass effect

Drugs absorbed along the gut are collected in the network of capillaries and mesenteric veins which meet to form the hepatic portal vein that drains the liver before entering the systemic circulation (via the inferior vena cava). Many drugs are therefore removed by the liver before reaching the systemic circulation. This is termed the 'first-pass effect'. It has been estimated that up to 75% or more of the drug may be removed by the first-pass effect. Elderly people have been estimated as having 50% of the first-pass effect when compared with younger adults, allowing more drug to enter the systemic circulation.

The gut wall has the capability of metabolising certain drugs before the drug reaches the liver. One classic example is the anti-Parkinson drug, levodopa. This drug undergoes metabolism during absorption by an enzyme (dopa decarboxylase) in the gastric mucosa. Elderly people have a reduction in dopa decarboxylase and therefore there is a substantial increase in the absorption of levodopa (three-fold increase).

Table 4.2 gives examples of drugs which have altered drug absorption in the elderly.

Table 4.2 Drugs with altered drug absorption in elderly people.

Drugs with increased absorption	Drug with decreased absorption
Chlordiazepoxide	Ampicillin esters
Labetalol	Iron compounds
Levodopa	Ketoconazole
Metoprolol	Prazosin
Propranolol	
Verapamil	

Drug distribution

Diminishing cardiac output with advancing age influences the rate of distribution of drugs which enter the body. In many older patients, this decline in cardiac output is accompanied by an increase in peripheral vascular resistance (less blood flow to the extremities) and a proportional decrease in hepatic and renal blood flow.

The main alteration in the distribution of drugs in elderly people is attributed to the ratio of fat/water. While body weight remains relatively constant up to the age of 65–70 years, the proportion of total body fat increases by 25% by the age of 75. At the same time there is a reduction in total water content from 61% to 53%. Thus, the volume of distribution (V_d) of drugs that are distributed primarily in body water or lean body mass (e.g. lithium or digoxin) is decreased in older patients; unadjusted dosing can result in higher plasma levels in older people. Conversely, drugs of high lipid solubility (anaesthetics or benzodiazepines) would enter the increased fat stores to a greater degree (i.e. have a higher V_d) than in the young person and persist longer in the body after the drug is stopped. The reservoir of fat soluble drug in the body may accumulate with continued use and possibly lead to toxic effects, as seen with long acting benzodiazepines (e.g. nitrazepam).

Protein binding of drugs

Factors which may affect binding with special applicability in older patients include protein concentration, disease states, co-administration of other drugs, and nutritional status.

There are two main proteins which bind to drugs in the body, albumin and alpha-1-acid glycoprotein. The former is the more important and is therefore described in more depth. Serum albumin concentrations fall progressively for each decade beyond 40 years of age, reaching a mean of 3.58 g/dl (normal 4gm/dL) in those older than 80 years (Koda-Kimble & Young, 1995); therefore the binding of certain drugs also decreases, e.g. phenytoin and digoxin. This can have an effect of increasing the unbound (active) fraction of drug, causing increased therapeutic and toxic effects. For these drugs the administered dose should be reduced.

Hayes *et al.* (1975) found that although plasma protein binding of phenytoin was decreased in older people, the clearance of phenytoin was enhanced as more unbound drug was presented to the elimination system.

The list below shows drugs which are affected by reduced protein binding to albumin.

- Clobazam
- Diazepam
- Lorazepam
- Naproxen
- Phenytoin

- Salicylic acid
- Sodium valproate
- Theophylline
- Tolbutamide
- Warfarin

Increases in levels of alpha-1-acid glycoprotein, with advancing age affects the binding of basic drugs such as lignocaine (lidocaine), chlorpromazine and propranolol. For these drugs a decreased amount of unbound (active) drug would result in reduced therapeutic effectiveness.

Metabolism

Beyond the age of 50 years, the mass, overall function and blood flow to the liver decrease by approximately 1% per year. Therefore the number of enzyme units available for metabolism is reduced, as is the rate at which the drug is presented to these enzymes. The elderly patient's hepatic clearance has been estimated to be about one-fifth that of a young person for many drugs (Woodhouse & Wynne, 1992). However, large inter-individual variation in liver metabolism exists for any given drug, and in most cases may be more important than the changes associated with ageing.

When we talk about the metabolism of drugs, we are referring to two main processes (Phase 1 and Phase 2), which occur in the liver. Phase 1 metabolism (reduction, oxidation, hydroxylation, demethylation) modifies the drug so that it becomes more water soluble. In doing this the unique structure of the parent drug is lost, although the metabolite(s) may still have active properties. The group of enzymes responsible for drug metabolism are termed cytochrome P450. Phase 2 metabolism (conjugation, acetylation, sulphonation, glucuronidation) adds large units to the drug molecule, making it very water soluble and therefore more likely to be excreted by the kidney. Any reduction in the metabolic capacity of the liver will ultimately lead to more drug becoming available to the systemic circulation after oral dosing (reduced first-pass effect), and a reduced clearance of the drug and its metabolites. This becomes more important for drugs which are chiefly broken down by the liver, such as nitrates, barbiturates, lignocaine (lidocaine), morphine and propranolol.

With few exceptions it is the phase one processes that are most adversely affected by age. As a consequence of this the drug's half-life is increased, prolonging its action, which may lead to escalation in drug plasma levels on further dosing. For drugs that are affected significantly by this, the prescriber should choose an alternative drug or, if this is not possible, start with a lower dose of drug, and possibly lengthen the dosing interval.

Table 4.3 shows the effect of volume of distribution and half-life on the total clearance of certain commonly used drugs in the elderly.

Table 4.3 Volume of distribution, half-life and total clearance of some drugs in elderly people.

Drug	Volume of distribution	Half-life	Total clearance
Amitripyline	↓	↑	↓
Ampicillin	Unchanged	↑	↓
Chlordiazepoxide	↑	↑	↓
Cimetidine	↓	↑	↓
Diazepam	↑	↑	↓
Digoxin	↓	↑	↓
Propranolol	↓	↑	↓
Tolbutamide	↓	↑	↓
Warfarin	Unchanged	↑	↓

Renal elimination

Age related changes in renal function have been well documented, and are probably the single most important physiological factor resulting in adverse drug reactions. Glomerular filtration rate and renal plasma flow decrease about 1% per year after the age of 30 years (Lindeman *et al.*, 1985).

Even in healthy elderly patients the renal function will still have declined, although significant variability can occur. Age related changes in renal function are measurable through increases in serum creatinine levels. Appendix 3 in the *British National Formulary* (*BNF*) (Mehta, 1997) gives guidance to the prescriber of the action which needs to be taken for a particular drug in the event of reduced renal function. (Please refer to the section in this chapter on renal failure for further information.)

Reduced kidney function in elderly people can lead to drugs having a prolonged half-life and elevated plasma concentrations. The highest risk drugs are those that depend entirely upon the kidney for elimination. For drugs such as gentamicin and vancomycin, that have a narrow window between therapeutic and toxic levels in the plasma (therapeutic window), it is important to assess renal function before commencing administration. Failure to check renal function for these drugs may lead to inappropriate doses being prescribed, resulting in ototoxicity and nephrotoxicity.

The list below shows drugs which are predominantly renally excreted.

- ACE inhibitors
- Allopurinol
- Amiloride
- Aminoglycosides
  (streptomycin, neomycin,
  gentamicin, amikacin)
- Amphotericin B
- Atenolol
- Bleomycin
- Ceftriaxone
- Chlorpropamide
- Cimetidine
- Ciprofloxacin
- Cisplatin
- Digoxin
- Fluconazole
- Imipenem
- Lithium
- Loop diuretics, e.g. frusemide
  (furosemide)
- Methotrexate
- Metoclopramide
- Phenobarbitone (phenobarbital)
- Penicillamine
- Ranitidine
- Trimethoprim
- Thiazide diuretics
- Vancomycin

Pharmacodynamic changes

Pharmacodynamic changes are defined as changes in concentration–response relationships or receptor sensitivity. The increased susceptibility of elderly people to adverse drug reactions is partly due to an increased sensitivity to that drug and also to the prescribing of multiple drugs (polypharmacy). Impairment of the body's ability to regulate blood flow and failure to maintain adequate cerebral blood flow on standing (baroreceptor function) leads to orthostatic hypotension. This is aggravated by drugs which affect the nervous system (sympatholytic action), e.g. tricyclic antidepressants, by volume-depleting drugs (diuretics) and by vasodilating agents (nitrates and alcohol).

The ageing brain becomes more sensitive to the effects of certain drugs, especially to sedating drugs and those which affect mental function (cause confusion). This may be due to alterations in the blood–brain barrier allowing a greater proportion of the administered dose to reach the brain. Drugs with anticholinergic properties (hyoscine, amitriptyline) are particularly notorious for inducing mental fuzziness and confusion in older patients.

The heart is also affected by the ageing process, leading to a blunted response to beta-blockers in older people. Clotting factor synthesis is inhibited to a greater extent in older than in young patients at equivalent warfarin concentrations. The dose of warfarin required to give the desired international normalised ratio (INR) will be generally lower in the elderly than in younger adults.

Thermoregulatory responses are often compromised in elderly people. Hypothermia can be produced by direct drug effects on temperature control, as well as by a reduction in mobility and cognition. Phenothiazines, such as chlorpromazine, are the prime culprits for drug induced hypothermia.

Pregnancy

The most important aspect of drug therapy in pregnant women is, of course, the effect of the drug on the fetus. Most manufacturers of drugs will usually not recommend the drug to be used in pregnancy. Therefore drugs are best avoided unless the benefits outweigh the risks. It has been estimated that nearly 40% of women in the UK take at least one drug during pregnancy, excluding iron, vitamins and drugs used during delivery. For many conditions (hypertension, diabetes, epilepsy, thyroid disease) drug treatment must be continued throughout pregnancy, as the impact of the disease on the developing fetus would be greater than the potential risk of the drug. This part of the chapter examines how pregnancy alters drug pharmacokinetics.

Pregnancy can alter the rate of elimination of certain drugs. It has been postulated that the change in steroid levels in the body can increase and decrease the activity of some cytochrome P450 enzymes. A recognised example of this is the increase in seizures during pregnancy due to increased elimination of antiepileptic drugs (e.g. phenytoin, phenobarbitone (phenobarbital), carbamazepine). The doses of these drugs would therefore need to be increased during pregnancy.

Table 4.4 shows the physiological changes that take place during pregnancy and their impact on drug pharmacokinetics.

The placenta, uterus, amniotic fluid and fetus increase significantly in size and weight during pregnancy. These tissues and fluids comprise a complex and changing compartment, into and out of which drugs distribute to differing degrees throughout pregnancy. The ease with which drugs penetrate the placental barrier governs their relative distribution. Those drugs which penetrate easily may reside in the fetus and act as a drug reservoir for the maternal blood, prolonging the action of the implicated drug. Examples of drugs in which the placental concentration is greater than the maternal concentration are sodium valproate, ketamine, cefuroxime and diazepam. This accumulation may be advantageous when treating amniotic infections with cefuroxime.

Appendix 4 of the *BNF* (Mehta, 1997) gives information on drugs in pregnancy, and Appendix 5 provides information on the impact of breast feeding on drugs.

Renal failure

The kidney represents one of the major routes of drug elimination. A decrease in normal function can influence the clearance of drugs and their metabolites that would normally be cleared by the kidneys.

Factors that need to be considered when selecting a drug for patients with renal failure are the following:

Table 4.4 Physiological changes in pregnancy and their impact on drug pharmacokinetics.

Parameter	Effect on drug pharmacokinetics
40% increase in plasma volume	Increase in V_d for water soluble drugs
30–50% increase in renal blood flow	Increased drug elimination. Clearance of ampicillin doubles in late pregnancy. Drug dosage may need increasing
Decreased albumin level in last trimester by 20%	Increased unbound (active) fraction of acidic drugs (diazepam, phenytoin, sodium valproate)
Increased alpha-1-acid glycoprotein levels of up to 100%	Decreased unbound (active) fraction of basic drugs
Increased blood flow to skin	Increased absorption following transdermal application, and from subcutaneous injections
Basal metabolic rate increased by 13%	Enzyme activity increased. Increase in drug elimination, e.g. carbamazepine
Increase in hormone secretion, e.g. thyroxine, insulin, glucocorticoids	For people with deficiencies of any of these hormones. Dose increments likely
Decrease in gastrointestinal transit time	Increased absorption for poorly soluble drugs (digoxin). For drugs absorbed in small intestine, delay may lengthen time to reach peak concentration Decrease in the absorption of drugs that undergo metabolism in the gut (chlorpromazine)
Emesis and oesophageal reflux during early pregnancy	Reduced oral drug absorption

Adapted from data from Roberts and Silbergeld (1995)

- Degree of renal impairment
- Fraction of the dose that is renally excreted
- Activity of metabolites that are excreted by the kidneys
- Therapeutic window of the drug.

In general, the dosages of drugs that rely on renal clearance need reducing in patients with renal disease; these patients will require lower dosages or less frequent administrations, or both. For many drugs there is a certain degree of renal failure that the body can cope with in clearing drugs before any alteration in dose needs to be undertaken. Company literature, the *BNF* (Mehta, 1997), or other sources of information will indicate the degree of renal failure required before action needs to be taken. Renal function is expressed as glomerular filtration rate (GFR) or as creatinine clearance (CL_{cr}). GFR is calculated as shown in Chapter 3. The degree of renal failure is expressed as mild, moderate, and severe.

Mild renal failure CL_{cr} = 20–50 ml/min
Moderate renal failure CL_{cr} = 10–20 ml/min
Severe renal failure CL_{cr} <10 ml/min

Drugs with a narrow therapeutic window (e.g. gentamicin, vancomycin) will require a large alteration in dosage if administered to a patient with mild to moderate renal failure. However, drugs with a large therapeutic window (cephalosporins) only need dose adjustment in severely impaired renal disease. Diuretics such as frusemide (furosemide) and bumetanide are an exception to the rule of reduced dosage in renal failure. These drugs require excretion into the nephron of the kidney to become active. A reduced capacity of the kidneys to perform this role means that higher concentrations of the drug are required in the blood. Metformin is a drug that should be avoided in patients with renal disease as it can lead to lactic acidosis.

Protein binding

The concentration of proteins (e.g. albumin) decreases in severe renal disease, because the kidneys lose the efficiency of filtering proteins before excretion. This will alter the degree of protein binding of drugs and increase the unbound (active) fraction of the drug in the plasma. For example, the normal range for phenytoin in the plasma is 10–20 mg/l, which represents total (bound and unbound) drug. In renal failure the amount of free drug increases; therefore the corrected range calculated will be about 5–10 mg/l in severe renal failure.

Renal failure can also alter tissue sensitivity. Opiates (morphine), barbiturates such as phenobarbitone (phenobarbital), and benzodiazepines (temazepam, diazepam) all show greater central nervous system effects in patients with renal failure compared to those with normal renal function. Antihypertensive agents show an increase in the incidence of postural hypotension in patients with renal failure.

Liver disease

The liver is the single most important site of drug metabolism in the body. Drugs can also be metabolised in the skin, intestines, kidney and lungs, but overall these tissues make only a small contribution to drug metabolism.

The rate at which the liver metabolises drugs depends upon the flow of blood through the liver (i.e. presentation of drug to liver cells) and the metabolising capacity of the liver cells themselves. Any damage or change in these two factors will undoubtedly affect drug metabolism.

Patients with liver disease may not be capable of metabolising drugs to the same extent as a normal person, making them particularly susceptible to drug toxicity and side effects. Because the liver produces albumin and other plasma proteins, the reduction in albumin levels which follows liver damage may affect plasma drug–protein binding.

First-pass metabolism

'First-pass metabolism' refers to the metabolism of drugs before they reach the systemic circulation following oral or rectal dosing. The extent of this initial metabolism directly influences the drug's overall bioavailability. Other routes of administration (intravenous, intramuscular, subcutaneous, inhaled, sublingual, buccal, nasal, ocular, transdermal) bypass the liver on first entry into the circulation and therefore their doses will usually be smaller than oral dosing.

Hepatocyte drug metabolism

The function of hepatocytes is to make a drug molecule more water soluble, so that it can be eliminated by the kidney or through the bile. This metabolism usually inactivates but occasionally activates drugs, and in the process may produce toxic, inactive or active intermediate substances termed metabolites.

Fig. 4.2 shows the common metabolic pathways of several benzodiazepines. This shows that some metabolites may themselves be marketed as drugs in their own right.

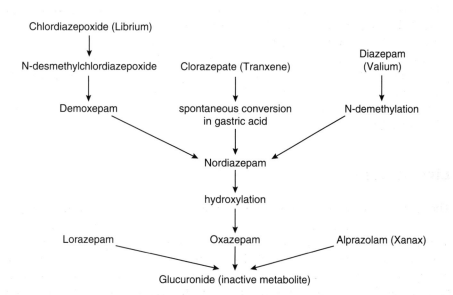

Fig. 4.2 Metabolic pathways of benzodiazepines. (Adapted from data from Koda-Kimble & Young (1995) and Bowman & Rand (1980).)

There are two phases of drug metabolism (phase 1 and phase 2). Phase 1 reactions mainly involve oxidation, reduction, hydrolysis and hydration. These are carried out by the hepatic enzymes, most notably the cytochrome P450 enzyme system. This is a family of enzymes capable of metabolising a large spectrum of drugs, and will usually be quoted if you read further textbooks on drug metabolism. Phase 1 metabolism chemically modifies the drug molecule, rendering it more water soluble. The drug is then either excreted from the body or undergoes phase 2 metabolism if it is still insufficiently water soluble.

The quantity of cytochrome P450 enzymes in the liver varies considerably in the general population, and is influenced by genes, age, sex, pregnancy, nutrition, smoking, alcohol and by other factors. The genetic split gives rise to slow and fast acetylators. Slow acetylators show greater therapeutic responsiveness and toxic adverse effects than do fast acetylators.

Enzyme induction and inhibition

The cytochrome P450 enzymes are capable of being influenced by chemicals which either increase their numbers (inducers) or deplete their numbers (inhibitors). Because the effect of inducers depends upon new enzymes being produced, the effect may take several days to become clinically noticeable. Induction results in an increased rate of metabolism of both the inducing drug and any other drug that is metabolised by the same enzyme system. Conversely, inhibition results in a decrease in the rate of metabolism for the inhibiting drug and any other drugs, thereby increasing their therapeutic and toxic properties. The effect of enzyme inhibition is rapid and can lead to rapid elevation in drug levels. Table 4.5 shows some common enzyme inducers and inhibitors.

Table 4.5 Enzyme inducers and inhibitors.

Enzyme inducers	Enzyme inhibitors
Alcohol	Erythromycin
Carbamazepine	Fluconazole
Food preservatives	Itraconazole
Griseofulvin	
Nicotine	
Phenobarbitone (phenobarbital)	
Phenylbutazone	
Phenytoin	

Examples of interactions of clinical significance include the following:

- A common phenomenon encountered is the enhanced metabolism and hence reduced effectiveness of oral contraceptives (oestrogens) in women who have received P450-inducing agents such as phenobarbitone (phenobarbital) or rifampicin.

- The clearance of theophylline, a drug that undergoes hepatic P450-mediated metabolism, is decreased after administration of ciprofloxacin or erythromycin.

As has already been mentioned, the metabolic rate of the liver depends upon blood flow to the liver and the number of hepatocytes. The following sections will address these factors.

Liver blood flow

Total blood flow to the liver is reduced in advancing age, due to the reduction in the total cardiac output. Chronic liver disease can result in shrinking of the liver with subsequent reduced blood flow. In patients with severe liver disease and in alcoholic liver disease there is a tendency for the portal blood supply to be shunted away from the liver, giving rise to a condition known as portal hypertension. Reducing the blood supply to the liver reduces the presentation of drug to the liver for metabolism. For drugs which have a high extraction ratio for the liver (lignocaine (lidocaine), nicardipine, dextropropoxyphene, morphine, pethidine, nortriptyline, propranolol), the rate of metabolism is proportional to the rate of blood flow. Therefore they are likely to be influenced by changes in blood flow.
Below are examples of drugs which need dose adjustment in liver disease.

- Analgesics – morphine, pethidine
- Anti-arrhythmics – verapamil, diltiazem
- Antidepressants – imipramine, amitriptyline
- Beta-blockers – propranolol, metoprolol, labetalol.

Below are recommendations for the use of drugs in liver disease.

- Paracetamol is best used as pain relief
- Drugs which reduce cognitive awareness should be avoided as they interfere with cognitive tests for encephalopathy (e.g. opiates, long acting benzodiazepines)
- Hypoglycaemic drugs readily induce coma (reduce glycogen stores). Avoid long acting diabetic drugs (e.g. chlorpropamide, glibenclamide)
- Drugs which have direct hepatotoxic side effects should be avoided (e.g. methotrexate, isoniazid)
- NSAIDs are best avoided as they can irritate oesophageal varices and lead to fluid accumulation.

Drug hepatotoxicity

A reduction in the number of functional liver cells greatly reduces the metabolism of low-hepatic extraction drugs (caffeine, diazepam, warfarin, paracetamol, chlorpromazine, fluoxetine and theophylline). These are unaffected by changes in liver blood flow, but their metabolism is governed directly by enzyme activity. Liver damage can be caused by direct drug toxicity, immunological susceptibilities to certain drugs and other biochemical factors.

Paracetamol is probably the most noted of drugs that can cause liver damage when taken in overdose. Most other drug-induced liver damage is poorly understood, and the idiosyncratic nature of most drug hepatotoxicity makes it difficult to investigate. Many hepatotoxicities arise as a result of toxic metabolites which are formed by liver metabolism of a certain drug.

Studies have shown that in patients with cirrhosis of the liver, the disease affects individual cytochrome P450 enzymes differently, so that in the same person there may be different degrees of impairment of the metabolism of different drugs and of different metabolic pathways for the same drug.

Pharmacodynamic changes in patients with liver disease which are clinically significant include increased cerebral sensitivity to strong analgesics, anxiolytics and sedatives, and decreased sensitivity to diuretics and beta-blockers (McLean & Morgan, 1991).

Because the liver is the main site for blood clotting factor synthesis, cirrhosis of the liver leads to a reduction in vitamin-K-dependent clotting factors, enhancing the effect of oral anticoagulants such as warfarin.

Prodrugs

The successful use of a prodrug relies on its conversion to the active moiety, usually in the liver. Failure to convert the drug to its active form means reduced clinical benefit in most cases. For several angiotensin converting enzyme (ACE) inhibitors (enalapril, lisinopril, cilazapril), the metabolism into their active metabolites is substantially reduced in cirrhosis. However, with the exception of cilazapril, this seems to be of no clinical significance in their anti-hypertensive effect. In cirrhosis, the conversion to methylprednisolone of the prodrug methylprednisolone hemisuccinate is halved. The cytotoxic drug cyclophosphamide is the prodrug for several metabolites which produce the pharmacological effect. Many drugs, including imipramine, propranolol and diazepam, are themselves active but also have metabolites which contribute to the overall effect of the drug.

Other factors

Oedema

Many diseases are associated with the formation of oedema of various degrees of severity. Examples are congestive cardiac failure (CCF), decompensated liver cirrhosis and chronic renal failure. Certain drugs, such as non-steroidal anti-inflammatory agents (NSAIDs), can cause salt retention leading to oedema. The retention of large quantities of water can affect the distribution of drugs in the body. This effect is greatest on drugs with a relatively small volume of distribution (V_d). Liver disease can lead to the formation of ascites which may additionally affect drug distribution. The influence of oedema is not confined to distribution. Absorption of drugs is also greatly affected. The rate and, to a lesser degree, the extent of absorption of frusemide (furosemide, a diuretic) is decreased in the presence of an oedematous gut. Bumetanide is affected to a lesser extent than frusemide and may be a better choice of oral diuretic for severely oedematous patients, especially those with CCF. Several other drugs have been implicated as being affected by oedema, but their clinical significance has not yet been shown (lignocaine (lidocaine), ACE inhibitors, verapamil, digoxin and theophylline).

Cancer

It has been suggested that a primary malignancy may itself cause changes in drug metabolism independent of coexisting liver metastases, and that liver metastases from different primary malignancies might affect drug metabolism in different ways. The large number of drugs taken by cancer sufferers also increases the likelihood of drug–drug interactions.

Thyroid disease

Thyroid disease may affect drug pharmacokinetics partly by effects upon the rate of drug metabolism and partly via changes in renal elimination.

Digoxin

It has been shown that patients with thyroid disease have an altered response to digoxin. Hyperthyroid patients are relatively resistant to digoxin and require large doses, whereas patients with hypothyroidism are extremely sensitive to its effects. The reason behind this is twofold: Firstly the V_d of digoxin decreases in hypothyroidism and increases in hyperthyroidism, and secondly hypothyroidism increases the sensitivity of digoxin receptors in the heart. Therefore in patients taking both thyroxine (levothyroxine) and digoxin, a change in thyroxine (levothyroxine) dose may require a change in digoxin dose depending on clinical symptoms.

Oral anticoagulants

Hyperthyroidism causes an increase in catabolism of vitamin-K-dependent clotting factors, leading to an increase in the prothrombin time and increased sensitivity to oral anticoagulants such as warfarin.

Shock syndrome

In a patient with shock, the body undergoes redistribution of blood to maintain adequate blood flow to essential organs (e.g. brain, heart and lungs). Blood is diverted away from the periphery (skin) and from the gastro-intestinal tract. This movement of intravascular fluid can have a large impact in drug pharmacokinetics. Table 4.6 shows the effect of shock on drug pharmacokinetics.

Table 4.6   Effect of Shock On Drug Pharmacokinetics

Parameter	Effect On Drug Pharmacokinetics
Reduced blood supply to gastrointestinal tract	Oral absorption greatly reduced. Should not be used as a route of administration in a shocked patient
Reduced blood supply to skin and muscle mass	Transdermal, intramuscular and subcutaneous absorption of drugs significantly reduced
Albumin loss during certain types of shock (burns)	Reduced protein binding for certain drugs (digoxin, diazepam, penicillin, warfarin). Increase in unbound (active) drug in plasma
Renal insufficiency leads to excretion of proteins	As for albumin loss
Renal failure	Leads to drug accumulation
Impaired liver function	Reduced hepatic metabolism of active and prodrugs

Because the effect of shock is so variable, drug dosages are best gauged from actual plasma levels. However, this is expensive for all drugs, so only those drugs with a narrow therapeutic window (aminoglycosides) should be monitored. For the rest of the drugs, clinical improvement or toxicity is an indicator of drug dosage. Shock patients treated in intensive care units (ICU) are usually administered large numbers of drugs (15–20 drugs per patient per day), thus increasing the likelihood of pharmacokinetic and pharmacodynamic drug–drug interactions.

Gastrointestinal diseases

Any condition that affects the gastro-intestinal system is likely to alter drug absorption and bioavailability. Table 4.7 shows some conditions that can influence gastric emptying.

Table 4.7 Conditions that can influence gastric emptying.

Decreased gastric emptying	Increased gastric emptying
Gastric ulcer	Coeliac disease
Intestinal obstruction	Duodenal ulcer
Labour	
Migraine (slows absorption of painkillers)	
Pain	
Trauma	

Coeliac disease

In coeliac disease there are many factors that can affect absorption of drugs from the gastro-intestinal tract:

- Reduction in the absorptive surface of the small intestine
- Altered rate of gastric emptying and intestinal transit time
- Decrease in reabsorption of bile (enterohepatic circulation)
- Increased permeability of the gut wall
- Intestinal drug metabolism is decreased.

The outcome of all these factors on drug absorption is complex. Drugs such as amoxycillin (amoxicillin) show a decreased absorption, while cephalexin shows increased absorption.

Crohn's disease

As in coeliac disease, the absorptive surface area of the small intestine is markedly reduced by both the disease and by the surgical resections of the bowel that will need to be performed throughout its history. The gut wall which is damaged becomes thickened, hindering absorption of drugs. Surprisingly, clindamycin absorption is increased in this disease.

Cystic fibrosis

The reduced pancreatic enzymes and bile flow which result from this condition can reduce the absorption of highly fat soluble drugs, as well as cause deficiencies in the fat soluble vitamins A, D, E and K.

Cigarette smoking

The effect of smoking on the pharmacokinetics of other drugs has been researched, but many people are still unaware of the adverse effects this may have. Cigarette smoking may alter drug response. Cigarette smoke is a mixture of over 3000 different chemicals, each with a potential to cause problems. It was first thought that nicotine may have been the main culprit; however, a group of chemicals known as polycyclic aromatic hydrocarbons (PAHs) have been implicated in enhancing drug metabolism through the induction of cytochrome P450 enzymes (Schein, 1995).

Like drug–drug interactions, not all smoking–drug interactions are of clinical significance, but the effect of smoking on drug pharmacokinetics is clearly observed in patients taking theophylline, insulin and benzodiazepines.

Theophylline

The enhancement by cigarette smoke of the liver metabolism of theophylline almost doubles the rate of elimination of the drug from the body, with the consequence that larger doses are required. Patients who stop smoking need to reduce the dose of theophylline after several weeks (depending on the number of cigarettes smoked), to allow for the reduction in enzyme activity to normal levels. Lee (1987) showed that within 7 days of abstaining from tobacco, the clearance of theophylline declined by an average of 35%. Non-smokers taking lower doses of theophylline products experienced fewer side effects than smokers on larger doses. Nicotine gum and patches have little effect on theophylline levels because the PAHs are absent from these preparations.

Insulin

Some investigators have reported that patients with insulin-dependent diabetes and who smoke require larger doses of insulin compared to non-smokers. Madsbad *et al.*, (1980) concluded that average smokers with diabetes required 15–20% more insulin than non-smokers, and 30% more if they smoked heavily. Clinicians should consider this to be a contributing factor to poor diabetic control.

Benzodiazepines

One study has shown that drowsiness was less likely to occur in smokers than non-smokers when they were given the same dose of a benzodiazepine (diazepam or chlordiazepoxide). The mechanism of action was thought to be the arousal effect of nicotine acting on the central nervous system, rather than an acceleration of metabolism and reduction of the concentrations of these drugs in the brain (Boston Collaborative Drug Surveillance Program, 1973). Clinicians should be aware that larger doses may be required to achieve a sedative effect in smokers as opposed to non-smokers.

Obesity

Obesity is common enough to constitute a serious medical and public health problem. Drug prescribing for the obese patient is difficult because drug dosage recommendations are based on pharmacokinetic studies in normal weight individuals. The majority of obese people have a larger absolute amount of lean body mass as well as fat than normal individuals of the same sex, height and age. However, the percentage of lean tissue and water is reduced per body weight and the percentage of fat increased. Table 4.8 shows the effect of obesity on drug pharmacokinetics.

Table 4.8 Effect of obesity on drug pharmacokinetics.

Parameter	Effect on drug pharmacokinetics
Drug absorption not affected	No effect
Increase in V_d of highly lipophilic drugs	Benzodiazepines (nitrazepam, temazepam) have an increased V_d and increased half-life
Total blood volume increased	Also increased V_d for water soluble drugs
Blood flow per gram of fat is less than in non-obese individuals	Lack of correlation for altered drug clearance
Increased renal clearance for some drugs	Aminoglycosides and cimetidine

For drugs distributed in lean mass and partly in fat tissue (aminoglycosides), loading doses should be based on ideal body weight (IBW). For some drugs V_d is decreased (cyclosporin (ciclosporin), propranolol), suggesting that factors other than lipid solubility intervene in tissue distribution.

Gender

There are a number of examples of gender differences in drug pharmacokinetics and pharmacodynamics. These have yet to become clinically significant. However, for drugs with a narrow therapeutic window this may be an important consideration for the clinician. Clinical trials should have an equal split of male and female volunteers to eliminate the effect of gender.

Differences in drug handling between the genders is mainly due to differences in body composition and liver metabolism.

Body composition

Men tend to weigh more than women, having more muscle mass and less fat, i.e. a higher ratio of water/fat. Blood flow to organs will thus be different. Drugs with a high affinity for adipose tissue (i.e. diazepam) are therefore likely to have a larger initial volume of distribution and a lower serum concentration in women. With long term administration concentrations would build up, potentially leading to a prolonged half-life and higher incidence of side effects. In obese female patients this is of greater clinical significance. Women have a lower volume of distribution (V_d) for alcohol, and a higher V_d for diazepam, than do men.

Liver metabolism

The relative proportions of cytochrome P450 enzymes have been put forward as an explanation for gender differences in drug pharmacokinetics. The clearance of the benzodiazepines oxazepam, temazepam and chlordiazepoxide, is higher in men than women. In contrast, no gender differences were found in the clearances of nitrazepam and lorazepam (Harris *et al.*, 1995).

Researchers have found that an important P450 enzyme (CYP3A4) is more plentiful in the liver of women than men (Wrighton, 1992). This enzyme metabolises many drugs, including erythromycin, cyclosporin (ciclosporin), quinidine, midazolam, dapsone and lignocaine (lidocaine). Not all of these drugs show gender differences in overall clearance. Erythromycin is cleared more rapidly from the body in women than in men by as much as 25%. Prednisolone and methylprednisolone are cleared more rapidly from the body in women than men. Midazolam is cleared 20–40% faster by women.

In contrast the following drugs are metabolized by different P450 enzymes and show greater clearances in men than women: clomipramine, desipramine, propranolol, ondansetron, digoxin and paracetamol.

Other differences

- Women empty solids from the stomach more slowly than do men.
- Women secrete less gastric acid than men.
- Stomach alcohol dehydrogenase efficacy may be considerably lower in women than men, causing gender differences in alcohol metabolism.
- Aspirin is found to be absorbed more rapidly in women, but bioavailability remains the same.
- Men have greater muscle mass, which may influence the absorption of IM injections.
- After the menopause certain P450 enzymes (CYP3A4) are reduced. It has been shown that a woman's ability to metabolise alfentanil is reduced after the menopause.
- Large variations in hormone levels throughout the menstrual cycle may influence drug pharmacokinetics: the maximum plasma theophylline concentration was found to be highest at mid-cycle; phenytoin clearance is highest at the end of the menstrual cycle; the absorption of alcohol and salicylates appears to be slowed at mid-cycle.

Clinical significance

The clinical significance of many gender differences in drug pharmacokinetics remains to be determined. Gender differences in drug metabolism may become an important factor in determining the dosage of drugs that have a narrow therapeutic window. Female-specific issues such as pregnancy, menopause, oral contraceptive use and menstruation may also have profound effects on drug pharmacokinetics. Women appear to respond differently and experience more adverse effects from cardiovascular drugs than do men. However, few trials have specifically looked at gender differences within this class of drugs.

Food–drug interactions

The bioavailability of a number of drugs (e.g. penicillins, erythromycin, rifampicin and thyroxine (levothyroxine)) is reduced by food. In such cases it is recommended that the drug be taken half an hour before meals. Some drugs, however, including aspirin, levodopa, metformin, metronidazole and NSAIDs (diclofenac, naproxen), cause gastric irritation or sickness if taken on an empty stomach. Taking them with food helps prevent stomach irritation. However, taking drugs at the same time as food may in some cases delay the onset of action of that drug (aspirin, paracetamol, frusemide (furosemide)). Taking disodium etidronate and similar drugs with food can totally abolish the drug's action by interacting with salts within the stomach.

The increase in concentrations observed for many drugs when administered concomitantly with grapefruit juice has been attributed to inhibition of cytochrome P450 enzymes by naringenin, a chemical found in grapefruit juice. The change in bioavailability of certain calcium channel blockers (felodipine and nifedipine) due to interaction with grapefruit juice has been studied. Bailey (1993) showed that grapefruit juice produced a marked and variable increase in felodipine bioavailability.

The properties of food in the stomach greatly influence the gastric emptying time. As already mentioned, the gastric emptying times can affect drug levels. Increasing the gastric emptying time will allow poorly soluble drugs (nitrofurantoin, spironolactone) to dissolve. However, keeping acid-labile drugs in the stomach longer will reduce their absorption. Hot drinks generally shorten the gastric emptying times, whereas fatty foods increase it. Table 4.9 shows the impact of food on drug absorption.

Interaction of monoamine oxidase inhibitors with tyramine

Monoamine oxidase inhibitors (MAOI) are a class of antidepressant drugs which have a potentially serious interaction with food containing the amino acid tyramine. Tyramine in foods is normally metabolised by monoamine oxidase in the gastrointestinal wall and liver before reaching the systemic circulation. In the presence of MAOI, excessive amounts of tyramine may reach the systemic circulation, resulting in a hypertensive reaction.

Table 4.9 Impact of food on drug absorption

Increased absorption	Decreased absorption	Delayed absorption
Carbamazepine	Amoxycillin (amoxicillin)	Aspirin
Griseofulvin	Aspirin	Digoxin
Lithium citrate	Bisphosphonates	Frusemide (furosemide)
Nitrofurantoin	Cephalexin (cefalexin)	Glibenclamide
Propranolol	Erythromycin	Paracetamol
Spironolactone	Levodopa	
	Rifampicin	
	Tetracyclines	
	Thyroxine (levothyroxine)	

Below is a list of common foods and drink that contain tyramine.

- Avocados
- Bananas
- Beans, broad (especially pods)
- Beer, imported and non-alcoholic
- Bovril
- Cheese, fermented
- Figs
- Fish, dried or pickled
- Marmite
- Oxo
- Soy sauce
- Wine, Chianti, champagne
- Yeast, brewer's yeast, vitamin supplements

Interactions with antacids

Antacids can influence the absorption of drugs if taken concomitantly. In some cases, for example tetracyclines, antacids lead to reduced absorption. Neuvonen and Kivistö (1994), however, demonstrated enhancement of drug absorption with the commonly used antacids magnesium hydroxide and sodium bicarbonate, but not with aluminium hydroxide. Their results showed that magnesium hydroxide and sodium bicarbonate can increase the rate and sometimes the extent of absorption of certain NSAIDs (e.g. mefenamic acid and ibuprofen), sulphonylurea antidiabetic agents (e.g. glipizide, glibenclamide and tolbutamide), and the oral anticoagulant dicoumarol. The antacids in question, by increasing the pH of the stomach, increased the solubility of these sparingly soluble drugs. The clinical significance of this interaction is unknown but could possibly lead to alterations in glucose levels with sulphonylurea drugs, and INR with dicoumarol.

The sodium content of sodium bicarbonate and other over-the-counter antacid preparations can lead to sodium overload causing fluid accumulation. This may compete with the beneficial water loss caused by diuretics in heart failure. Secondly the sodium ion Na^+ competes with the drug lithium for renal excretion in the kidneys, thereby elevating lithium levels causing toxicity.

Influence of fat on drug absorption

Zhi *et al.* (1995) studied the effects of dietary fat on drug absorption. It is very difficult to quantitatively measure the effects of fat, because dietary fat consists of complex organic compounds and includes triglycerides, phospholipids, sterols, hydrocarbons and waxes. Ingestion of fat causes the formation of an emulsion in the stomach which increases the absorption of lipid soluble drugs. Also the presence of fat in the stomach stimulates the secretion of gastric acid and bile which further influences drug absorption. The following are examples of drugs for which absorption is increased by fat: fat soluble vitamins A, D, E and K, analogues of vitamin A (isotretinoin, acitretin), cyclosporin (ciclosporin), griseofulvin, atovaquone.

Drug interactions involving alcohol

Alcohol is a CNS depressant, and additive effects are seen when consumed while taking other CNS depressant drugs, such as antihistamines and benzodiazepines. Alcohol also has the capacity to induce liver P450 enzymes, so increasing the metabolism of other drugs. Alternatively drugs which inhibit the metabolism of these liver enzymes (MAOIs) will increase the effect of alcohol.

Summary

Caution is always advised in prescribing for neonates. Since clinical trials carried out by manufacturers do not generally include neonates, expert reference guides are recommended. The reduced liver capacity to metabolise drugs, along with the reduced renal capacity, results in a decreased clearance and prolonged half-life of drugs in the neonate. Therefore lower doses are generally employed with a longer dosing interval than that usually seen in the adult patient. As a general rule, using surface area to calculate drug dosage is more accurate than using weight.

There is a large intra-patient and inter-patient variability in maturation of organs that are responsible for the elimination of drugs. This puts the neonate, infant and young child at risk of both toxic and sub-therapeutic concentrations of drugs. The prescribing clinician is advised to consult reference sources for drug dosages as many drugs are not licensed in children. Drugs that have been proven to be safe in adults may produce unexpected toxicity in paediatric patients.

Because elderly people are more sensitive to the effects of drugs and because they handle the drug slightly differently, the prescriber should, when possible, choose drugs which will not be greatly affected by age, i.e. temazepam instead of diazepam. If this is not possible, then the smallest initial dose should be initiated and the dose carefully increased. The nurse is in a position to routinely monitor the success of a given drug and closely watch for the emergence of toxic effects. Drugs with long elimination half-lives, such as piroxicam, should be avoided because they are more likely to cause toxicity in the elderly.

In patients with renal failure it is best to avoid, if possible, drugs that are mainly eliminated by the kidneys, those which are nephrotoxic (aminoglycosides, cyclosporin (ciclosporin), penicillamine), those that lead to increased fluid retention (NSAIDs) and those which can increase urea levels (tetracyclines except doxycycline).

The liver's drug handling mechanisms are altered sufficiently in chronic liver disease with cirrhosis to warrant dosage reduction, but not sufficiently to warrant dosage reduction if cirrhosis is absent. Unlike the measurement of creatinine clearance and GFR in renal disease, there is no simple test that can predict with certainty how a drug will be handled in liver failure. The levels of liver enzymes (alkaline phosphatase, aspartine transaminase), of bilirubin, and a prolonged prothrombin time indicate damage to the liver. Appendix 2 of the *BNF* (Mehta, 1997), gives some guidance to the clinician on drugs which are affected by liver disease.

This chapter has provided an insight into the very complex factors that can affect both the drug's blood concentration and the drug's effect on the body. It is not meant to be an exhaustive list of factors, and I would recommend that the references listed at the end of this chapter be used to gain more in-depth information. The nurse has a key role in drug usage, and with the increased patient contact is more likely to see both therapeutic and any toxic effects of an administered drug. The nurse's knowledge of how drug levels are affected will help in preventing drug interactions and drug toxicities and ultimately provide better patient care.

References

Bailey, D.G. (1993) Grapefruit juice–felodipine interaction: mechanism, predictability, and effect of naringin. *Clin. Pharmacol. Ther.* **53**, 637–42.

Boston Collaborative Drug Surveillance Program (1973) Clinical depression of the central nervous system due to diazepam and chlordiazepoxide in relation to cigarette smoking and age. *N. Engl. J. Med.* **288**, 277.

Bowman, W.C. & Rand, M.J. (1980) *Textbook of Pharmacology*, 2nd edn. Blackwell Scientific Publications, Oxford.

Choonara, I. (1994) Percutaneous drug absorption and administration: *Arch. Dis. Child.* **71**, F73–4.

Harris, R.Z., Benet, L.Z. & Schwartz, J.B. (1995) Gender effects in pharmacokinetics and pharmacodynamics: *Drugs* **50**, 223–36.

Hayes, M.J., Langman, M.J.S. & Short, A.H. (1975) Changes in drug metabolism with increasing age. Phenytoin clearance and protein binding, *Br. J. Clin. Pharmacol.* **2**, 73.

Koda-Kimble, M.A. & Young, L.Y. (1995) *Applied Therapeutics. The Clinical Use of Drugs.* 6th edn. Chapter 101–3, Applied Therapeutics Inc. Vancouver.

Lee, B.L. (1987) Cigarette abstinence, nicotine gum, and theophylline disposition. *Ann. Intern. Med.* **106**, 553–5.

Lindeman, R.D., Tobin, J. & Shock, N.W. (1985) Longitudinal studies on the rate of decline in renal function with age. *J. Am. Geriatr. Soc.* **35**, 278–88.

Madsbad, S., McHair, P. & Christiansen, M.S. (1980) Influence of smoking on insulin requirement and metabolic status in diabetes mellitus. *Diabetes Care* **3**, 41–3.

McLean, A.J. & Morgan, D.J. (1991) Clinical pharmacokinetics in patients with liver disease. *Clin. Pharmacokinet.* **21**, 42–69.

Mehta, D.K. (1997) *British National Formulary No. 34,* British Medical Association and Royal Pharmaceutical Society of Great Britain, London.

Neuvonen, P.J. & Kivistö, K.T. (1994) Enhancement of drug absorption by antacids. *Clin. Pharmacokinet.* **27**, 120–8.

Roberts, J.S. & Silbergeld, E.K. (1995) Pregnancy, lactation, and menopause. *M. Sinai J. Medi.* **62**, 343–55.

Saltzman, J.R., Kowdley, K.V. & Pedrosa, M.C. (1994) Bacterial overgrowth without clinical malabsorption in elderly hypochlorhydric subjects. *Gastroenterology* **106**, 615–23.

Schein, J.R. (1995) Cigarette smoking and clinically significant drug interactions. *Ann. Pharmacother.* **29**, 1139–47.

Walker, R. & Edwards, C. (1994) *Clinical Pharmacy and Therapeutics,* Churchill Livingstone, Edinburgh.

Woodhouse, K.W. & Wynne, H.A. (1992) Age-related changes in hepatic function. Implications for drug therapy. *Drugs Aging* **1**, 243–55.

Wrighton, S.A. (1992) The human hepatic cytochromes P450 involved in drug metabolism. *Crit. Rev. Toxicol.* **22**, 1–2.

Zhi, J., Rakhit, A. & Patel, I.H. (1995) Effects of dietary fat on drug absorption. *Clin. Pharmacol. Ther.* **58**, 487–91.

Chapter 5
The Patient's Role in Optimising Treatment

Margaret Ling

Introduction

Understanding patient views about both the form and function of medications in a social rather than biomedical context has important consequences in optimising treatment. Based on studies with a sociological and anthropological focus, this chapter explores some ideas on lay perceptions of medication.

Consideration will be given firstly to what is meant by self medication and to the social context within which medication is taken. The chapter then considers social attitudes to medicines and the influence that the ethnic or cultural context exerts. Having established the social and cultural framework within which medication operates, the chapter then explores the often contentious and problematic nature of patient adherence to or compliance with medication.

Self medication

In this chapter no distinction is made between medication purchased over the counter whether from pharmacists or from other retailers, and medication obtained on prescription. Rather, Britten's (1996) definition of self-medication is adopted:

> 'All medicine taking outside institutional care is self-medication in the sense that the individual decides whether or not to take the drug, when, where and in what quantities.'

Such a definition highlights the fact that taking medicines occurs, not within a vacuum, but in a specific sociocultural context. Indeed, increasing reliance upon care provided in the community rather than within institutions can lead to problems for the role of medication as part of the therapeutic process of care. Such problems may occur when the emphasis shifts from direct medical care to a form of patient or carer management. This may happen when patients leave the institutional setting of the hospital to return to their own homes, or when a patient has to live with and manage a chronic condition.

Thus, it is important for nurses to be aware that patients are not 'blank sheets' (Donovan *et al.*, 1989). Account must be taken of the different experiences and structures which give relevance to people's lives and so to their experiences of medication. Hence, the patient's role in optimising treatment requires consideration of patients' own beliefs, concerns and patterns of behaviour.

The following sections explore a range of the experiences and structures which people use in making decisions about health and illness, and how medication is perceived by patients who are involved in the process of treatment.

The social context of medication

Medication is perceived by those who use it as possessing various attributes. Many people are concerned about experiencing symptoms which affect their ability to perform their social roles and relationships effectively. People suffering from acute or chronic conditions often worry about their ability to undertake the tasks involved in maintaining a home and family life. Those in employment may become concerned about their ability to sustain the demands of their job, or about how they are perceived by employers and fellow employees because of the symptoms of their illness. Such worries and concerns influence people's attitudes to medication, both because of the medicine's impact on their symptoms and because of their perceptions regarding taking or being seen to take medication. An informative way of understanding these concerns is to explore both the uses to which medicines are put and the properties they are perceived to have by the people who use them. To do this several studies with a social focus will be considered.

Although such studies explore aspects of peoples' use of medication and their perceptions of the social environment, apart from Britten's work (1994), which focuses on patients within the general population, most studies have been concerned with exploring the views of patients who are taking medication for forms of chronic illness. Such work is nevertheless relevant, since it raises important issues about sociocultural meanings of medication from the patient's point of view.

Medication as a form of social benefit

An example of people's use of medication to try and exert control over difficulties in their lives was recorded by Engels in 1844. Godfrey's cordial, a substance containing laudanum, was administered to infants and young children to quieten them. The children had to be sedated to ensure that mothers and carers could carry on without interruption the paid work they took in to do at home (Berridge & Edwards, 1981). Although by current standards this use of Godfrey's cordial may seem both inappropriate and undesirable, by nineteenth century standards it was an acceptable practice which offered the women the opportunity to sustain an income for their family's benefit.

More recently, of those who choose to take medicines because of the benefits their use offers to themselves and their families, many emphasise the sub-ordination of pharmacological power to the personal power of the individual taking the medicine. Thus different medications are viewed as helping to maintain a variety of social roles.

Control of roles at work

For many people, there is an apparent and direct link between the effect of medication and their ability to maintain their work-role. The use of medication to ensure that there will be no impediment to performing their role at work, particularly when others' expectations of their performance is an issue, may be illustrated by the following quotation:

> Last Wednesday I took an antihistamine for the first time in many years ... I had an important presentation to make.
>
> (Britten, 1994)

For the person in the example above, ensuring effectiveness at work would appear to have been a significant influence in their decision to use medication which would relieve symptoms.

However, in a study on men with chronic asthma, Hewett (1994) includes the views of one participant who explained that, although others (clients and colleagues) apparently considered he fulfilled his role as a solicitor effectively, he was less certain. The participant explained that when he required relief from his symptoms, he took medication in the form of Ventolin (salbutamol). Although his asthma was then controlled, and he could appear in court and deal with his clients, he nevertheless felt that he was 'not quite as sharp' as he should have been.

Control of everyday worries

Similar episodic use of medication was also reported in a study of women over 60 years of age (Helman, 1981). These women viewed their medicine (benzo-diazepines) as a 'tonic', because like a 'tonic' it was taken episodically only when the women required aid in maintaining effective social roles within their homes. These women took full responsibility for its use, viewing the medicine positively and not as a crutch to support a failing or difficult relationship. The medication thus gave more power and control to those using it.

Another positive use of medication as a means of limiting personal worries and emotional distress was recorded by Gabe & Lipshitz-Phillips (1982) and by

Gabe & Thorogood (1986). They described similar patterns of use regarding tranquillisers and antidepressants However, they respectively used the terms 'intermittent users' and 'standby users' to describe people for whom tranquillisers served as a means of gaining control over personal worries. For these patients, it was the calming effect of the medication, together with the effective control they were then able to exert over worries, which was deemed important.

For those experiencing forms of chronicity, medication also operates as a means of controlling the difficulties and worries associated with their personal and social roles. Nearly all of the men in Hewett's (1994) study of chronic asthma reported that the disease had consequences in their personal and social lives. They reported that some types of food, cigarette smoke and alcohol could trigger an attack of asthma. However, when their attitudes to the medication they used were explored in greater depth, the men in this study made a clear distinction between two different ways of using their medication.

Medication as preventer or reliever

When these men used medication as a 'reliever' of their condition, Hewett (1994) reported that they '...felt that asthma had had little impact on their families, and there was little evidence of dependence on wives, girlfriends, mothers or other members of the immediate family.' However, when medication was taken preventatively, a rather different picture emerged. Preventative medication was regarded as far less important in helping them to maintain their social effectiveness than was relieving medication, which resulted in a clear amelioration or eradication of undesirable symptoms.

A study of chronic heart failure (Mair *et al.*, 1996) illustrates how preventative medication, in the form of angiotensin converting enzyme (ACE) inhibitors, was viewed with a marked degree of reservation by the patients for whom it was prescribed. As with the men experiencing chronic asthma, there were reservations about the value of preventative medication, with patients reporting their perception that the medication had only a marginal impact upon their condition.

Testing medication

However, despite such a belief, the majority of the chronic heart failure patients continued to follow some form of the prescribed regimen, although several patients did admit to stopping their medication or else dramatically curtailing the amount they took. Such patients described this action as 'testing' their medication. It was only after rather dramatic and undesirable changes in their symptoms that they resumed the prescribed regimen.

In Hewett's study (1994) one patient explained how he decided to stop taking his medication to see if he really did need to take it. However, having stopped taking the oral steroids he was prescribed, the effects of this action were so 'terrible' he resumed his original drug regimen very quickly.

One elderly woman patient suffering from chronic heart failure (Mair *et al.*, 1996) adopted a somewhat different form of testing. She described how, after failing to understand the doctor's instructions regarding alteration in the amount of medicine she was prescribed, she decided to resolve the problem herself. The resolution involved the woman systematically reducing the dosage of her medication until she felt 'well again'. By this approach she discovered for herself the dosage of the medication she was able to tolerate. Apparently she had not considered stopping taking the medicine entirely.

Control of worry about symptoms

Medication can also act to control worry about symptoms experienced by patients suffering from a particular illness or disease. Patients suffering from hypertension (Morgan, 1996) acknowledged their limited understanding of their condition, but saw prescribed medication as a means of allaying any of their concerns about their illness. The following comment was made by one such patient:

> No I wasn't worried. He [the doctor] gave me tablets and said they would keep it down a bit. No I wasn't worried.

A similar view of the efficacy of prescribing tablets for some patients was described in a study on diabetes by Posner (1977). In a discussion Posner had with one doctor, about the often undesirable effects some tablets had on the patients taking them, the doctor justified the continued prescription of such medications with the following comment:

> ... doctors and patients feel that by giving tablets you're practising real medicine ... by putting someone on a diet you're not practising real medicine.

Thus medication may be regarded as a visible means of expression that care, however inappropriate, has been offered to the patient.

Living a normal life

Some patients, however, see their medication as a means of expressing their autonomy. They achieve autonomy by establishing the normality of their roles. Normality may result from weighing the risks and benefits associated with taking prescribed medication.

A woman suffering from a chronic disease (post-viral inflammatory arthropathy) explained her rationale for taking medication:

> I don't like taking [tablets]. I'd much rather not, but I'm not prepared to give up and stop working and stop living just because I've got something wrong

with me. If taking painkillers is a way of living a normal life, I want to live it to the full and so I take them.

(Donovan & Blake, 1992)

This patient came to the conclusion that overall 'the tablets' had a positive rather than negative influence on her ability to maintain an effective social role.

A rather different view of the use of medication, but to the same effect – to maintain an effective social role – is offered by MacIntyre & Oldham (1977). In a paper about coping with migraine, they describe their actions to attain normality. Normality is achieved, not by weighing risk, but by behaving creatively and pragmatically with regard to the medicalisation of their symptoms.

MacIntyre (MacIntyre & Oldham, 1977) achieves her aim because she becomes an 'expert patient', who is characterised by: 'knowing exactly what I want and using the GP partly as a resource to supply me with those drugs that I want, but which are on prescription.'

Oldham (MacIntyre & Oldham, 1977) is even more pragmatic in his approach to using medication to normalise the role migraine plays in his life. He talks of 'borrowing' drugs from friends and relatives. This enables him to 'top up' his prescribed medication, unknown to his GP, so that he can ensure that he, himself, treats the condition effectively. For Oldham, 'medicalising' his condition is the most effective way of allowing himself to achieve a 'normal' social status. However, it is Oldham who controls much of the treatment and not the professional. This is a somewhat different model to that traditionally associated with medicalisation, where the process hinges on professional control of everyday reality.

Medication as nourishment?

The effectiveness of the medication for some women patients occurred because the tablets they took (benzodiazepines) were viewed as representing either 'fuel' because they were taken at specific times when needed, or 'food' because they were essential to nourish and aid the survival of relationships (Helman, 1981). Thus, again patients may use medicines to fulfil similar functions, but regard them as possessing different properties.

Helman's (1981) symbolisation of the medicines, into 'tonic', 'fuel' and 'food' can be seen to convey that the participants considered they were not taking 'real drugs' rather they were consuming growth promoting nourishment with its attendant benefits of repairing and improving their damaged relationships.

By contrast, the participants in Gabe & Lipshitz-Phillips' (1982) study attributed a very different meaning to benzodiazepines. Using Helman's typology, the authors of the paper reported that the medicine was regarded as '...bad food, gritty fuel and nasty tonic.... Our patients seemed to feel that at best the Benzodiazepines maintained them, but they did not mistake Benzodiazepines for growth-promoting food.'

The examples cited in this section illustrate very clearly that people take medicines, particularly for example tranquillisers, in order to reap some form of social benefit for themselves and their families. However, in all the studies cited in this chapter, the majority of patients, even those women included in Helman's work (1981) who emphasised the nutritional aspects of benzodiazepines, expressed some form of reservation about the medicines they had taken or were taking. Such reservations may be attributed to either or both the patient's perception of the properties of their medication or the patient's orientation towards medication in general. These issues are discussed later in this chapter, in the section on factors affecting adherence.

While exploration of patients' experiences of medication is an important aspect of its social context, so too are the structures which are used in decision-making about health and illness and which are thus active in shaping views on medication.

Managing cultural beliefs

Awareness of the explanatory frameworks and treatments derived from differing cultural systems is another area of importance.

Ethnicity

As Morgan (1996) states, '... despite ... recognition of the importance of patients' meanings and the ways in which such meanings are shaped by the broader lay culture and patients' own circumstances and resources, little attention has been paid to the meanings of prescribed drugs held by ethnic groups in the UK.'

Consideration therefore has to be given to whether or not the social context of medication for any ethnic group remains within its traditional cultural framework or is regarded as an important aspect of the wider culture of the 'other' often larger and usually more powerful group.

In her study which included 'Afro-Caribbean and white hypertensive patients', Morgan (1996) discovered that the Afro-Caribbean patients reinterpreted the disease categories for which their medication was given. Morgan attributed this to two factors. The first concerned the perceived pharmacological power of the modern medicine as opposed to the milder traditional remedy. Powerful medication was regarded by this group as appropriate for managing acute bouts of illness, but it was certainly inappropriate for managing chronic conditions, especially if they were asymptomatic.

The second factor is that many of these patients preferred to take what they considered were readily available herbal remedies rather than taking medication only available from pharmacists in the form of pills. These attitudes were accounted for by 'the significance they attached to symptoms in assessing the need for treatment.' Symptoms thus required a response, whereas an absence of symptoms did not.

Rationality

Morgan's account (1996) emphasises the importance of understanding such differences as a form of reasoned decision-making rather than as any type of irrationality. She also comments on how such concerns are also to be found in lay culture and among patient groups in apparently western medical systems. Indeed amongst a group of patients in a rural area of Virginia, USA, Nations *et al.* (1985) found lay beliefs about hypertension which differed from orthodox medical explanations.

Similarly, in the study about patient perceptions of chronic heart failure based in a family practice centre in Middle America, it was discovered that patients often held medically unorthodox views of their symptoms (Mair *et al.*, 1996). Despite having a confirmed diagnosis of chronic heart failure and receiving diuretics and ACE inhibitors, one patient accounted for her condition as resulting from 'an enlarged heart' and the fact that her body was retaining fluid which happened because '...I messed up my sciatic nerve and then it started swelling, my legs started swelling and then they had to increase the dose [of medication].'

Another patient with chronic heart failure attributed the tiredness she constantly experienced to 'coeliac sprue, a form of malnourishment', and did not see herself as suffering from anything apart from 'just old age'. That patient's account of her condition as arising from 'just old age' suggests that she had adapted to her state of discomfort and therefore failed to notice the limitations she was experiencing as a result of the chronic heart failure. Because she did not regard her symptoms as resulting from ill health, she saw no need to use medication.

As patients' use of medication is often a vital factor in optimising treatment, consideration will now be given to the conceptual basis of their involvement within the treatment process.

Adherence or compliance?

In this section, the term 'adherence' rather than 'compliance' is used when referring to patients' involvement with medication as part of their therapeutic care. The reason for choosing to use 'adherence' stems from an attempt to emphasise the importance of accepting that both medical and lay patient views are based upon reasoned decision-making. Thus a patient's involvement with medication is active and cannot be governed solely by professionally or scientifically derived norms and values. Some consideration of that individual's norms and values must be included when medication and treatment are prescribed.

The inclusion of a patient's own norms and values or beliefs about medication, when prescribing or planning treatment, helps to ensure that any departure from treatment by the patient is not regarded simply as failure on a passive patient's part to understand medical views and rationales (Williams, 1984). As the report from the Royal Pharmaceutical Society of Great Britain & Merck, Sharp & Dohme (1997) suggests, implicit within such an attribution of error is the ascription of blame.

In order to avoid ascription of blame and in an attempt to adopt a broader view of patients' involvement with medication, this report (Royal Pharmaceutical Society of Great Britain & Merck, Sharp & Dohme, 1997) suggests using the term 'concordance' to replace the terms 'adherence' or 'compliance' stating that:

> Concordance is based on the notion that the work of the prescriber and patient in the consultation is a negotiation between equals and that therefore the aim is a therapeutic alliance between them.

Traditional medical/professional approaches have usually focused on non-adherence. Heidel & Wiffen (1996) in their paper reviewing the literature on patient adherence with medication and particularly randomised controlled trials on adherence, consider that non-adherers may be divided into two groups: (1) 'those who find it difficult to follow their prescribed regimen due to, for example, forgetfulness, a complex regimen or because they received insufficient information' and (2) 'those who intentionally choose not to follow their treatment instructions for other reasons such as side-effects, general dislike of taking medication, perceived improvement or no perceived improvement of symptoms.' Their paper concludes that randomised controlled trial evidence suggests that the main professional interventions which can improve adherence involve a reduction in the frequency of the daily dosage, more patient-friendly packaging and access to a pharmacist who will provide advice on how to take medicines.

Other approaches have targeted attempts to make the medical rationale comprehensible to the passive patient, assuming that greater understanding or knowledge by the patient will facilitate their improved adherence.

It has been suggested that, because complete adherence with a treatment regimen may not be necessary to achieve the desired therapeutic effect, some lower threshold of adherence at which the therapeutic effect is achieved could be adopted as a basis for defining adherence (Meichenbaum & Turk, 1987). However, such a view, although allowing for the imperfections of patient behaviour, retains an essentially medicalised view of adherence. It also substitutes for perfect behaviour a threshold of adherence which is perhaps arbitrary or at best generalised, taking no real account of the views or circumstances of the individual patient.

The limitation of such professionally oriented approaches is apparent from their relative lack of success. Although adherence rates are difficult to determine, within the medical literature typical rates are estimated at between 30% and 60%. However, since many people are willing to expend time and money in purchasing over-the-counter medication, amounting according to Rosenstock

(1985) to the expenditure of 'enormous sums of money', it appears that there is no obvious general hostility to the use of medication to control illness. Rather, the issue lies with how medication is viewed and the nature of the various factors influencing its use.

The term adherence has therefore been used within this chapter in recognition of the importance of the patient's active involvement in optimising treatment. The chapter thus provides explanations of adherence to medication that make clear the importance of both professional and lay perspectives.

Factors affecting patients' adherence to medication

In addressing the factors related to adherence or non-adherence to medication and the ways in which medication is used, it is useful to consider a number of themes associated with patients and with their perceptions of their symptoms and of the treatment available to them.

Patients' characteristics

Very little success has been recorded regarding the use of patient characteristics as a means of predicting likely non-adherence to treatment. Demographic variables such as age, sex, or social class would generally seem to have little predictive value regarding adherence to medication (Royal Pharmaceutical Society of Great Britain & Merck, Sharp & Dohme, 1997). These variables, whether used alone or in combination as some form of sociodemographic profile, are only weakly correlated with adherence. Such relationship as does exist would seem most likely to arise as a consequence of the association between sociodemographic characteristics and the prevalence of multiple health problems.

Studies of patients' attitudes or behaviour in the context of various medical conditions, e.g. chronic heart failure (Mair *et al.*, 1996), asthma (Hewett, 1994) and diabetes (Drummond & Mason, 1990), have shown that patients who also have other medical problems are more likely to experience problems with taking their medication. These other medical problems may result from their primary condition, or may be unassociated with it.

There appear, however, to be some exceptions to the generally accepted conclusion regarding the weak relationship between sociodemographic characteristics and adherence to medication. Meichenbaum & Turk (1987), when discussing the issue of patient characteristics and adherence comment that, 'This conclusion, however, does not exclude the possibility that under certain very specific treatment conditions patient and sociodemographic variables may indeed be implicated.' They then cite several examples from research results which support such a conclusion. These supporting examples include a study by Kasl (1975) describing how there is poor compliance among older men and younger women patients suffering from tuberculosis and taking their medication at home; and a study by Martin & Dubbert (1986) which offers a sociodemographic profile of men who tend to drop out of exercise pro-grammes.

Patients' beliefs

As the examples discussed in the section on the social context of medication convey, patients as a group exhibit many different rationales with regard to how they perceive medication.

Unnaturalness

A common concern expressed by patients was the 'unnaturalness' they asso-ciated with most prescribed medication. Patients offered descriptions of medicine ranging from 'a factory made chemical' which could cause damage or harm to a person's immune system, to 'an alien force' which acted as an intruder upon an individual's body (Britten, 1994). The most extreme description was that medication often was a 'form of poison' (Fallsberg, 1991).

According to the patients offering these descriptions, the 'unnaturalness' arose because medicines were created in a laboratory rather than created and grown 'naturally'. Such views were expressed by patients who were suffering from a variety of forms of illness extending from chronic to acute conditions.

Another consideration regarding patients' beliefs about medication is awareness that the advice offered by any professional forms a very small part of the patient's decision regarding adherence. When the decision-making process of the patient, regarding adherence to medication, differs from the professional involved in offering treatment, two explanations may be considered. Non-adherence may represent an attempt by patients to establish control of over both the condition and its treatment, or there may be variation in patients' expectations about their condition, its aetiology, development, prognosis and treatment.

Control

Regarding medication as a means of control, there are many examples of the use of tranquillisers, antidepressants and antihistamines which illustrate how important perceptions of control are to many patients. Medication can be used to exert a positive influence over unpleasant episodes of a condition such as anxiety, depression, or hay fever, in order that patients' lives can proceed without undue interruption.

However, for many patients, particularly those with chronic conditions such as epilepsy (Conrad, 1985), medication is seen as exhibiting an undesirable degree of control over a patient's life. The control is seen as arising from dependency upon a medication which has been created without regard to the individual's need.

Expectations

Closely linked to ideas about control is the way symptoms are regarded by many patients as an indicator to determine when they should adhere to medication. The different approaches patients exhibited to drugs used in the treatment of hypertension (Morgan, 1996) chronic heart failure (Mair *et al.*, 1996), or asthma (Hewett, 1994) illustrate how patients use their symptoms to decide whether or not it is appropriate for them to take drugs. Such a decision is often considered necessary when patients are either asymptomatic or else lulled into a false sense of security because their medication controls their symptoms so well that they see little reason for its continuation. Patients then use their symptoms as a gauge against which their need to use medication can be judged.

Patients' treatment

Connected to patients' perceptions of their medication is the patient's orientation towards medication in general. By orientation is meant the patient's attitudes towards taking any form of medication. Patients' choices regarding medication may thus be represented upon a continuum ranging from positive to negative views of the validity of medication in the management of illness.

Medication as a continuum

While some patients consider taking medication at the first sign or symptom of illness, others resort to taking medicine only when they feel there is no other alternative available.

Britten (1994) offers such an example when she describes how pain is very often 'a trigger for taking medication particularly for those who were otherwise opposed to medication taking in general.'

The middle path

A middle path is taken by many patients. They typically express distrust about the medication they have had to take, whilst often having a hearty dislike of the idea of taking any such substance; yet they nevertheless accept that medication is an effective way of addressing their particular health needs.

Others pursue a middle path by viewing habitual taking of medication as a normal part of their lives. Hewett (1994) describes how the group of men participating in his study on chronic asthma used inhalers 'automatically' and said that at night they thought they used them 'almost in their sleep'. Apparently by integrating medication in such a way so that it became 'habitual and automatic rather than something that needed even occasional thought, concern or worry', this particular group of men were able to avoid much of the 'uncertainty' (Weiner, 1975) and gradually worsening symptoms experienced by those with other forms of chronic illness.

Negative views

Patients with a negative orientation towards medication often state their preference for tolerating a health problem and not taking any medication at all. By adopting such a course of action they feel that they are able to maintain control over their health. Apparently any form of treatment can be regarded as symbolising an abrogation of personal responsibility, with the attendant possibility of such diminution of control seeping into other areas of their lives.

Closely related to negative views of medication is the issue of stigma. For many patients, having to take medication or any form of treatment produces such feelings. However, for those patients suffering from chronic conditions such as asthma, many ensure that the invisibility of the disease, produced by the control that medication can bring, is re-enforced by the invisibility of treatment which they conduct in private.

Medication and paradox

An interesting example of the often paradoxical nature of control within the context of medication is provided by Rajan (1996) in her work on pain relief for women in childbirth. The following description is of a woman's view of epidural anaesthesia:

> I was not prepared for the pain of the contractions... Having had the epidural I felt marvellous, so relieved to be pain free and in control and able to enjoy the labour.

Yet as Rajan (1996) indicates:

> Of all methods of pain relief, apart from the general anaesthetic (which was regarded by the women more as a surgical procedure than a method of pain relief), epidural anaesthesia renders the woman the most helpless.

The views expressed by the patient in Rajan's study offer a clear indication of the complexity inherent in many patients' perceptions of their treatment.

Complexity is also a characteristic of medication regimens, and can militate against effective use of medication, a problem often compounded by the advanced age of patients. For many older people multi-medication is required, which in turn leads to confusion. Confusion may arise when instructions about treatment regimens are unclear to patients. Several aspects of confusion ranging from the meaning of the term 'take the drug four times a day' to 'keep your leg elevated most of the day', have been identified by Zola (1981). Complexity and confusion may thus militate against patients' autonomy and control over their condition or disease.

The patient's condition/disease

While issues about control and the need to play an active part in their treatment are important for many patients and do affect patients' adherence to medication and treatment, for others more emphasis is placed upon factors associated with the disease or condition.

Although many patients use medication to establish normality, others regard the use of medication as an inappropriate source of relief for certain conditions. As Morgan (1996) describes, the use of powerful drugs to control the often asymptomatic condition of hypertension was avoided by many in her study group. Like some of the patients experiencing chronic heart failure (Mair *et al.*, 1996), the use of long term medication was inappropriate because for many of these patients 'real illness' only ever took an acute form. Similarly, as Hewett's study of adult males suffering from asthma conveys more directly, medication taken to relieve a condition is often viewed more positively and prescribed use adhered to more strictly by patients, than is medication taken preventatively.

Another aspect of 'normality' which is important in assessing patients' likelihood of adhering to medication, concerns the way in which so many patients who suffer from chronic conditions adapt to the symptoms they experience. If adaptation has been well achieved by patients, and their condition is assimilated into their everyday lives, they then become unaware that others do not experience similar sensations. Such patients then consider themselves healthy, or as in the case of those who are elderly, suffering from nothing more serious than 'just old age'.

Symptoms thus play a very important part when exploring issues which affect adherence. However, as was explained when discussing patient characteristics, it is the specificity of the symptoms and the particularity of the context together which require consideration, not the wider and more general characteristics. With regard to adherence to medication, it is therefore patients' subjective assessment of their condition which is of importance, rather than any objective measure of the disease or condition.

Medication may be perceived as insensitive to patients if it is seen to offer '... uniform treatment for all problems, in other words not being tailored to the needs of the individual' (Britten, 1994). Perhaps, most importantly many medications are regarded as treating symptoms rather than addressing their causes.

There are, however, in the cases of conditions such as diabetes or schizophrenia, additionally associated characteristics such as confusion, visual impairment or an inability to judge time which can affect the patient's ability to take medication as prescribed.

Patients' relationships with professionals

Studies, not directly related to adherence, have emphasised the importance of the quality of the interaction between health care professionals and patients in terms of the improvement which takes place in positive health outcomes for the patient. The role of the doctor–patient relationship as a means of achieving adherence to medication has been identified by Ley (1988). He describes such adherence as resulting from the creation of effective communication and patient satisfaction.

The influence on adherence is not restricted to the professional relationships and communication between doctors and patients. All health care professionals can influence patients' attitudes to their medication and treatment, especially when they act as members of the health care team. In their guidebook for health care providers, Meichenbaum & Turk (1987) describe one of the features of the lay–professional encounter which has been identified generally as important with regard to adherence:

> It probably goes without saying that a caring attitude and a warm, approachable, personalized treatment approach can significantly enhance patient satisfaction and treatment adherence.

However, although the value of creating a good rapport within the interaction is very important in terms of patients' adherence to medication and treatment, so too is the information exchanged within the interaction.

Information provision

It is clear from numerous studies (Ley, 1982; Busson, 1986; Weinman, 1990) that various aspects of information provision have important influences upon adherence to medication. The form in which information is given, especially whether it is written or verbal, has been shown to significantly affect the level of patients' knowledge about their medication. Patients express a general preference for written rather than verbal information (Morris & Groft, 1982).

Whilst improved knowledge would appear to increase patients' levels of satisfaction, it is less certain whether it also improves levels of adherence (Ley, 1988), although Weinman (1990) concludes that if the needs of the patient are met by the provision of adequate information, both knowledge and adherence can be addressed effectively. Adequacy of information comprises both technical correctness, an aspect particularly valued by patients with higher levels of educational achievement, and realisation of patients' expectations, attitudes and beliefs about treatment and medication. Thus, the nature of the information, and in particular the balance between positive outcomes to be expected from the medication and negative aspects (e.g. side effects), are deemed important by many patients.

There has been much debate about the influence of information regarding side effects on patients' adherence to their medication and treatment. Work by DiMatteo & DiNicola (1982) revealed that discussion about possible side effects, with both patients and significant others, served to enhance rather than reduce adherence. Patients were particularly receptive if the style of communication was informative rather than instructive. Work by Berry et al. (1995) reports that most patients request information about the possible side effects of their medication, if they are not given such information during their interaction with the professional. However, another study by Berry *et al.* (1997) indicates a possible effect on adherence of 'negative information', indicating the need for further exploration of this issue.

Patients' organisational and practical needs

Although patients' beliefs and the nature of their relationship with health care providers are most often the focus of research and literature on adherence, the influence of organisational and practical factors is also important.

Continuity of care and carer

For many patients, particularly those experiencing forms of chronic illness, being able to see the same professional at successive clinic visits in familiar surroundings, can have a positive effect upon adherence. Meichenbaum & Turk (1987) assert that '... nurses are more likely to provide greater continuity of care than physicians in medical clinics.' They conclude that this, together with nurses' greater concern for patients' social problems, results in improved adherence to treatment and medication by patients.

Appointments

The way appointments with professionals are organised may also have an effect upon patients' attitude to medication and treatment, and to their subsequent adherence. By making individualized appointments rather than block bookings, patients are often saved waiting time. Reduced waiting time thus encourages patients to feel that their needs are indeed important, and contributes to re-enforcing caring as an intrinsic aspect of patient treatment.

It is also important for health care professionals such as nurses to be aware of the mechanisms which may help to minimise any barriers to adherence likely to be encountered within a particular treatment regimen. Such barriers may be encountered either in obtaining the medication or in its effective use.

Cost

Cost is a factor that is mentioned by some patients, both in terms of the medication itself and with regard to obtaining the medication. Harrison (1983) describes how in Inner London, when patients have seen their general practitioner, this is only the first hurdle they have to overcome.

Taking a prescription to the pharmacist, where there may be fewer dispensing in poorer outlets than in more affluent areas, often requires having to spend time and money travelling to find such a service. In the evening, because of the limited number of pharmacies open, time and cost may increase further, so making adherence to treatment less likely.

Customisation of medication

When the treatment regimen is first introduced, suggesting that taking medication should coincide with events within the patient's everyday experience, such as time of getting up or going to bed, toothbrushing or bathing, or meal times, can be an effective way of integrating treatment into a patient's everyday routines. It is important, however, not to presume that all patients necessarily follow typical daily routines. Thus, those prescribing or instructing on the use of medication should discuss with the patient how the timing of doses required is best related to their particular lifestyle and daily routine. Not only does such integration act as a form of customisation for the patient, and so overcome the problem many patients had with treatment not 'tailored to the needs of the individual' (Britten, 1994), it also can serve as a reminder to take medication.

Presentation of medication

A variety of devices have been developed to assist patients in following the prescribed medication regimen. Their effectiveness is almost wholly dependent upon the patient actively wishing to adhere to the prescribed treatment regimen. Thus they largely address those barriers to adherence associated with regimen complexity and patient forgetfulness; they thus act primarily to facilitate compliance by patients who are already mindful to adhere.

Typically such devices act to remind patients of the prescribed dosage, to actively or passively remind them to take the medication, or to deliver the medication in a readily accessible form. A review of devices aimed at creating improved patient compliance is given in a monograph by Berg *et al.* (1993) which is based largely upon American practice.

Their list includes relatively simple devices, such as prescription label scratch-offs where the patient removes a dot on the bottle label as each dose of medication is taken, and counter caps which advance automatically when the patient opens and closes the container to indicate the day of the week and the number of doses of medication taken that day. Many forms of packaging can be designed to present the medication in dosage units and can be printed with numbering or days of the week in order to facilitate accurate usage.

More complex aids to compliance can involve electronic or computer based devices that may be programmed to sound an alarm when a dose is due or when a repeat prescription is required and which can maintain a record of the amounts of, and times at which, doses were taken. An advanced form of such devices can communicate automatically with a terminal at a professional's office to report persistent non-adherence.

The packaging of medication can directly influence adherence both by unit-of-use and calendar packaging, and by delivering the medication in an easily storable and readily accessible form, such as bubble packs. However, a trade-off exists between providing ease of use, especially by elderly patients or those with manipulative disabilities, and designing packaging to protect against accidental overdose or misuse, especially by children. Furthermore, these more user-friendly forms of packaging often involve additional costs in the production or distribution of medication.

Conclusions

The material presented in this chapter has illustrated the multifaceted and complex nature of the concept of adherence to medication and treatment. Thus consideration of how professionals may adapt their practice in order to improve patient adherence requires a holistic approach to both patients' rationales and to the role of the health care provider.

It is therefore necessary to address the individual patient's attitudes and beliefs regarding their condition and the treatment being offered, and to focus the relationship with the patient and the treatment regimen in the context of that individual. This in turn requires an integrated approach to both interaction and medication, and involves the whole of the health care team, particularly nurses, pharmacists and doctors.

While more traditional biomedically oriented approaches have emphasised the need for medication and treatment to reflect professional rationales, it has become clear that it is possible to achieve only limited adherence within such a context.

Although more integrated approaches to both patient–professional interaction and medication have been implemented, as the report from the Royal Pharmaceutical Society of Great Britain & Merck, Sharp & Dohme (1997) states:

> '... we conclude that multifactorial strategies are most likely to be effective. But effective in pursuit of what goal?'

The report identifies the goal as 'concordance'. While the terminology used is perhaps of only limited significance, of greater consequence is the underlying ethos and anticipated outcome attributable to the concept of 'concordance'. The report also attributes many of the problems of adherence to a completely 'misleading model of the clinical encounter'. Instead, it is suggested the only way that 'taking medicines to the best effect' can be ensured, is by bringing about 'a fundamental shift in the balance of power in the clinical encounter'.

It would seem likely that cases involving acute conditions require rather different approaches to those appropriate to cases involving chronicity. For acute conditions, once the patient has obtained medication which is both acceptable to and clearly understood by them, the immediacy of the treatment and the usual presence of symptoms to which the patient is unaccustomed act to prompt adherence to the medication. The emphasis in achieving effective treatment therefore lies in effective communication between the patient and the health care team at the outset of treatment, coupled with efficient user friendly delivery of the medication during the course of treatment.

These issues are, of course, also important for cases involving chronicity. However, for these conditions medication and treatment need to become part of patients' everyday lives. Perhaps therefore, parallels can be drawn with the Changing Childbirth initiative (Department of Health, 1993), a prime objective of which is the transformation of pregnancy from a highly medicalised condition to a state of normality. Thus, the issues of choice, control and continuity, highlighted in the Changing Childbirth initiative, may be regarded as important in achieving effective treatment of chronic conditions.

In the context of medication, choice embodies both patient involvement in the establishment of the original treatment regimen, and patient initiation of treatment review. Patients may wish to choose whether or not to follow a particular course of treatment and where possible to be involved in selecting the form, dosage and brand of medication used. For example, a patient may prefer a particular medication because it is easier for them to take, easier for them to obtain, or seems to have fewer undesirable side effects. Such issues are not just pharmacological: ease of use may be a matter of packaging; particular medication may only be available from certain, perhaps less convenient outlets; and side effects might include whether taking medication in a particular form is more or less acceptable to work colleagues and family members.

When involving patients in choice, it is important that their choices be informed ones. Informed choice requires both clear communication of information and a respect for the autonomy of the patient. Patients will vary in the extent to which they wish to be involved in the selection of their treatment. Some will welcome close involvement and may tend to reject treatment which they feel has been imposed upon them. Others, who do not wish to make choices for themselves, may resent what they perceive to be the professionals' abrogation of responsibility for their treatment, and then mistrust the medication offered to them. It is therefore important for health care providers to tailor their approach to the needs and preferences of the particular patient.

Whilst involvement in the choice of medication provides one aspect of control, other aspects require patient involvement throughout the process of treatment so that they may take effective ownership of it. Thus, for example, patients should be given the maximum opportunity to influence, if not decide, the timing and location of monitoring check-ups, the frequency and methods of obtaining repeat prescriptions, and the form of delivery of the medication itself. Naturally, pharmaceutical and medical factors will also have an influence, but the decision-making process should be managed in such a way that the patient feels in control of the medication rather than the medication acting as a control over the patient.

The importance of continuity of health care providers has already been mentioned. Continuity facilitates the establishment of dialogue and the building of trust and confidence. These in turn help to ensure effective communication not only from the health care providers to the patient, but also, and perhaps more importantly, from the patient to the members of the health care team.

Effective communication and patient involvement can thus be seen as the centrepiece of achieving effective treatment through adherence to appropriate medication. As Meichenbaum & Turk (1987) in their text which they wrote to 'provide practical clinical guidelines and techniques for HCPs (Health Care Providers)' emphasised:

'Lack of adherence is likely to be a major cause of therapeutic failure, and therefore it interferes with our ability to determine the effectiveness of our treatments.'

Summary

Medication, as part of the therapeutic process of care, operates within a sociocultural context. Understanding the many different aspects of such a context, which involves patients' everyday lives, is complex, but is important in order that patients may be offered effective treatment and care. The terms compliance and adherence, and most recently concordance, have been used when seeking to convey a range of ideas regarding patients' participation in and treatment with medication. Common and recurrent themes associated with each of these terms are those of patient knowledge and the patient–professional relationship. By developing understanding about patient knowledge and the patient/professional relationship, professionals are able to help patients become active participants in, rather than passive recipients of, therapeutic care. Patients are enabled to become active participants when professionals accept the validity of patients' views about medication and treatment, and involve patients in the management of their own condition. Patients thus become more knowledgeable and proactive and so optimise their treatment.

References

Berg, J.S., Dischler, J., Wagner, D.J., Raia, J.J. & Palmer-Shevlin, N. (1993) Medication compliance: a healthcare problem. *Ann. Pharmacother.* **27** (9), S5–S19.

Berridge, V. & Edwards, G. (1981) *Opium and the People.* Allen Lane, London.

Berry, D.C., Gillie, T. & Banbury, S. (1995) What do Patients Want to Know? An Empirical Approach to Explanation Generation and Validation. *Expert Syst. Appl.* **8**, 419–29.

Berry, D.C., Michas, I.C., Gillie, T. & Forster, M. (1997) What do patients want to know about their medicines and what do doctors want to tell them? A comparative study. *Psychol. Health* **12**, 467–80.

Britten, N. (1994) Patient's ideas about medicines: a qualitative study in a general practice population. *Br. J. Gen. Pract* **44**, 465–8.

Britten, N. (1996) Lay views of drugs and medicines: orthodox and unorthodox accounts. In: *Modern Medicine: Lay Perspectives and Experiences* (eds S.J. Williams & M. Calnan). UCL Press, London.

Busson, M. (1986) Patients' knowledge about prescribed medicines. *Pharm. J.* **236**, 624–6.

Conrad, P. (1985) The meaning of medications: another look at compliance. *Soc. Sci. Med.* **20**, 29–37.

Department of Health (1993) *Changing Childbirth: Report of the Expert Maternity Group*, HMSO, London.

DiMatteo, M.R. & DiNicola, D.D. (1982) *Achieving Patient Compliance: The Psychology of the Medical Practitioner's Role*, Pergamon Press, New York.

Donovan, J.L. & Blake, D.R. (1992) Patient non-compliance: deviance or reasoned decision-making? *Soc. Sci. Med.* **34** (5), 507–13.

Donovan, J. L., Blake, D.R. & Fleming, W.G. (1989) The patient is not a blank sheet: lay beliefs and their relevance to patient education. *Br. J. Rheumatol* **28**, 58–61.

Drummond, N. & Mason, C. (1990) Diabetes in a social context: just a different way of life in the age of reason. In: *Readings in Medical Sociology* (eds S. Cunningham-Burley & N.P. McKeganey). Tavistock/Routledge, London.

Fallsberg, M. (1991) Reflections on medicines and medication. A qualitative analysis among people on long-term drug regimens. *Linkoping Studies in Education*, Vol. 32, Linkoping University, Sweden.

Gabe, J. & Lipshitz-Phillips, S. (1982) Evil necessity? The meaning of benzodiazepine use for women patients from one general practice. *Soc. Health & Illness* **4**, 201–9.

Gabe, J. & Thorogood, N. (1986) Prescribed drugs and the management of everyday life: the experience of black and white working-class women. *Sociol. Rev.* **34**, 737–72.

Harrison, P. (1983) *Inside the Inner City*. Pelican, London.

Heidel, B. and Wiffen, P.J. (1996) Improving patient compliance with medication: a review of randomised control trials. *Eur. Hosp. Pharm.* **2** (1), 13–16.

Helman, C.G. (1981) "Tonic", "fuel" and "food": social and symbolic aspects of the long-term use of psychotropic drugs. *Soc. Sci. Med.* **15B**, 521–33.

Hewett, G. (1994) Just a part of me: men's reflections on chronic asthma. *Occasional Papers in Sociology & Social Policy*, Vol. 1, South Bank University, London.

Kasl, S.V. (1975) Issues in patient adherence to health care regimens. *J. Human Stress* **1**, 5–18.

Ley, P. (1982) Satisfaction, compliance & communication. *Br. J. Clin. Psychol.* **21**, 241–54.

Ley, P. (1988) *Communicating with Patients: Improving Communication, Satisfaction & Compliance*. Croom Helm, London.

MacIntyre, S. & Oldham, D. (1977) Coping with migraine. In: *Medical Encounters* (eds C. Davis & G. Horbin). Croom Helm, London.

Mair, F.M., Ling, M.S. & Faimon, G. (1996) Patient perceptions of chronic heart failure. Proc. 24th Annual Meeting, The North American Primary Care Research Group, Vancouver, paper 65.

Martin, J.E. & Dubbert, P.M. (1986) Exercise and health: the adherence problem. *Behavioral Med. Update* **4**, 16–24.

Meichenbaum, D. & Turk, D.C. (1987) *Facilitating Treatment Adherence: A Practitioner's Handbook*. Plenum Press, New York & London.

Morgan, M. (1996) Perceptions and use of anti-hypertensive drugs among cultural groups. In: *Modern Medicine: Lay Perspectives and Experiences* (eds S.J. Williams & M. Calnan). UCL Press, London.

Morris, L.A. & Groft, S. (1982) Patient packet inserts: a research perspective. *Drugs Ther. Bull.* **30**, 191–217.

Nations, M.K., Camino, L.A. & Walker, F.B. (1985) 'Hidden' popular illnesses in primary care: residents' recognition and clinical implications. *Culture, Med. Psych* **9**, 223–40.

Posner, T. (1977) Magical elements in orthodox medicine. In: *Health Care and Health Knowledge* (ed. R. Dingwall). Croom Helm, London.

Rajan, L. (1996) Pain and pain relief in labour: issues of control. In: *Modern Medicine: Lay Perspectives and Experiences* (eds S.J. Williams & M. Calnan). UCL Press, London.

Rosenstock, I.M. (1985) Understanding and enhancing patient compliance with diabetic regimens. *Diabetes Care* **8**, 610–16.

Royal Pharmaceutical Society of Great Britain & Merck Sharp & Dohme (1997) *From Compliance to Concordance: Achieving Shared Goals in Medicine Taking.* RPSGB, London.

Weiner, C.L. (1975) The burden of rheumatoid arthritis: tolerating the uncertainty, *Soc. Sci. Med* **9**, 97–104.

Weinman, J. (1990) Providing written information for patients: psychological consequences. *J. R. Soc. Med.* **83**, 303–5.

Williams, G. (1984) The genesis of chronic illness: narrative reconstruction. *Soc. Health Illness* **6** (2), 175–200.

Zola, I.K. (1981) Structural constraints on the doctor–patient relationship: the case of non-compliance. In: *The Relevance of Social Science for Medicine* (eds L. Eisenberg & A. Kleinman). Reidel, New York.

Chapter 6
Factors Influencing Prescribing

Simon T. Gelder

Introduction

Prescribing is a very complex process requiring many skills. Factors which can influence prescribing, either positively or negatively, are many and varied. This chapter will provide the reader with an overview of the subject and will cover the more important points in detail. The references and further reading provided should be used if further detail is required.

Increasingly medicines are being deregulated so that other professionals, besides doctors, can prescribe a greater number of more powerful medicines. It is vitally important that all professionals concerned with prescribing, either directly or indirectly, master the skills necessary for good prescribing. It cannot be emphasised too strongly that prescribing is a very serious process.

Skills used in prescribing

Prescribing has been put increasingly under the spotlight over the last few years, more often than not in an attempt to reduce expenditure on drugs. Drugs expenditure constitutes an enormous portion of the NHS budget. As described in Chapter 1, many government-sponsored initiatives have been set up with the aim of making sure that this money is well spent.

Good prescribing should be appropriate, safe, effective and economic. This definition is a worthy aim, but in practice compromises are necessary and so an attempt to balance these must be made (Barber, 1995). Fig. 6.1 illustrates the factors which need to be balanced for each patient.

Maximise benefit

Firstly, the clinician must decide which drug is likely to have the best-desired effect in the patient being treated, and must ascertain what the effect is so that it can be monitored. In some cases the effect may be an end effect such as a cured

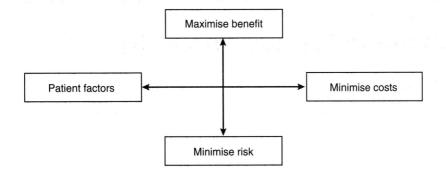

Fig. 6.1   Factors to be balanced in prescribing.

infection, or in other cases will be a surrogate effect such as reduced diastolic blood pressure. The decision to treat a patient with a drug which causes a surrogate effect should be based upon evidence that this will benefit the patient and improve outcome. In a hypertensive patient the reduction in diastolic blood pressure should reduce the likelihood of a stroke and renal failure, and reduce mortality. A reduction in a raised systolic blood pressure is also important.

The correct dosage must be chosen with respect to the patient's characteristics e.g. age, weight, renal and hepatic function, and other drugs. In addition a suitable formulation must be chosen that can be administered to the patient. Overly complicated dosage regimens may also reduce compliance and therefore prevent the patient from benefiting from the treatment.

An end point should be considered if it is not appropriate to continue the prescription indefinitely. If the prescription must be continued, then suitable intervals for monitoring the treatment must be chosen.

Minimise risk

Any substance administered to a patient presents them with some element of risk of causing an adverse effect. Attempts should be made to reduce risk by reducing polypharmacy and prescribing only when there is likely to be a real benefit. Often, especially in the age of computer generated repeat prescriptions, it is easier to initiate a prescription than to review and discontinue an existing one. Common sense suggests that the greater the number of drugs a patient is prescribed the more likely they are to suffer an adverse effect from at least one of them.

Risk is always relative and must be balanced against the likely benefit of treatment. Relatively trivial adverse effects such as drowsiness can be intolerable when the drug is used to treat a minor disorder, e.g. older antihistamines used for the treatment of hay fever. The reduction in mental ability caused in such cases may be dangerous if the patient performs complicated tasks, e.g. pilots, lorry drivers. A serious or life-threatening adverse effect of a treatment, which is used to treat a minor disorder, is likely to be totally unacceptable if safer alternatives are available, even if the effect is uncommon. A recent example of this is terfenadine, a non-sedating antihistamine, causing sudden death through prolongation of the QT interval i.e. the time elapsing between ventricular depolarisation and repolarisation (Committee on Safety of Medicines, 1997a,b).

Penicillins carry a risk of spreading resistance and allergy, including life-threatening anaphylactic shock. The incidence of this is considered acceptable in the light of the benefits of successful treatment of infections. However, the use of penicillin inappropriately, such as in viral infections, exposes the patient to an unnecessary risk. Anticancer treatments have very serious side effects including neutropenia and induction of tumours themselves. However, the side effects are often well known and can be minimised if anticipated. They are considered acceptable as the drugs are used to treat life-threatening conditions.

It is vitally important that wherever possible patients are informed of the risks of the treatment. In nearly all cases the patient takes the prescribed treatment voluntarily and should give their consent to the treatment. A common complaint in the media is that the doctor didn't tell the patient or his/her guardians of the risks of the treatment. These cases are often the subjects of litigation.

Patient factors

The decision to prescribe a drug should be taken on the basis that each patient is an individual and as such has individual needs. The balance of the expected benefit versus the anticipated risk has been discussed above. A risk, which the prescriber considers acceptable, may be unacceptable to the patient and vice versa. The patient may have individual opinions and preferences which need to be taken into account. It must be remembered that the patient chooses whether or not to take the medicine as prescribed.

Compliance with treatment is of paramount importance. In some cases the prescriber may have to prescribe more expensive, proprietary medicines to patients who insist that the generic versions do not help them. The prescriber thus cannot be inflexible, and if willing to listen to the patient, may ensure improved compliance. A common example is when a patient insists that Distalgesic helps their pain but co-proxamol or co-dydramol does not, despite having the same or similar constituents. There may well be an element of placebo effect with Distalgesic. This can be accepted and then prescribed in such cases. If the pain is treated successfully with Distalgesic it will avoid or delay the need for morphine or alternative strong analgesics and their associated side effects. It also helps the prescriber to gain the trust of the patient, as they know that their views are listened to and acted upon.

There will always be some cases where such flexibility is inappropriate. This could be when a patient demands treatment when none is appropriate. The drug addict demanding methadone or codeine linctus is an example.

Minimise cost

Money saved by economical prescribing may be used elsewhere. Initiatives such as incentive schemes for GP fundholders have demonstrated that with adequate encouragement savings are often possible. It is of interest to all tax-payers that NHS money is not wasted.

Money saving can be done in many ways. The best known is probably the encouragement of generic prescribing. When a proprietary drug's patent expires, other companies can manufacture the drug. These products are usually much cheaper than the original proprietary drug, as the generic manufacturers do not need to conduct the research needed to gain the product licence for the drug.

In many cases the cost of the medicine can be high, but if it reduces the need for hospitalisation or surgery, then it will save money overall. The use of modern antiulcer treatments, including histamine H-2 antagonists and proton pump inhibitors, has made the need for surgery uncommon. New anti-psychotic drugs, such as clozapine, are often effective where other treatments fail. These drugs are very expensive to prescribe but can result in in-patients being managed less intensively or even as out-patients and thus may save money in the end.

Successful drug therapy can be seen to be a great deal more than just choosing the right drug. It requires psychosocial skills as well as technical skills.

The prescriber must be able to exercise wisdom and judgement in order to balance the often conflicting requirements.

Factors influencing prescribing

There is an enormous number of factors which can influence the prescriber: this section will summarise some of the more important ones (see Fig. 6.2).

Policies and guidelines

Examples are formularies, antibiotic policies, post-myocardial infarction guidelines for treatment, headlice policy. These may either be produced locally by a practice, speciality or policymaking group, e.g. drug and ther-apeutics committee (DTC), or can be produced nationally, e.g. British Thoracic Society guidelines for the treatment of asthma. Ideally they should be evidence-based or reflect current expert opinion. Policies and guidelines should guide practice and ensure the best standards of treatment are practised. If the policy is produced locally then additional benefits are seen in improved communication between prescribers and in education. If accepted guidelines are not followed then there may be legal consequences if there is an adverse patient outcome.

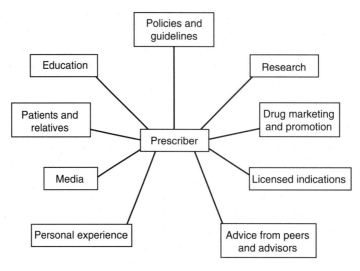

Fig. 6.2 Factors influencing prescribing.

Research

Ideally all prescribing should be based on strong, well-conducted, independent, published research. In practice this is not always possible. Good research and reviews of studies can change practice and set new standards.

Unfortunately much published research is of low quality, and the results of such should be interpreted with caution. The prescriber should always question the quality of the study carefully before accepting its findings. Research published in quality medical journals such as the *British Medical Journal, Lancet* and *New England Journal of Medicine* is usually, but not always, of a high standard. Caution should always be taken with unpublished research such as 'data on file' quoted in manufacturers' literature or free journals containing a high proportion of adverts. This topic was introduced in Chapter 2 in the context of drug information sources.

Patients and relatives

Patient factors include the clinical condition of the patient, their age, weight, sex, renal and hepatic function, concomitant drugs and other diseases or problems. These factors are often not under the control of the patient.

Patients or their relatives may have strong opinions including fears regarding various treatments. They can be influenced in these by personal experience, the media, friends and relatives, self-help groups, books and magazines.

Patients often expect to come away after an appointment with a prescription and feel let down if they do not. They often do not want to give up their unhealthy lifestyle (smoking, obesity) but still expect successful cures. Patients remember failures and accidents but take success for granted. This can put a lot of pressure on prescribers, limiting the treatments which may be used. Patients take treatment voluntarily so must always consent to the treatment. In order to make informed consent, time must be taken to explain the treatment adequately, informing the patient of the goals of the treatment and any possible problems it may cause.

Peers and expert advisers

Junior prescribers may often be instructed to prescribe a particular drug by a more senior colleague; in many cases this is satisfactory. Prescribers must still be aware that when they write a prescription, they are responsible for it, whether or not they were ordered to prescribe the medicine. They still have a duty as a professional to question choices with which they disagree. This is fundamental and is a natural part of the training process. It also provides the opportunity for the more senior prescribers to reconsider their own practice.

It is impossible for the prescriber to be an expert in all areas, and occasionally they will need to ask for opinions and advice regarding some clinical situations. This may be from peers or from external advisers such as drug information pharmacists or drug company medical information departments. Sometimes these advisers will give specific advice, but often they will provide further information to help the prescriber consider their options.

Personal experience

This is often based on anecdotes and situations in which the prescriber has been previously involved. There is obviously no substitute for experience, but it must be remembered that practice should be based on sound evidence not anecdotal experience.

Experience of dealing with certain situations often gives the prescriber more confidence. This may be the confidence to prescribe a particular drug or it may be to question a senior colleague's recommendations.

It is impossible to remember enough details about all drugs to be able to prescribe them without reference to information sources such as the *British National Formulary* (BNF). Most prescribers will limit their prescribing to a limited number of drugs with which they are familiar and which they know in detail.

Education

Education plays a large part in forming the basic practices of prescribers. It can be from formal courses at university or college through undergraduate and postgraduate training. It can also be less formal in the form of ward rounds, grand rounds, lectures and symposia. Prescribers are obliged to maintain up to date knowledge in their clinical areas, so postgraduate training and continuing education are essential.

Product licences

The product licence specifies the indications for which a drug may be prescribed. A drug company can only promote the use of its products for licensed indications. Drug companies are liable for harmful effects of their products if they are prescribed correctly as specified in their data sheets or summaries of product characteristics.

Prescribing strictly to licensed indications can be severely limiting in some situations, e.g. paediatrics, pregnancy and rare disorders. It is unusual for a drug to be licensed for use in special groups such as these, especially if it is a new drug. Prescribing outside the product licence confers liability on the prescriber who must be aware of the extra responsibility this entails. The considerations which should be made in these circumstances are listed below.

If a drug is prescribed outside its licensed indications the prescriber should check that:

(1)   No other drug is licensed for the required indication.
(2)   The drug is accepted for the treatment of the required indication by experts in the field.
(3)   There is good evidence that the drug is effective for the indication.
(4)   The benefit outweighs any potential risk.
(5)   The patient is informed and consents to the treatment.

The media

The media include television, radio and newspapers. Health is a topic of great interest to many of us, and this is reflected in the amount of coverage it receives in the media. Unfortunately the media are not well regulated and can produce articles that are highly biased.

The aim of the media is often to sell as many papers as possible, or to achieve high viewing ratings. Extreme views are often represented without appropriate balance, and anecdotes proliferate. Scoops and sensational headlines abound. Often these put the prescriber in difficult situations, such as having their image tarnished, having advice criticised, or reducing compliance through increasing fear of side effects.

Clinical examination

Drug history

An accurate drug history is an invaluable aid to planning future treatment. It is often difficult and time consuming to obtain, and in many cases is inadequately performed.

The drug history may highlight inadequacies in previous therapy such as:

- Subtherapeutic doses
- Insufficient duration of previous treatment before the next drug tried

A good drug history:

- Aids choice of next step in therapy
- Prevents repetition
- Prevents the use of poorly tolerated drugs
- Reduces delays in appropriate treatment

Care must be taken to obtain an accurate and comprehensive drug history. This will require asking patients whenever appropriate about over-the-counter medications, herbal and alternative remedies, and the oral contraceptive pill. It is also important to question the patient about drugs used in the recent past as some have very long half-lives and can cause problems even after they have been discontinued, e.g. amiodarone, fluoxetine.

It is a great help to other prescribers and health professionals caring for the patient if an up to date patient medication record is carried by the patient or is available in their notes. This can be either a simple card with current treatment written on, a printout from the practice computer, or smart card technology.

Clinical examination

Before prescribing a drug a thorough clinical examination is vital, not only to confirm the diagnosis but to define a baseline from which the drug's effects can be measured objectively.

Cautions and contra-indications to drugs need to be considered in the light of the examination, e.g. allergies, history of gastro-intestinal bleeding, asthma. The parameters to allow objective monitoring of the therapy should be chosen. These should include a direct measure of the desired therapeutic effect, e.g. reduced blood pressure, improved peak expiratory flow rate. They may also include a measure of adverse effects, e.g. monitoring liver function tests with carbamazepine, monitoring renal function with ACE inhibitors. In some cases it may be necessary to monitor plasma concentrations of the drug if it has a narrow therapeutic index, e.g. gentamicin, lithium.

Drug marketing and promotion

The role of the pharmaceutical industry is the same as any other manufacturing industry, namely to sell its products and make profits. It is vital that companies sell their products, otherwise they would go out of business. Medicines should not be viewed as anything more than products that are sold to a specialist market. Accepting these basic facts will help the prescriber to assess information provided by pharmaceutical companies more critically.

The purpose of drug marketing and promotion is primarily to encourage prescribers to prescribe or patients to buy specific drugs. Many millions of pounds are spent to achieve this aim. Much of the money is spent on the familiar forms of promotion such as adverts, glossy brochures, representatives, sponsored meetings, etc. These methods ensure that prescribers are familiar with the promoted products, know the claimed advantages over existing treatments and have adequate information to prescribe the drug. The free pens, Post-it notes, mugs and other material given out assist in this process.

Free samples

Free samples are often used to provide the prescriber with the opportunity to conduct a perceived low-cost, no commitment, open, uncontrolled, non-comparative single centre, low power clinical trial. For obvious reasons, decisions to use particular drugs should be based on sound, scientific evidence. The uncontrolled use of samples is generally undesirable. A major marketing objective has been achieved when the prescriber can be made to start prescribing the drug. Free samples are one way of achieving this aim.

Meetings

Educational meetings, symposia and conferences are often company sponsored. Usually the material presented at such meetings is produced by well-known local or national experts. It is vital, however, to remember that the meeting is company sponsored. It is highly unlikely that the presenters at such meetings will be critical of the sponsoring company's products.

The company representative

Drug company representatives are familiar to many health professionals. They provide the personal point of access to information from the company. They are the providers of the detailed information required on the products they are promoting and of the familiar gifts. Usually representatives will organise meetings, educational/promotional videos and presentations, free lunches/meals.

Drug company representatives are usually highly trained professionals who are very knowledgeable about their products, their competitors' products and the disease areas in which the products are used. It must be remembered that their livelihood is dependant on persuading prescribers to prescribe or recommend their product rather than a competitor's. If you are not a prescriber then their aim is to obtain information on local prescribers and their practices in order to facilitate their aims. It will probably be known if you have the capacity to exert an influence on these prescribers regarding their choices of drugs. Drug promotion is a very serious, very sophisticated, highly targeted process with huge sums of money at stake. The needs of the drug company are not necessarily compatible with the needs of the prescriber, patient or health care organisation.

By becoming familiar with the local representative, receiving assistance to organise meetings, receiving materials, sponsorship of posts, e.g. nurse specialists, it becomes more difficult to make objective choices on drug use. It would be naive to think that drug promotion does not have an effect on prescribing. Remember that there is no such thing as a 'free' gift or a 'free' lunch.

Written materials

In order to attempt to meet the needs of their customers, material may be presented in different forms. Examples include detailed product monographs, non-glossy presentations for drug information pharmacists. Health economic, outcome measures and quality of life research and reviews are provided more frequently, reflecting the needs of the companies' customers.

Interpretation of company provided support material

Even in detailed monographs it is unusual to read about research with negative findings. Information on the advantages of the promoted drug against its competitors will be presented to make it look as good as possible. Below is a checklist for use when reading this material.

When presented with information on products which has been prepared by or sponsored by a drug company always:

(1) Check that the product is licensed for the required indications.
(2) Check for well-conducted studies directly comparing the drug with its competitors in equivalent dosages.
(3) If an advantage is claimed is it of clinical relevance? Has the advantage been proven in clinical trials?
(4) Are there any outcome measures, e.g. reduced mortality?
(5) Is there any guidance on using the drug in special patient groups, e.g. children, elderly or renally impaired people, in pregnancy?
(6) Check for information on drug interactions.
(7) Look for information on drug safety and adverse effects. How many patients has the drug been used in? How long has it been used for?
(8) Read data presented carefully, especially graphs. How many patients were in the trials? What was the size of the difference between the groups (rather than just if it was clinically significant)?
(9) Check that any references used are from reputable sources.

The pharmaceutical industry

The pharmaceutical industry is a multibillion pound, highly successful industry. The UK industry exported £2.7 billion more than was imported in

1996, thus contributed significantly to the UK economy (ABPI, 1996). The UK industry invests £2 billion per annum into research and development. It also employs nearly 75 000 people.

Manufacturers can be split into two broad groups:

(1) Research-based companies
(2) Generics manufacturers

Research-based companies

These invest huge resources into identifying and developing new drugs and innovations. They will rely on the new products in future to provide profits and further money to invest into research and development. The cost of developing a new drug is enormous (approximately £100 million per drug that reaches the market). Because of the huge costs, we rely heavily on the industry to provide us with the cures for diseases in the future. There will always be a tendency for investment to be made into the potentially more lucrative disease areas occurring in the developed world. Work on diseases in the developing world, a little researched field, is actively encouraged by governments and organisations such as the World Health Organisation.

Generics companies

These companies specialise in the manufacture of medicines that were originally developed by research-based companies. Generic products are usually much less expensive than proprietary products because their manufacturers do not need to invest in drug development to the same extent. The quality of generic medicines is often perceived to be less than that of proprietary products. The licensing bodies, such as the Medicines Control Agency in the UK, control and regulate the manufacture of all medicines and ensure that minimum standards for quality are met. As a result generic medicines can usually be substituted for their proprietary equivalents without any problems. With the exception of those medicines specified in Chapters 3 or 12, the use of generic medicines is essential in the minimisation of expenditure on drugs.

Because of the importance of the pharmaceutical industry to the UK economy, there is close liaison between the industry and the government. An important component of this is the Pharmaceutical Price Regulation Scheme (PPRS) which agrees the profits which may accrue from medicines prescribed on the NHS. The PPRS recognises the needs of both the industry to make profits and the government to minimise health-sector expenditure.

Association of the British Pharmaceutical Industry (ABPI)

Many companies in the UK industry are members of this organisation. It acts both as a representative body for the industry in the UK and as a self-regulatory body. The ABPI has a code of conduct and standards for the promotion of medicines. A system is in place to deal with breaches in this code, e.g. unfair claims of benefits of one medicine over another in an advert.

Role of the media

- Newspapers
- Books
- Magazines
- Television
- Radio
- Internet

Health care is heavily covered by the media, reflecting high public interest in the subject. It is not unusual to hear of new drug breakthroughs, scares about side effects or tales about prescribing errors. There are numerous programmes covering medical topics in detail, e.g. Watchdog, Tomorrow's World. A look in any good bookshop will reveal many books from family health guides to the latest alternative health craze. The Internet now provides access to enormous amounts of health-related material simply by using a personal computer and a modem.

In a free, democratic society access to information by the public is a basic right. Unfortunately there is no way to ensure that this information is presented in a fair, accurate and responsible manner. In many cases it is clear that material is sensationalised, unbalanced and irresponsible.

Adverse effects

A recent example of an adverse effect, which was reported extensively, concerned studies which had revealed that certain brands of the oral contraceptive pill increased the risk of thrombo-embolism more than others (Guillebaud, 1995; MacRae & Kay 1995). This information made headlines during 1995 before the majority of prescribers were aware of the findings of the studies. It would be unfair to criticise solely the media for premature and irresponsible reporting. Some blame must be apportioned to the government who were slow to distribute advice and information to prescribers. Three studies, which were at that time unpublished, were found to show that oral contraceptive pills containing desogestrel and gestodene increased the risk of venous thrombo-embolism from 15 cases per 100 000 to 30 cases per 100 000 as compared with older formulations. During the year following the scare the British Pregnancy Advisory Service reported that abortions carried out in the UK could have risen by up to 10% as a result (Dillner, 1996). In many cases women had stopped taking their contraceptive pills and not consulted their doctors regarding their concerns or alternative contraception. The fact that the risk of thrombo-embolism in pregnancy is double the risk presented by even the oral contraceptive pills concerned in the scare was not made clear.

New treatments

It is not uncommon for clinicians to be asked by patients for treatments which they have heard of or read about via the media. This can sometimes put the prescriber in a difficult situation as the patient can be given false hopes and expectations. Examples of diseases and drugs which have received much media attention recently include:

- Beta-interferon and multiple sclerosis
- Riluzole and motor neurone disease
- Donezepril and Alzheimer's disease

The facts that these treatments are not cures, have limited effects and may only benefit sub-groups of patients, are often not made clear or are not registered by the patient.

It is important for the prescriber to be aware of topics concerning medicines in the media. Where these topics concern research into major changes of practice or important side effects, the prescribers should ideally be forewarned before the media publishes or broadcasts the information. This allows time to consider appropriate responses to questions raised. The prescriber may then need to take time to explain to patients their response in order to maintain trust and confidence.

Evidence-based practice

Evidence-based practice may be defined as the process of systematically finding, appraising, and using contemporaneous research findings as the basis for clinical decisions (Rosenberg & Donald, 1995). The aim of evidence-based practice is to close the gap between research and everyday practice, and ensure that clinical decisions are based on the best available scientific evidence. The idea of evidence-based practice is certainly not new. It is, and has been, common practice when confronted with a clinical problem to consult the literature in search of guidance.

Evidence-based practice involves a formal approach to dealing with questions. It requires the use of explicit frameworks to answer clinical questions rather than the traditionally less formal approach. It requires clinicians to develop skills in tracking down new types of strong and useful evidence, distinguish it from weak and irrelevant evidence and put it into practice. Fig. 6.3 details the steps required to undertake evidence-based practice.

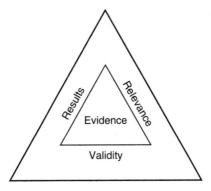
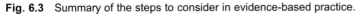

Fig. 6.3   Summary of the steps to consider in evidence-based practice.

The pursuit of evidence-based practice involves four steps:

(1)   Formulation of a clear clinical question to be investigated
(2)   A literature search for relevant clinical articles
(3)   Evaluation of the evidence for its validity and usefulness
(4)   Implementation of the findings in clinical practice

The practice of these four steps requires time, skill and thoroughness.

Appraisal of the evidence

Critical appraisal enables decisions to be made on whether articles can be relied upon to give useful guidance. Unfortunately much published research lacks either relevance or sufficient methodological rigour to be reliable enough to answer questions (Altman 1994). Table 6.1 shows a set of critical appraisal questions for evaluating articles about treatment.

Acting on the evidence

Once evidence, which is valid and relevant, is identified it can be used directly in a patient's care or to develop protocols or guidelines. The results of a number of studies may be pooled and analysed using meta-analysis. This technique can be used to produce conclusions from pooling the results of small, inconclusive studies. It is vital that expert statistical advice is sought for meta-analysis and that the results of negative as well as positive studies are used so that bias can be minimised.

Clinical trials

Before a drug may be marketed for use in clinical practice it has to undergo formal clinical trials. Clinical trials:

Table 6.1 Checklist for The appraisal of the evidence (kindly reproduced from Guyatt *et al.*, 1993, 1994)

	Yes	Can't tell	No
Are the results valid?			
Was the assignment of patients to treatments randomised?			
Were all patients who entered the trial properly accounted for and attributed at its conclusion?			
Was the follow up complete?			
Were patients analysed in the groups to which they were randomised?			
Were patients, health workers, and study personnel blinded to the treatment?			
Were the groups similar at the start of the trial?			
Aside from the experimental intervention were the groups treated equally?			
What are the results?			
How large was the treatment effect?			
How precise was the treatment effect?			
Will the results help me care for my patients?			
Can the results be applied to my patient care?			
Were all the clinically important outcomes considered?			
Are the likely benefits worth the potential harms and costs?			

- Convert the ideas of research workers into safe and effective therapeutic agents
- National drug regulatory bodies set formal requirements for trial design and conduct (the Medicines Control Agency (MCA) in the UK)
- The majority of clinical trials are funded and performed by the pharmaceutical industry

Because of the complexity of clinical trial design and conduct this section can only give the reader an overview of the subject. It is extremely important for the clinician to have a reasonable understanding of the drug development and clinical trial process. Clinical trials, reviews of clinical trials and articles quoting trials form the basis of the majority of the medical literature and promotional material. They are mandatory for drugs to receive product licences. Good basic understanding of clinical trial design and conduct enables the clinician to critically assess the medical literature and to decide whether practice should change or be questioned as a result. This is fundamental in the implementation of evidence-based practice.

In order to be aware of all the processes involved in drug development the following stages of drug development will be overviewed:

(1) Discovery
(2) Pre-clinical studies
(3) Clinical trials
(4) Post-marketing studies

Discovery

This involves the identification and isolation of a drug. It may come about by a number of means:

(1) From screening chemicals for biological activity
(2) By chance (serendipity)
(3) By design

- Discovery and development of a new drug costs approximately £100 million
- It takes more than 10 years to complete
- Patent from time of discovery is valid for about 20 years.

Pre-clinical studies

These aim to establish the pharmacology and toxicology of the drug in animals to support its use in man. It is a usual requirement to test the drug in at least two species of animals. In practice drugs are tested in many species of animals. It is often difficult to test the drug on an adequate model of the disease state which occurs in humans. Caution must be taken with the results of these studies as lack of toxic effects does not mean there is no risk in humans. Because of the ethical problems with conducting clinical trials on pregnant humans, animal studies may be the only information available on safety in pregnancy when the drug is licensed.

Clinical trials

Clinical trials are studies which are carried out in humans. There are a number of stages of clinical trials:

Phase I
- Typically carried out with 20–50 subjects
- Usually use healthy volunteers
- Establish a drug's pharmacology in humans, e.g. drug effects and suitable dosages

Phase II
- Typically carried out with 50–300 patients
- Confirm the drug's pharmacology in patients with the disease state rather than healthy volunteers
- Establish evidence of safety and dose range

Phase III
- Can involve 250–1000 plus patients
- These are formal therapeutic trials
- Efficacy and safety is established
- The drug being studied is compared with placebo and/or with other drugs

Post marketing studies

Post-marketing surveillance
- Data are gathered on adverse effects of the drug in clinical practice
- Long term safety data are sought
- Involves many more patients than during the clinical trials
- Often relies on passive reporting and is less formal than clinical trials

Phase IV clinical trials
- Further studies are often performed to investigate the drug's effects in other indications
- May also compare with drugs licensed for the same indication to establish if it is superior
- Conducted as formal clinical trials as with Phase III studies

Clinical trial conduct

This will be considered under the following headings:

(1) Aims of the trial
(2) Clinical trial design
(3) Subjects
(4) Analysis of data
(5) Ethical considerations

In practice these are all inter-related and need to be considered and/or specified before a trial begins.

Aims of the trial

The aims of the trial should be clearly defined. They will usually be in the form of a limited number of questions to be answered or hypotheses which are to be tested, e.g. is drug X effective in lowering blood pressure? Trials will usually be designed around these aims. Results or conclusions which were not part of the aims of the study should be interpreted with caution.

Clinical trial design

Good design is fundamental to the conduct of good research in any discipline and is especially so in clinical trials. Under this heading the method of conducting trials will be discussed. In reality the design of a trial will include selection of subjects, analysis and ethical considerations in addition to the methods.

Blindness. Both the researchers and patients are subject to bias. This is a fact of life. The researchers would not go to the trouble of organising a trial if they thought that it would not produce their hoped for result. The patient who knows that they are being administered placebo is not going to appear foolish by saying that it is helping their symptoms. Wherever possible trials should be double blind, that is neither the researcher nor the patient knows which drug is being administered. In some cases the drug has a distinct effect which impairs the ability to blind the study, e.g. drug A colours the urine red. If possible attempts should be made to maintain blindness. Double blind studies are more complex and expensive to organise than other studies.

In some cases single-blind studies can be acceptable. In a single-blind study either the researcher or the patient is blinded but not both. Single blind studies should rely on objective measurements of drug effects which are not subject to placebo or suggestive effects, e.g. measurement of full blood count in an unconscious patient in an intensive care unit. Wherever possible the researcher who interprets the results should be blinded to the treatment which has been administered.

Open trials are when neither the researcher nor the patient is blinded to the treatment(s).

Randomisation. Randomisation is another process that is aimed at reducing bias. It prevents the researcher selecting the patients for a particular treatment group and not another. Ideally randomisation should be carried out immediately before the treatment is commenced. There are a number of different randomisation processes varying in complexity. In practice the researcher entering a patient in a study will have to enter the patient on a code list. Each code will determine the treatment to be given, which remains blind until the code is broken. The treatments allocated to each code are selected randomly.

Use of placebos. Placebos are inactive treatments or 'dummies' which should match the active treatment in order to maintain blindness. The use of placebos is useful to distinguish between pharmacodynamic and psychological effects of treatment. They can also be used to distinguish between drug effects and fluctuations in the underlying disease. Placebos help greatly in the avoidance of making false conclusions. However, no matter how desirable placebo use may be from a study design point of view, it is not ethical to deprive patients of seriously effective treatment, e.g. in a trial of an antibiotic for the treatment of a serious infection. In this case it would be more appropriate and perhaps more useful to compare the drug with an accepted standard treatment for the condition.

Controlled trials. These are studies where two or more groups are compared. These can be either the active treatment versus placebo or drug A versus drug B if the use of placebo is inappropriate (see Fig. 6.4).

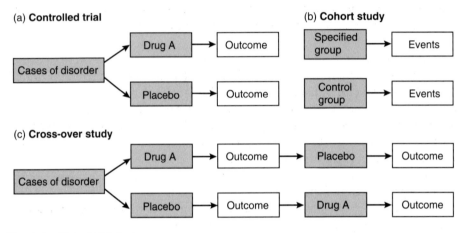

Fig. 6.4   Clinical trial design.

Cross-over studies:
• The patient is used as his/her own control
• May only be used in chronic stable disease
• Can only be used for palliative, symptom relieving treatment, not curative treatment
• A washout period is essential between treatments to avoid carry-over of effects from the previous drug
• The order of treatment may affect patients' perception of effects
• May be used in smaller numbers of patients than parallel group studies
• Prospective in design

Parallel Group Studies:
• Require more patients than cross-over studies
• The 'normal' way trials are conducted
• Fewer potential problems than with cross-over studies eg. washout between treatments
• Prospective in design

Observational studies such as cohort studies and case-control studies may be performed in the looser conditions of true clinical practice.

Cohort studies:
- The patients all have all same attribute, i.e. they are all on the same drug
- The patients and controls are then followed for a period of time and observed for events occurring, e.g. adverse effects of the drug
- Prospective in design
- Need large numbers of patients
- Take a long time to perform
- Selection of an appropriate matched control group is difficult
- An example would be a study following women who have taken the oral contraceptive pill for evidence of increased risk of breast cancer

Case control studies:
- A group of patients with the same disease is assembled along with a control group with similar characteristics
- Complete drug histories are taken from all participants
- The groups are then followed up retrospectively to determine the proportion in each group who have taken the suspect agent
- Need not be as large as cohort studies
- Take a relatively short time to conduct
- Retrospective in design
- An example would be a study of cases of abnormalities in pregnancy to determine if any particular drugs have been taken

Subjects

The selection of adequate numbers of appropriate patients to be entered into the study is second in importance only to the elimination of bias. Clinical trials must detail explicitly the inclusion and exclusion criteria for entering patients into the trial. In practice this means that patients taking part in clinical trials are highly selected and often have fewer problems or complicating factors than patients who are seen commonly in everyday practice. For example it is common for clinical trials to exclude children, elderly patients, patients with liver or renal impairment and patients with concomitant medical disorders. The groups within a clinical trial should be matched so that they have similar characteristics, e.g. age, sex, race, severity of disease. This is vital.

The number of patients entered into a trial must be adequate to allow any differences between the groups after treatment to be demonstrated. The size of a clinical trial:

- Depends on the difference the investigator regards as clinically important and the number of patients available

- Should follow the advice of a medical statistician and be specified before it is commenced
- Be adequate to prevent
  Type I error – finding a difference when none exists in reality
  Type II error – finding no difference when in reality the groups differ
- Should be calculated by determining the power required. See section on analysis of results.

The numbers of patients entered into a clinical trial can be fixed or variable.

Fixed sample trials:
- The number of patients to be treated is determined before the trial is commenced
- False differences such as type I or II errors are minimised as long as adequate numbers of patients are entered
- The end results, however, may be disappointing, especially if a non-significant difference between the groups was demonstrated. Entering more patients into the study may allow a significant difference to be shown. This would increase the risk of type II errors occurring

Variable number trials:
- The number of patients to be entered into the trial is not defined in advance
- This allows continuous or intermittent assessment of the results
- The trial will stop when a statistically significant result is reached or becomes unlikely
- It is essential for the trial to be stopped at a predetermined point otherwise false positive results may be generated. Sometimes there may be pressure to stop a trial early for non-scientific reasons such as publicity, marketing pressure, finance
- The advice of a medical statistician is essential to prevent type II errors

Analysis of data

It is common when following the debate and correspondence after the presentation or publication of a clinical trial for criticisms to be aired regarding the statistical analysis and validity of the results. Statistics is a highly specialised discipline and it would be foolish for a researcher to commence conducting a clinical trial without obtaining detailed advice from a statistician beforehand when designing the study. A number of statistical terms will be commonly seen when reviewing studies. Here is a brief explanation of some of these:

Statistical significance. This is a widely used term and is usually presented in the form of a probability or 'p' value. It is generally acknowledged that if there is less than a 1 in 20 chance ($p < 0.05$) of no difference existing between the groups there is probably a real difference between them. This is termed a statistically significant difference.

The null hypothesis. The null hypothesis is that there is no difference between the groups in a study. The statistical analysis then performed on the results is based on determining whether or not the null hypothesis is likely.

Confidence interval
- This is the range of values over which we have 95% certainty that the true value lies
- The confidence interval is the mean plus or minus two standard deviations
- A broad range indicates that there is uncertainty about the true value and that the study may have been too small
- A narrow range indicates that there is relative certainty about the true value
- If the confidence intervals for the results of two groups overlap they indicate that the study has failed to find a difference between the groups

Power. The power of a study is the probability of detecting a defined statistically significant difference, should a difference between the groups really exist. A power of 80–90% is regarded as being an appropriate range. Calculation of power enables the study designer to calculate the number of subjects required to be entered into the study to achieve a target result.

Withdrawals. The statistical handling of data from withdrawn patients should be clearly defined when designing a clinical trial. Most clinical trials should be analysed on an intention to treat basis. Bias can arise if one of the treatments causes an increased number of withdrawals from a study and these patients are not included in the analysis. Because the 'intention to treat' approach tends to decrease the size of the differences between groups, the sample size may need to be increased.

End-points in clinical trials. It is important for the clinician to look for the end-point in a clinical trial. Equally it is crucial that the researcher designing a clinical trial defines a suitable end-point. End-points can be defined that are of varying usefulness. It should always be questioned whether the result is clinically significant even when it may be statistically significant. End-points may be either:

(1) The therapeutic effect itself, e.g. sleep, cure of infection, reduced mortality
(2) A factor related to the therapeutic effect or a surrogate effect, e.g. reduction in blood lipids or blood pressure. We presume that by reducing raised lipids that we will reduce mortality from coronary heart disease.

Ethical considerations

Consent. All potential research subjects have the right to choose for themselves whether or not they will participate in research. They should be given all the information and explanation necessary to make informed consent. An adult patient may validly consent to participate in a clinical trial if they are competent to understand what will be undertaken. The legal position is unclear regarding patients who cannot give consent for some reason, e.g. they are unconscious or are incompetent.

Research and ethics committees

These committees are set up to scrutinise clinical research proposals and to advise on whether or not they consider them to be ethical. Research on patients within the NHS in the UK is denied without the prior approval of each local research and ethics committee where the trial will be conducted. These committees are usually made up of doctors, nurses, pharmacists and lay members of the public. Their principal responsibility is to ensure that that each patient entered into a clinical trial should be no worse off than if they had been in the hands of a reasonable and competent physician. The issues of informed consent and patient safety are the principal factors addressed. The *Declaration of Helsinki* gives formal recommendations regarding research on humans which are applied by research and ethics committees (World Medical Association, 1964).

Clinical audit

Clinical audit is the comparison of current clinical practice with known standards. It should be carried out with a view to modifying that practice, if necessary, to ensure that the desired standard of care is achieved. Clinical audit is a systematic and cyclical process (Fig. 6.5).

Usually clinical audit looks at the processes used for diagnosis, care and treatment of patients. It should examine how associated resources are used and investigate the effect care has on the outcome and quality of life for patients. It must be emphasised strongly that re-audit or closing of the audit loop is vital for successful audit once an initial audit and change of practice has taken place.

In its methods, clinical audit is similar to clinical research. Lack of adequate care when planning the audit will cause meaningless results to be produced. Research, however, breaks new ground by seeking the answers to questions such as 'what is the best way' or 'does this work'. Research helps to set the standards which can then be used in clinical audit.

Formal review is the review of all cases to show what is happening at a given point in time. It can be used to help to set standards or can be turned into an audit. If it aims to compare practice to set standards then it would become

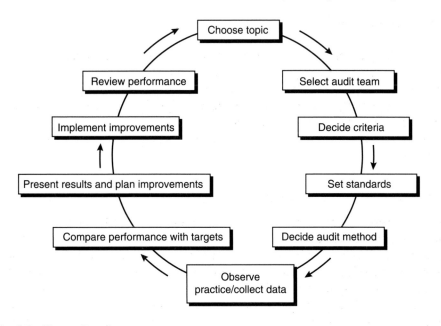

Fig. 6.5 The audit cycle.

audit. Informal review is a snapshot of a small number of cases. Informal review may be helpful to indicate whether or not a formal review or audit is necessary.

Successful clinical audit is usually:

- Multi-professional
- Patient focused
- A method of developing a culture of continuing education and improvement of clinical effectiveness

Advantages of clinical audit

- Encourages formal review of practice
- Establishes and records what is actually done as opposed to what it is thought is done
- May show areas which have been ignored or omitted but which need attention
- Establishes and clarifies standards
- The comparison with standards is implicit in the clinical audit cycle
- The standards used should be quantifiable and explicit for successful audit to be performed
- Standards which are used should ideally be evidence-based
- Ultimately standards of practice will be raised

Disadvantages of clinical audit

- It can be very time consuming
- It can be expensive in both manpower time and equipment to gather data and analyse results
- Staff may view it as just another management tool which takes up valuable practice time

Summary

This chapter provides an insight into the complexity of the prescribing process. It is unfortunately easy, because of this complexity, to lose sight of the prime aim of all prescribing; that is, to cure, or to relieve the symptoms of disease if cure is not possible, in each patient under a prescriber's care. The focus of all prescribing must be on the patient as an individual. What is correct generally for patients with a specific disease may not be appropriate in some individuals.

The prescriber must keep up to date with new developments and be receptive to new evidence or debate. There is much temptation to prescribe new drugs or to modify practice following promotional activity. To balance the sometimes overly positive and enthusiastic claims made by drug companies about their products the prescriber should adopt a sceptical approach. Why should they change their practice from that which is established, has been proved to work and has a proven safety record? The skills of critical analysis of clinical trials and evidence-based medicine will help the prescriber to reach informed, objective and rational decisions on which drugs should be prescribed. The clinical audit process can then reinforce this by highlighting areas of practice where improvements can be made to benefit patients further.

It is strongly recommended that the reader makes use of the references and further reading section to broaden their knowledge of the skills used in prescribing.

References

Altman, D.G. (1994) The scandal of poor medical research. *Br. Med. J.* **308**, 2283–4.

Association of the British Pharmaceutical Industry (1996) *ABPI Annual Review*. ABPI, London.

Barber, N. (1995) What constitutes good prescribing? *Br. Med. J.* **310**, 923–5.

Committee on Safety of Medicines (1997a) Terfenadine: now only available on prescription. *Curr. Prob. Pharmacovigilance* **23**, 9.

Committee on Safety of Medicines (1997b) Terfenadine: information for doctors and pharmacists. *Letter to Doctors and Pharmacists*, April.

Dillner, L. (1996) Pill scare linked to rise in abortions. *Br. Med. J.* **312**, 996.

Guillebaud, J. (1995) Advising women on which pill to take. *Br. Med. J.* **311**, 1111–2.

Guyatt, G.H., Sackett, D.L. & Cook, D.J. (1994) User's guides to the medical literature: How to use an article about therapy or prevention II. *J. Am. Med. Assoc.* **271**, 59–63.

Guyatt, G.H., Sackett, D.L. & Cook, D.J. (1993) User's guides to the medical literature: How to use an article about therapy or prevention I. *J. Am. Med. Assoc.* **270**, 2598–2601.

MacRae, K. & Kay, C. (1995) Third generation oral contraceptive pills. BMJ, 311, 1112.

Rosenberg W. & Donald A. (1995) Evidence based medicine: an approach to clinical problem-solving. *Br. Med. J.* **311**, 1112.

World Medical Association (1964) The declaration of Helsinki. The World Medical Association Inc, (Amended 1975, 1983, 1989).

Further reading

Asscher, A.W., Parr, G.D. & Whitmarsh, V.B. (1995) Towards the safer use of medicines. *Br. Med. J.* **311**, 1003–6.

Consumers' Association (1983) Getting good value from drug reps. *Drug Ther. Bull.* **21**, 13–5.

Consumers' Association (1991) Helping patients to make the best use of medicines. *Drug Ther. Bull.* **33**, 1–2.

Consumers' Association (1995) Risk:benefit analysis of drugs in practice. The doctor, the patient and the Licensing Authority. *Drug Ther. Bull.* **33**, 33–5.

Fowkes, F.G.R. & Fulton, P.M. (1991) Critical appraisal of published research: introductory guidelines. *Br. Med. J.* **302**, 1136–40.

Grahame-Smith, D.G. & Aronson, J.K. (1992) *Oxford Textbook of Clinical Pharmacology and Drug Therapy*, 2nd edn, Oxford University Press, Oxford.

Grisso, J.A. (1993) Making comparisons. *Lancet* **342**, 157–60.

Horton, R. (ed) (1997) Good manners for the pharmaceutical industry. *Lancet* **349**, 1635.

Kayne, S. (1996) The legal and ethical protection accorded to persons participating as subjects in clinical trials. *Pharm. J.* **256**, 425–7.

Laurence, D.R. & Bennett, P.N. (1992) *Clinical Pharmacology*, 7th edn. Churchill Livingstone, London.

McInnes, G.T. & Murray, G.D. (1992) Clinical trials. *Med. Int.* **101**, 4216–20.

McNamee, D. (1994) Stopping trials early. *Lancet* **344**, 327.

Medicines Resource Centre (1995a) An introduction to assessing medical literature. *MeReC Briefing* **9**, 1–8.

Medicines Resource Centre (1995b) Evidence based medicine. *MeReC Bulletin* **6**, 45–8.

Sackett, D.L., Rosenberg, W.M.C., Gray, J.A.M., Haynes, R.B. & Richardson, W.S. (1996) Evidence based medicine: what it is and what it isn't. *Br. Med. J.* **312**, 71–2.

Shenton, D. (ed) (1991) Symposium: drug development and clinical trials. *Prescr. J.* **31**, 219–57.

Wiffen, P.J. (1995) Clinical trials: a guide to the licensing system. *Hosp. Pharm.* **2**, 15–21.

Chapter 7
Non-prescription Medicines

Ross Lynton Groves

Historical Perspective

Medicines have been freely available to the general public for several centuries. Some of our most potent drugs are derived from plants, which can grow wild, and folklore was the original 'evidence base' for the use of such remedies. In Britain, itinerant vendors of potions for every ill could be seen at mediaeval village fairs or the castles of the wealthy, promoting their wares. Not all of the 'cures' sold were effective. Indeed, some were potentially fatal. Little has changed!

As commerce and trade developed as a vital part of our social structure, heavily populated areas began to see the need for specialism in the provision of materials. This included medicaments. Apothecaries became commonplace and, later, barbers and druggists continued the trade. By the mid-nineteenth century, 'Chemists and Druggists' were to be seen in most retail environments.

There was a mystery surrounding the treatments available from these outlets. The pharmaceutical chemist would compound preparations either on the prescription of a doctor or to his own formula. Tinctures, mixtures, pills and powders were originally prepared 'on site' in the dispensary. The basic ingredients were, however, coming under much closer scrutiny than previously. It had been found that the actions of many traditional remedies were due, not to the raw material as a whole, be it plant or otherwise, but to a single ingredient. The advances in chemistry had made it possible to isolate and purify many such chemicals.

Attempts to classify and standardise medicinal compounds had been made over the years. Ancient Chinese writings contain references to the healing properties of various plants. Monasteries were the original seats of learning and writing in Europe from the beginning of this millennium, and the monks produced booklets about the herbs that they grew to be used to heal the sick.

Such *'Materia Medica'* became the *British National Formulary (BNF)* of their era. As knowledge became more detailed and subject to more rigorous scrutiny, reference texts which detailed the appearance, properties and uses of compounds became commonplace. The *British Pharmacopoeia* (*BP*) and *British Pharmaceutical Codex* (*BPC*) were much used and updated as new compounds were discovered and new information became available. We would think that the gap of 13 years between the 1885 and 1898 editions of the BP was overlong, but the rate of change in recent times has made revision of reference texts a continuous process.

It is interesting to note that some issues that concern us about the sale of drugs had been documented 100 years ago. White's *Materia Medica* of 1898 includes a monograph on the dried leaves of *Nicotiana tabacum*, the tobacco plant (White, 1898a). It notes that nicotine is one of the most powerful and rapid poisons known, that it is never used therapeutically and that smoking may produce 'catarrh of the pharynx' 'even in those who are used to it'. The monograph on hops (White, 1898b) notes that 'many people find the soporific influence of beer very well marked'! Both nicotine and alcohol are on sale to the public today and, although restricted by law to some degree, are not treated as drugs. Their detrimental effects, both to individuals and society as a whole, seem to be tolerated by successive governments because of their tax raising potential.

Legal classification and ethical issues

Before discussing the actual preparations available for over the counter (OTC) sale in detail, there are a number of factors that warrant consideration. Exactly what is it that determines the level of access that the general public has to a particular medicine? Having thought about that issue, do individuals then have an absolute right to purchase an OTC medicine whenever they want to? Should health care professionals have a role in advising people on the suitability or otherwise of a particular treatment that has been advertised in the media?

Legal status

The legal classification of a product determines whether or not it can be sold in the first place (see Table 7.1). It is important to remember that movement between the legal categories is possible. Amendments to classification occur frequently enough to mean that the current status of a product should be confirmed before giving information about its availability to a patient.

Drugs are divided into three main categories as regards the public's access to them. Drugs or products in the first of these are termed prescription only medicines or POM. As the name implies, they can only be supplied on the receipt of a prescription written correctly, by an appropriately qualified individual. This is usually because it is considered that the effects of a preparation could be detrimental to health unless the supply is carefully monitored. Doctors, dentists, opticians and nurses are all allowed to prescribe certain

Table 7.1 Legal classification of medicines.

Classification	Restrictions to availability
Prescription only medicines (POM) includes controlled drugs (CDs)	Must be prescribed by an appropriate practitioner. If a CD the prescription must be written correctly before dispensing can take place
Pharmacy only (P)	Can only be sold from registered pharmacy premises under the supervision of a pharmacist
General Sale List (GSL)	None

categories of drugs or appliances. Prescriptions may be either under the auspices of the National Health Service (NHS) or given privately. For NHS prescriptions, a charge is made for each item, unless the patient falls within one of the categories for exemption. Patients pay the actual retail cost of drugs prescribed on private prescriptions.

The second category is termed pharmacy only: the symbol P is used for items that fall into this class. Sales of such products may be made from registered pharmacy premises under the supervision of a registered pharmacist. They are, therefore, OTC preparations. The basis of this classification is not uniform. In some instances, the amount of a particular substance in a product determines the category. In others, the pack size is the determining factor.

We are all familiar with the availability of medicinal products from retail outlets other then pharmacies. This is possible because the third classification of medicines is the General Sale List (GSL). The strength of a drug or the quantity in a particular pack are, again, two of the determinant factors. Some preparations are thought to be so innocuous as to come within this category. Again, some of these products may be prescribed, thus complicating the public perception of the legal categories.

It should be recognised that there are national variations in availability of medicines. The UK system is by no means universally recognised. The increase in foreign travel has meant that patients often request a product that they have purchased abroad. Frequently, there are equivalents available but some will only be available on prescription in Britain, as many countries have a less restrictive approach to drugs. The community or hospital pharmacist is a useful reference source in such instances. They will be able to identify possible alternative products and advise as to the legal status in this country.

Ethical dilemmas

Whatever their legal classification, all drugs have adverse effects on the body as well as their beneficial ones. Using a drug in the treatment of an illness or condition means the balancing of the positive effects it will have on the patient with the negative ones. Ideally, the positives should outweigh the negatives by some margin so that the patient feels better without suffering any side effects. Unfortunately, we live in the real world and such drugs are rare. The sufferer will still, however, expect an instant cure with little or no additional discomfort.

For many years, the prevailing public perception of products available for sale has appeared to be that they are all safe for anyone to take at any time. The fact that many products are advertised reinforces the perception of safety. If a product appears on television or in a magazine, it is felt that the statements made about it must be true and applicable to everyone. Of course, advertising is carefully regulated and no reputable manufacturer would use incorrect information in the promotion of one of its products. The problem remains that some people who see the advert think that the preparation will be suitable for them, whatever their medical condition or state of health.

Misconceptions about medicines are often due to a lack of knowledge about the subject. Adverts can be considered a form of education but, by their very nature, they can provide only a fraction of the information available about their topic. It would be unreasonable to expect that a 30 second slot on television or a page in a glossy magazine, designed to be eye-catching and imprint a product name and image in the mind of the target audience, should provide minute details about a product. Who, then, should provide information and advice on medicines to the public? Indeed, does the public want or need to be educated further when purchasing medicines?

The majority of medicines, both in hospitals and in the community, are obtained from a pharmacy. It is mainly in the community that OTC products are stocked in addition to the prescription items. Pharmacists have a legal and ethical duty to oversee medicine sales as well as supervising the dispensing process. Personal handling of every medicine enquiry is, therefore, impossible but they are well placed to answer any queries that people may have when purchasing medication. The products for sale are becoming increasingly potent and so, in recent years, the pharmaceutical profession has introduced protocols, to ensure that all prospective purchasers are subjected to a screening process.

Pharmacy staff are now trained to ask appropriate questions when requests for products are made. The format is not rigid but the intention is to standardise the procedures, as much as possible, throughout the country. One method of questioning in common use is the '2 WHAM' system:

W   Who is the medicine for?
W   What are the symptoms for which the purchase is being made?
H   How long have the symptoms persisted?
A   Action taken so far? (Any medicines tried?)
M   Medicines taken for other conditions? Allergies/difficulties experienced
          with any drugs?

If the answer to any of the questions does not fall within defined parameters, the pharmacist will become personally involved, if they have not already intervened. Further questioning will then take place and an appropriate course of action suggested. Sometimes this means that the product requested is sold but appropriate advice is also given. More frequently, reasons will be given as to why the medicine requested is unsuitable and an alternative offered if one is available. Sometimes no sale is made but advice is given and the patient may also be referred to their GP or the local hospital emergency department.

Many people now appreciate the time taken to ensure that they get the best product for their particular problem. Some individuals, however, become irritated and even abusive when asked questions regarding their purchase. There are several reasons why we too might feel aggrieved in a similar situation. Our society prides itself on the freedom of the individual and professes to encourage individual responsibility. These factors could be seen to give someone the right to purchase a product merely because it is available for sale. Self medication has always been common in this country, but few people consider whether or not it is sensible to self medicate when they are already receiving treatment for illnesses or conditions from a doctor.

Few people welcome intrusions into their personal affairs, and questions about their health can be regarded as private. They may not wish to see a doctor and, indeed, any adult has a legal right to refuse or not to seek medical treatment in the majority of cases. They do not perceive that the pharmacist has a professional responsibility to elicit relevant information to ensure that a medicine is used appropriately, and expect that a sale be made without delay. The expectation of a cure for every ill without adverse effects is common. Only by raising awareness of the possible dangers of medicines will the efforts made to protect the public from harm be appreciated fully.

The role of any health care professional as a dispenser of good advice on matters of health is only now developing. We have all been seen as providers of services on request and not as gatekeepers of the public health. Education regarding our health promotion roles is necessary if our advice is to be taken seriously. Communication between the professions is also of great importance. We must all give consistent messages so that patients do not become confused and distrustful of conflicting advice.

Disadvantages of OTC medicines

- Many commonly used OTC products are potentially lethal if added to an individual's current prescription medication, and legal status gives no indication of the potential for danger
- Overdosage may be a problem due to lack of knowledge about the ingredients of a preparation
- Inappropriate use of an OTC medicine may mask symptoms of a more serious problem

• A number of products that are available for sale have a potential for misuse

The problems with overdosage and interactions are related to the pharmacology of the drugs involved. Examples will be given in the following section that discusses some common drugs found in OTC products. The problem of inappropriate use and abuse are difficult to deal with as they often involve social and economic factors that complicate the issues involved. They merit mention here whilst law and ethics are fresh in our minds.

OTC drug abuse

As with any other type of drug misuse, OTC problems fall into two categories. These are intentional and unintentional misuse. Given the availability of medicines and the anomalies in the law controlling them, little can be done about those who intentionally misuse OTCs. Most will find an outlet from which to obtain supplies, legally or otherwise, and will probably vary their purchasing pattern to allay suspicion. There are those, however, who appear not to realise that regular purchases of certain products attract attention. They may use the same pharmacy on several occasions until a sale is refused, then move on to other premises until the pattern is repeated.

The protocols used when dealing with requests for OTC products work extremely well when the potential customer is open and honest in their replies. The system is, however, open to abuse. Someone determined to obtain a particular product can answer dishonestly once they are familiar with the responses necessary to prevent the refusal of a sale. The possible scenarios range from the relatively innocent to the downright deceitful. An asthmatic wishing to purchase ibuprofen, who has not got the time to explain that they are one of the 25% of sufferers who do not suffer a worsening of their symptoms when taking the drug, may omit to mention their condition. An anorexic may swear that the laxative they are purchasing is for a grandparent, who needs it to counteract the constipatory effects of an analgesic. Both instances mean that the pharmacist is unable to advise the purchaser accurately due to the erroneous information given.

The product groups which are abused vary from pharmacy to pharmacy, but there is a hard core of preparations which would be recognised as posing problems. Repeated requests for these products would arouse suspicion in most pharmacies, and the pharmacist may well handle all such requests personally. The ingredients which cause most concern include opioid derivatives, caffeine and other stimulants, laxatives and sedatives. Less obvious candidates for abuse are hyoscine, the volatile oils and rubs used for congestion, citric and ascorbic acid and unmarked tablets which can be passed off as Ecstasy. An increase in sales in any manner of products may indicate that the local population has discovered an alternative use for them!

Abuse does not necessarily involve ingesting the products involved. Drug injectors use citric acid to increase the solubility of the powdered substances that they use. Rubs and oils are used in an attempt to improve the 'high' or 'buzz' from other substances by evaporating on the skin and increasing the peripheral blood flow. Solvents are sniffed to give the 'high'. Most products are, however, taken or injected to produce the desired effect.

Drugs such as codeine have similar effects to those of their more potent opioid relatives, morphine and heroin. They do, however, have to be taken in large quantities because of the limited strength of OTC preparations. Combination analgesics are common and it has been known for attempts to be made to filter the codeine from such products for the purposes of injection. If the other ingredient is aspirin, the resultant powder will be poisonous as up to 70% of the aspirin will remain.

OTC preparations may be abused for many reasons. If an illegal substance of misuse is in short supply, OTC products may be used as temporary alternatives. Not all misusers are addicted to the so-called 'hard' drugs. Some people have discovered that they find relief from their mundane routine when taking a particular product. The effects may decrease tension or produce a pleasant, detached feeling as with the opioids and certain sedatives, or they may produce excitement, as in the case of the stimulants. Hallucinations may be a release from the stresses and strains of modern living, and drugs such as hyoscine and cyclizine can give the desired effect.

Social and economic factors have been cited as causes of drug misuse of all types. Deprivation may be the largest contributory factor, but misuse can occur in all social and economic classes. The motivation behind the misuse does not alter the fact that intentional misusers are unwilling to listen to advice on the subject and to accept that they may be causing themselves harm. In some cases, more afluent and articulate individuals are less amenable to questioning and information than their less well off neighbours. This factor will affect the input of all health care professionals to this problem. In the nursing sphere, OTC misuse may come to light by the discovery of large quantities of OTC medication in a patient's home or on admission to hospital. Determining the extent of the misuse is as difficult under those conditions as in a community pharmacy.

Unintentional drug misuse is also very common. It may be easier to tackle than intentional misuse, but there has to be a unified approach to the subject by all members of the health care professions. A major factor in such misuse is a lack of understanding, either of the medical condition that the OTC product is being used to treat, or of the mode of action or dosage regimen of the drug itself. To overcome this effectively, information provided to patients must be reasonably standardised and consistent, not contradictory.

The misconceptions which lead to the misuse of prescription medicines also apply to OTC products. 'If one does me good then two will be even better!' seems to be a common thought process. This can, of course, lead to overdosage with potentially serious consequences. Analgesics containing paracetamol are particularly implicated in such cases. Lack of information about the condition being treated may be reinforced by folklore. Many older people believe that it is necessary and desirable to produce one bowel movement each day. Unintentional laxative misuse may result. Names of products do not give an indication of the substances that they contain. Again, overdosage may result. Cold remedies and analgesics are the main culprits in this case.

All of the above can be rectified, if the individual concerned is receptive, by providing accurate information, both written and verbal, on a regular basis. Some people see the error of their ways immediately, and are grateful for the intervention and advice. Others may take time to be convinced of the correct way in which to take a product or the information regarding their condition. Much patience is required at times!

The ethical problems still remain for us as health care professionals. How much right do we have to interfere with another persons' way of life, even if it is obvious to us that their actions may be incorrect and not in their best interests. We are in danger of judging outcomes by our own standards and criteria, and have to constantly balance our duty of care towards an individual's physical health with the possible negative effects on their mental and emotional state which our intervention may cause. This can be as simple as destroying their belief in a remedy that was having a placebo effect which nothing else can replace. The effects are twofold. Self worth is diminished because they are shown to have an erroneous belief, and stress will increase due to the removal of the beneficial effect, psychological though it may have been.

Reference is made to the possible misuse potential of OTC ingredients in the section dealing with the common preparations. This is not intended to be exhaustive, but gives some idea of the products involved.

Inappropriate OTC use

Inappropriate use of OTC medication is linked to unintentional misuse. It occurs when a product is apparently being used correctly but is, in fact, masking symptoms which may indicate a more serious condition than that which it is being used to treat. Several of the products which have been deregulated from POM to P may require particular care on the part of the pharmacist to pick up any untoward events. Education of consumers is of paramount importance so that they understand the need to consult their GP if symptoms are not relieved or recur.

One of the most common symptoms to present is that of upper abdominal or chest pain. This is usually associated with a request for an antacid, and it has been common practice for several years to question the individual carefully to ensure that angina or heart failure was not the cause. The advent of OTC H_2 antagonists has complicated this issue. Now, gastric disease, including gastric cancer, has to be excluded, as well as any cardiovascular problem.

Vaginal thrush can now be treated using OTC preparations containing imidazoles. This is a great benefit for many women who no longer need to visit their doctor every time they require such a product. It is, however, necessary to refer those who suffer repeatedly to ensure that systemic infection is absent. Understandably, the potential inconvenience of a surgery visit is not always greeted with enthusiasm.

Few cough mixtures are now available on prescription. The value of many products is theoretically questionable due to the combination of ingredients present. Some seem to counteract themselves by including both a cough suppressant and an expectorant. The increased number of requests for OTC relief compounds the problem. After their limitations have been explained, the correct product for the type of cough in question must be determined if a customer insists on a purchase. Trying to explain that coughing is a necessary function can prove difficult, and dissuading the purchase of a suppressant when catarrh is present is another delicate communication skill.

Some of our best efforts are negated due to the availability of GSL medication. Unless sold on registered pharmacy premises, no advice is available for these medicines. They include antacids, cold remedies and analgesics, all of which can be misused or used inappropriately.

Overview of OTC preparations

For ease of reference, this section classifies the ingredients of OTC products into broad therapeutic groups and uses a tabular format to present most of the information. As time passes, the proprietary names of products may change and new compounds will be added to our repertoire. The drugs within them will, however, remain the same with the obvious exception of newly discovered preparations. Crystal ball gazing is uncertain, so only drugs in common use at the time of writing are included.

The basic information given for each drug is:

- Legal status
- Uses
- Side effects
- Overdose
- Common interactions/contra-indications
- Potential for misuse

Any additional information is in the form of text after the table for each therapeutic class.

Analgesics

These drugs account for a large proportion of OTC sales and are present in widely varying doses and combinations in many products. The only sure way to establish the constituents of a product is to read the label. This is difficult at times due to the small print used and may be impossible for those with poor eyesight or who are illiterate. The use of brand names does not always help to identify the actual drug being taken. The potential for duplicate dosing is obvious and is most serious in the case of paracetamol. The characteristics of some analgesics are shown in Table 7.2.

Paracetamol poisoning

Paracetamol is, potentially, the most dangerous of the OTC analgesics due to its narrow therapeutic index. The therapeutic index is the difference between a safe, effective dose and an overdose. The figures quoted vary from paper to paper but the following gives an indication of the number of tablets that may cause harm.

- Normal adult dosage   **Max** of 8 tablets per day (2 per dose)
- Lowest reported toxic dose   10 tablets in 24 hours
- Lowest fatal dose   20–30 tablets as a single dose
                8–10 per day on a long term basis

Anyone suspected of taking an overdose should be hospitalised without delay. The symptoms of overdose are not always immediately evident. Nausea and vomiting may be the only initial symptoms, whatever the dose, and will subside within 24 hours. Hepatic damage begins after 12 hours and is maximal after 3–4 days. Sub-costal pain is an indicator of hepatocellular necrosis. Renal tubule necrosis is a rare complication of paracetamol poisoning but has potentially fatal implications in itself. Metabolic acidosis and cardiac arrhythmias may or may not be present.

Metabolism of paracetamol occurs in the liver and kidneys. Mixed function oxidase enzymes convert a small proportion to *n*-acetyl-*p*-benzoquinoneimine (NABQI). This is a highly reactive compound but is usually detoxified by conjugation with glutathione. It is excreted as mercapturate and cysteine conjugates. Following an overdose, tissue stores of glutathione become depleted and the accumulation of NABQI causes cellular damage. This may result in thrombocytopaenia, variceal haemorrhage, encephalopathy, hypoglycaemia, cerebral oedema and, after an interval of about 2 weeks, death.

It is perhaps surprising to realise that chronic overdose (intentional misuse) may occur when an individual wishes to experience the 'purging' effects of the drug. This can lead to T cell defects. In Africa, cases of women using toxic doses of paracetamol as an abortifacient have been reported. Such scenarios, when considered in the context of the metabolic dangers, indicate the need for education in relation to the unwanted effects of commonly used medicines.

Treatment of paracetamol overdose

The effectiveness of treatment is largely dependent on the dose taken and the time lapsed after ingestion. Accident and Emergency departments follow their own protocols for most procedures, but a rough guide to the time-scales used in

Table 7.2 Characteristics of analgesics.

	Aspirin	Ibuprofen	Codeine	Paracetamol
Legal status	GSL for ⩽30 P for >30 Non-effervescent preparations GSL for ⩽16 P for 17–32 POM for >32	GSL for 200mg if ⩽12 (POM >12) P for some controlled release preps. P for some topical preps	POM usually but P in low dose (possibly in combination with other drugs or in liquid form)	GSL for ⩽30 P for >30 Non-effervescent preparations GSL for ⩽16 P for 17–32 POM for >32
Uses	Analgesic Antipyretic Anti-inflammatory Anticoagulant	Analgesic Antipyretic Anti-inflammatory	Analgesic Cough suppressant Anti-diarrhoeal	Analgesic Antipyretic (mild)
Side effects	Gastric irritation Nausea Dyspepsia Gastric bleeding Reyes syndrome	Gastric irritation Nausea Dyspepsia Gastric bleeding Allergic reaction	Constipation Drowsiness Nausea	Rashes Blood disorders Acute pancreatitis
Overdose	**Mild** Tinnitus Perspiration Vasodilation **Severe** Hyperventilation Deafness Coma Cardiovascular insufficiency Respiratory failure Death	Nausea Vomiting Gastric pain Vertigo Sleeplessness Ataxia Coma	Depression of autonomic functions Death	Nausea Vomiting Hepatic necrosis Sub-costal pain Renal tubule necrosis Metabolic acidosis Cardiac arrhythmias Death
Interactions	Warfarin Methotrexate NSAIDs	Baclofen NSAIDs	Other opioids	Metoclopramide Warfarin Cholestyramine
Contra-indications	Under 12s Pregnancy Peptic ulcer Asthma Haemorrhagic disease	Pregnancy Peptic ulcers Asthma Haemorrhagic disease	Pregnancy Under 12s Respiratory failure Hepatic failure	Hepatic damage Renal damage Alcoholism
Potential for misuse	Low	Low	High	Moderate

dealing with paracetamol overdose can be drawn up. If the time after ingestion is 0–4 hours, gastric emptying is employed. If it is 0–12 hours, methionine is given. Acetylcysteine can be used from 0 to 24 hours after ingestion.

The rationale behind the treatments is fairly straightforward, although treatment during pregnancy presents particular difficulties. A stomach pump or induced emesis will prevent the absorption of much of the dose taken. Methionine is used to conjugate with the toxic products of impaired metabolism, and acetylcysteine will assist the excretion process. Should these strategies be ineffective, liver transplantation may be the only option. This is an extreme solution, both in terms of trauma to the patient and cost to the health service. Serious thought and effort must be focused on the prevention of the problem.

Causative factors of overdose

There are four factors that can cause overdose: accidental, suicide, alcoholism and drug therapy. Accidental causes result from any products containing paracetamol, and this is not always obvious. Examples include 'co'-products. Suicide may be a 'cry for help' which can end tragically. Alcoholism and any condition which involves reduced liver function will render the individual susceptible to paracetamol overdose. With drug therapy, enzyme inducing drugs will increase the risk of poisoning with paracetamol.

Targeting the first two factors could, potentially, reduce the incidence of paracetamol poisoning quite markedly. Education about the drugs contained in OTC products means that patients are less likely to overdose. Advice from pharmacists, nurses and doctors about the ingredients in prescription medicines is also essential if the patient's health is to be safeguarded. This encompasses mentioning that a preparation contains paracetamol and not to take additional doses from other sources, and making patients aware of potential interactions between their medication and paracetamol.

Analgesic/antipyretic use in children

Paracetamol is an effective analgesic but has only mild antipyretic activity when compared to aspirin. After the link between Reyes syndrome and aspirin led to the removal of paediatric aspirin preparations from sale, paracetamol became the only OTC product licensed for children under 12 years of age. It is, therefore, used in childhood pyrexia. An ibuprofen product is now available, giving parents a choice of drug for their feverish offspring. It will, however, take time to convince the public of the benefits of the new preparation.

Several studies have suggested that the value of paracetamol is doubtful in reducing fever and associated symptoms. References which support this view include Kramer *et al.* (1991), who showed that there was no difference between the mean duration of subsequent fever after administration of paracetamol or placebo and Doran *et al.* (1989), who found that overall symptoms in chick-

enpox worsened after paracetamol administration and time to complete scab-
bing increased. The Joint Working Group of the Research Unit of the Royal
College of Physicians & the British Paediatric Association (1991) reported that
no-one in the group had evidence that paracetamol influenced recurrence of
febrile convulsions.

Despite the availability of evidence, tradition dies hard. Paracetamol does
reduce temperature to some degree and so will continue to be used as an
antipyretic for many years to come.

Antacids

This class of compounds again accounts for a large proportion of OTC sales.
Brand loyalty is high and this leads to patients taking long established and well
advertised products, even if they are not producing the desired effect. Suggesting that a change be made to an alternative product may be met with
resistance. Antacid characteristics are shown in Table 7.3.

Combination products may eliminate the side effects by cancelling each
other out. Aluminium with magnesium is somewhat longer acting and has less
effect on the bowel than the various compounds alone. The side effects are less
important with this combination. Sodium and calcium compounds are being
superseded by more effective preparations.

Table 7.3 Characteristics of antacids.

	Aluminium salts	Magnesium salts	Sodium salts	Calcium salts
Legal Status	GSL	GSL or P depending on strength and combination	GSL or P depending on strength and combination	GSL or P depending on strength and combination
Uses	Antacid	Antacid Laxative	Antacid	Antacid
Side effects	Constipation Nausea Vomiting	Diarrhoea	Stomach pain Alkalosis	Constipation Acid rebound Renal damage
Overdose			Heart failure	
Interactions		Iron	Lithium	
Contra-indications	Hypophosphataemia	Hypophosphataemia	Hypertension	
Potential for misuse	Low	High	Moderate	Moderate

Despite their status as GSL medicines, products containing magnesium are purchased for use by misusers. Anorexics and bulimics use the laxative effect to their advantage, or so they think. Intense or long term use in the doses necessary will cause damage to the bowel.

H_2 antagonists and other deregulated gastro-intestinal remedies

Several of the H_2 antagonists available on prescription are now licensed for OTC sale. It is important to remember that the doses involved are, approximately, only a quarter of the maintenance dose for alleviation of peptic ulcer disease. Patients often attempt to buy the products, the names of which are the same as their POM counterparts, believing that they are identical to the medication prescribed by their doctors. This presents the pharmacist with several difficulties, not the least that of convincing the individual of the differences involved. The licensed indications are also different. A patient who asks for the product by name, stating that it is for long term treatment of a recurring ulcer, cannot be sold the preparation, however much they may wish to avoid a trip to their doctor. Much ill feeling may be caused, but the refusal is both clinically and legally correct. The products may be appropriate for patients with severe heartburn or indigestion as they prevent acid production, but long term use may mask more serious conditions. The costs involved may be some deterrent to those with limited incomes. Various preparations are depicted in Table 7.4.

The second class of medicines in this field is those to treat irritable bowel syndrome (IBS). This time, a previous diagnosis of the condition is necessary before a sale can be made. It is impossible to diagnose IBS 'over the counter'. The doses are almost all identical to those in the POM parent. Small pack sizes mean that the patient is unlikely to use the OTC purchase as an alternative to visiting a GP for prescriptions on a long term basis.

Alginates, antiflatulents and antispasmodics

These compounds are generally used in combination with antacids, although a number of single ingredient preparations are now on the market.

Alginates are inert compounds that float on the surface of the stomach contents and prevent damage to the oesophagus by preventing acid reflux. Antiflatulents such as dimethicone are surfactants that break down the bubbles of gas within the stomach, thus reducing the pressure and discomfort. A particularly useful innovation has been the advent of effective products for infant colic. Both types of compound are relatively innocuous, and vigilance is only necessary insofar as the masking of more serious conditions is concerned.

Antispasmodics, such as hyoscine and dicyclomine (dicycloverine) , reduce spasm in smooth muscle. Their main OTC use is to reduce pain in gastro-intestinal disturbance, although hyoscine is also used for dysmenorrhoea. They are classified as P medicines due to their side effect profile. Drowsiness and

Table 7.4 Characteristics of various gastro-intestinal remedies.

	Cimetidine/ranitidine/famotidine	Hyoscine/peppermint oil/alverine/mebeverine
Legal status	P	P
Uses	Short term symptomatic relief of indigestion and heartburn	Relief of GI smooth muscle spasm and symptomatic relief of IBS
Side effects	Cimetidine: hepatic enzyme inhibitor All: rash, lethargy, bowel disorders, headache, confusional states, blood disorders, muscle pain	Hyoscine: drowsiness/visual disturbance Peppermint oil: heartburn, allergy Alverine: nausea, headache, dizziness, pruritis, rash
Overdose	Cimetidine: gynaecomastia, impotence All: interstitial nephritis, bradycardia, pancreatitis, AV block	Bowel disorders
Interactions	Cimetidine: theophylline, antiepileptics, anticoagulants, antiarrhythmics, cyclosporin (ciclosporin)	Any drug with antimuscarinic side effects
Contra-indications	Long term use Children under 16 Pregnancy and breastfeeding	Children (minimum age varies) Hyosine: glaucoma All: intestinal obstruction, pregnancy, breastfeeding, difficulty in swallowing, porphyria, paralytic ileus
Potential for misuse	High in those with an income, wishing to avoid visits to a GP	Low

visual disturbance may occur and hyoscine should not be used in patients with glaucoma as a dangerous build up of ocular pressure may occur.

Laxatives

Constipation is a common side effect of several drugs. It is common in elderly people, those who lack exercise and those who eat a diet low in fibre. It may be worth checking if prescribed medication is a causative factor, and lifestyle advice, particularly with regard to diet and fluid intake, should also be given. All types of laxative can affect fluid/electrolyte balance and, hence, the metabolism of other drugs. The characteristics of laxatives are detailed in Table 7.5.

Antidiarrhoeals

The treatment of diarrhoea is covered by World Health Organisation (WHO) guidelines. It is extremely difficult to convince the general public that rehy-

Table 7.5   Characteristics of laxatives.

	Stimulant laxatives	Bulking agents	Osmotic laxatives	Magnesium salts
Legal status	GSL or P dependent on pack size	GSL or P	P	GSL
Side-effects	Abdominal cramp	Flatulence Abdominal discomfort	Intestinal obstruction if insufficient fluid intake	
Overdose	Dehydration Electrolyte depletion Atonic non-functioning colon Hypokalaemia			
Interactions				
Contra-indications	Nausea Vomiting Abdominal obstruction Abdominal pain	Intestinal obstruction Difficulty in swallowing	Intestinal obstruction Galactosaemia	Renal impairment Elderly Hepatic damage
Potential for misuse	Moderate to high	Moderate to high	Moderate	High

dration therapy is the answer in most cases, and that they should not need the following products! If food poisoning is suspected, no medication should be used for the first 24 hours without medical advice. Fluids are doubly important in such cases.

The condition may have been precipitated by prescribed medication. It is important to discover if this is the case, as the situation may be rectified by a change of prescription. Conversely, this class of drugs may affect elimination of other drugs, although diarrhoea itself is probably a bigger culprit. Advice should be given to those patients whose well-being depends on regular medication. Other patients who need particular help when treating diarrhoea are those in the first and third trimesters of pregnancy. The characteristics of antidiarrhoeals are shown in Table 7.6.

This condition is another where consistent information from all health care professionals is important. Appropriate treatment often falls by the wayside due to advice from friends or family based on messages given many years ago. The fact that drugs may not always be the answer to a medical problem is a

Table 7.6 Characteristics of antidiarrhoeals.

	Loperamide	Morphine	Rehydration fluids
Legal status	P	P (in combination products)	GSL
Side-effects	Abdominal pain Bloating Skin reactions Paralytic ileus	Nausea Vomiting Drowsiness Addiction	
Overdose		Depression of autonomic functions Death	
Interactions		Other opioids	
Contra-indications	Under 12s Pregnancy	Under 12s Pregnancy Respiratory failure Hepatic failure	
Potential for misuse	Low	High	Low

novel and unwelcome one for a number of individuals. We all have a duty to see that everyone is fully informed as to the latest ideas on treatments.

'Cold' remedies

Many such remedies are combination products and contain analgesics. Paracetamol or aspirin overdosage may occur if questions are not asked regarding other medication. The characteristics of cold remedies' ingredients are shown in Table 7.7.

Decongestants are included for obvious reasons. They are a source of concern when patients present with other conditions, and refusal to supply may cause some consternation. Pseudoephedrine and phenylpropanolamine are the most common oral compounds used. Oxymetazoline and xylometazoline are used in topical products.

The reason for the inclusion of antihistamines is not immediately clear. They are usually sedative antihistamines, thus encouraging sleep. They may also help to prevent sneezing, but their antihistaminic actions would seem irrelevant in colds and 'flu. Cough suppressants or expectorants may be present but are dealt with separately.

Antitussives

These can be divided into two categories, expectorants and cough suppressants. When asked for 'something for a cough', it is important to determine

Table 7.7   Characteristics of ingredients of 'cold' remedies.

	Sympathomimetics	Antihistamines	Analgesics
Legal status	GSL or P	P or GSL	GSL or P
Uses	Decongestants	Sneezing Dry up secretions	Headache Systemic pain
Side-effects	Hypertension Headache Palpitations Insomnia Anxiety Restlessness Rebound congestion (for topical products)	Drowsiness Antimuscarinic effects	As for individual drugs
Overdose	Severe hypertension Vomiting Cardiovascular collapse		As for individual drugs
Interactions	MAOI antidepressants Beta blockers Bromocriptine	Alcohol	As for individual drugs
Contra-indications	Hypertension Pregnancy Diabetes mellitus Prostatic hypertrophy Hyperthyroidism Ischaemic heart disease		
Potential for misuse	High	Moderate	Variable

the type of cough involved. Productive coughs should not be suppressed, a fact which is sometimes difficult to communicate without offence, and dry, irritating coughs will not respond to an expectorant. Coughing is a symptom of an underlying condition and referral is necessary if the problem does not resolve itself within 7 days. The cause may vary from an infection to a side effect of captopril, an ACE inhibitor used in hypertension and other cardiovascular disorders.

The efficacy of OTC cough remedies has been questioned over the years. Combination products, sometimes containing both an expectorant and a cough suppressant, are no longer prescribable, but the public still requests them. Advertising, tradition and the placebo effect may all play a part in their commercial success as people swear that their condition improves, despite the theoretical therapeutic contradictions.

A sensible course of action when dealing with cough remedies is to discover the exact symptoms, give advice on the limitations of symptomatic treatment and recommend a safe, single component, product with instructions to contact the GP if symptoms persist or worsen.

The compounds used vary greatly. Simple demulcents are available to soothe the throat and are fairly innocuous preparations. At the other end of the scale are codeine and theophylline, both potent drugs with potentially dangerous side effects. Pharmacists are mindful of the abuse potential of the preparations containing the latter substances, and efforts are made to prevent misuse. In the case of codeine, the solution is simple. Pholcodine has similar effects with regard to cough, but without the problem of potential addiction. The dangers of theophylline mean that it is unlikely to be recommended. Its mode of action is the reduction of bronchospasm, but how this prevents cough is unclear. The characteristics of expectorants, suppressants and theophylline are given in Table 7.8.

Antihistamines

Table 7.9 shows antihistamines' characteristics. Several drugs in this category have recently been deregulated from POM to P, but terfenadine has reverted to POM. Some compounds have been licensed for the treatment of sleep disorders but they are more commonly used to treat allergic conditions including hay fever. The more recent products have had less sedative effects than their predecessors due to their peripheral rather than central action. Unfortunately, since the deregulation of two of the drugs, terfenadine and astemizole, reports of serious cardiac problems associated with their use have increased.

For some time, questions have been asked and advice given regarding the sedative potential of the older drugs, such as chlorpheniramine (chlorphenamine) and promethazine. Detailed questioning has also been necessary for the newer drugs in view of the potentially fatal side effects and interactions. All of those involved in health care must be involved in the information giving process in such cases. The treatment of hay fever may seem minor, and many sufferers believe that they should be able to purchase their favourite products without intrusion. This is one example, however, of the intervention of a pharmacist being potentially life saving. Continued education regarding the dangers of medicines may help to break down resentment by increasing understanding of the intention behind any questioning involved. Hypnotic anithistamines are described later in this chapter.

Topical muscular pain relief products

There appears to be something comforting about the effect of rubbing a preparation onto an area of the body which is sore or aching. The warming glow produced by increasing the blood supply to an inflamed area can, however, be caused by massage alone and the efficacy of topical preparations must

Table 7.8   Characteristics of ingredients of 'cold' remedies (continued).

	Expectorants	Suppressants	Theophylline
Legal status	GSL or P	GSL or P	P
Uses	Reduce viscosity of catarrh	Depress coughing centre in brain	Reduce bronchospasm
Side effects		Sputum retention Constipation Drowsiness	Agitation Gastro-intestinal problems Insomnia Palpitations
Overdose		Respiratory depression Depression of autonomic functions Death	Low therapeutic index – real risk of overdose Vomiting Tachycardia Haematemesis Convulsions Arrhythmias Hypokalaemia
Interactions		Other opioids	Cimetidine Antibiotics Fluvoxamine Antiepileptics Calcium channel blockers Sympathomimetics
Contra-indications		Hepatic disease Ventilatory failure	Heart disease Hypertension Hyperthyroidism Peptic ulcer Epilepsy Pregnancy/ breastfeeding Elderly Pyrexia
Potential for misuse	Low	High	High

be questionable. Many older preparations can only have had a placebo, or at best a rubefacient effect.

A number of products have been extensively prescribed for several years. Some were POMs but others fell into the category of P medicines whose cost meant that few people considered purchasing them. Newer P category topical products are, almost without exception, deregulated derivatives of frequently

Table 7.9   Characteristics of antihistamines.

	Sedating	Non-sedating
Legal status	P	P or POM
Side-effects	Antimuscarinic effects Drowsiness Headache	Arrhythmias (terfenadine/astemizole) Increased appetite (astemizole)
Overdose	Coma	Heart failure (terfenadine/astemizole)
Interactions		Macrolide antibiotics Imidazole antifungals Antiarrhythmics Sotalol Diuretics Cimetidine
Contra-indications	Porphyria	Liver disease Pre-existing QT prolongation
Potential for misuse	Moderate	Low

prescribed POMs. The pack sizes are smaller and indications for use more limited, but the product name is similar to that of its POM classified parent. Most community pharmacists can produce instance after instance of requests for such products stimulated by advertising, a reticence to ask the GP for something to 'rub on' or an unwillingness on the part of the GP to prescribe something to 'rub on'. Perhaps the most worrying are the requests motivated by the necessity to give back to a neighbour, friend or family member the tube of cream prescribed for them, which had been lent to the purchaser without reference to a doctor.

Several of the products contain NSAIDs and it is these that cause most concern. Absorption through the skin does occur and systemic side effects are theoretically possible. They may not occur in everyone, but a warning about overuse needs to be given, particularly if the purchaser is taking oral NSAIDs as well. The prevalence of prescribing initiatives promoting evidence based practice will further reduce the number of these products prescribed. Advertising will, however, ensure that the demand for the OTC alternatives will increase. Vigilance on the part of all health care professionals will be needed to ensure that appropriate use of the products is made. Patient education is essential. The characteristics of topical pain relief preparations are shown in Table 7.10.

Hypnotics

The prescribing of hypnotics has been widespread for many years. Benzodiazepines form a large proportion of the drugs available, but are now only

Table 7.10   Characteristics of topical pain relief preparations.

	Ibuprofen	Salicylates	Felbinac/ piroxicam	Ketoprofen
Legal status	P in small pack sizes	P	P in small pack sizes	P
Uses	Muscular pain relief	Muscular pain relief	Muscular pain relief	Muscular pain relief
Side effects	Gastric irritation Nausea Dyspepsia Gastric bleeding Allergic reaction	Gastric irritation Nausea Dyspepsia Gastric bleeding Reyes syndrome	Gastric irritation Nausea Dyspepsia Gastric bleeding Allergic reaction	Gastric irritation Nausea Dyspepsia Gastric bleeding Allergic reaction
Overdose	Nausea Vomiting Gastric pain Vertigo Sleeplessness	**Mild:** Tinnitus Perspiration Vasodilation	Nausea Vomiting Gastric pain	Nausea Vomiting Gastric pain
Interactions	Baclofen NSAIDs	Warfarin Methotrexate NSAIDs	NSAIDs	NSAIDs
Contra-indications	Broken skin Under 14s Pregnancy Peptic ulcer Asthma/allergy Haemorrhagic disease	Broken skin Children (mainly under 6 years) Pregnancy Peptic ulcer Asthma/allergy	Broken skin Under 14s Pregnancy Peptic ulcer Asthma/allergy Haemorrhagic disease	Some not for children under 15, others no restriction NSAID sensitivity Pregnancy

recommended for short term use. There have been preparations for sale which have been used as an aid to sleep but they have, until recently, been homeopathic or other alternative medicinal products. None was licensed medicines for insomnia. It is only in the recent past that certain sedative antihistamines have been licensed for OTC sale to induce sleep, and their characteristics are shown in Table 7.11.

Topical hydrocortisone

Topical preparations containing anything from 0.1% to 1% hydrocortisone, either alone or in combination, are now firmly established in the OTC market. The licensed indications cover many types of skin irritation ranging from insect bites, to contact dermatitis, to mild to moderate eczema. None is licensed for use in children under 10 years of age and should only be used for a maximum of 7 days. The legal status for hydrocortisone is either POM or P.

Table 7.11   Characteristics of hypnotic antihistamines.

	Diphenhydramine/promethazine
Legal status	P or GSL
Uses	Temporary relief of sleep disturbance
Side effects	Drowsiness, headache, rash, antimuscarinic effects, convulsions, psychomotor impairment, photosensitivity
Overdose	Paradoxical stimulation Arrhythmias Palpitations
Interactions	Alcohol Benzodiazepines Antimuscarinics
Contra-indications	Under 16s Epilepsy Glaucoma Urinary retention Prostatic hypertrophy
Potential for misuse	High

Problems arise when GPs advise patients to purchase the OTC products because they are cheaper than a prescription charge. If the problem is above the shoulders, the product licence does not allow a sale. The same is true for severe eczema or for broken skin. Handwritten notes frequently state 0.5% hydro-cortisone cream and there is no OTC product of this strength. The pharmacist must refuse to sell a product, and the patient often appears to think that this is due to an obstructive personality. It is, however, usually due to the vagaries of the licensing regulations.

Antifungals

Over the counter antifungals have traditionally been antiseptics that inhibited fungal growth but did not eradicate the organism completely. Their main use was in the treatment of athlete's foot. Many are still available, but several members of the imidazole family have been deregulated from POM to P and are becoming the preferred treatments. They are also indicated for vaginal thrush, fungal infections of the oropharynx, and nappy rash. One oral prep-aration is also now available for use in vaginal thrush. Its cost is, however, prohibitive to many prospective purchasers. Clotrimazole and miconazole are the most common ingredients of the topical imidazoles. Fluconazole is used in the oral preparation.

Most of the controversy surrounding these products is associated with the treatment of vaginal thrush. The licences state that only those women between the ages of 16 and 60 may be sold the products for this condition. Pregnancy, recurring episodes of the infection, systemic symptoms and vaginal bleeding would all preclude a purchase. The oral product cannot be used by women of childbearing age without adequate contraceptive precautions being taken. As with any other OTC, and particularly the deregulated products, every effort is made to safeguard prospective purchasers. The trust placed in the veracity of the individual involved cannot, sadly, always be justified.

Vitamins

Although vitamin preparations are sold through pharmacies, most are not licensed as medicines. They are classed as food supplements in the majority of cases and may contain varying quantities of an assortment of vitamins and minerals. Although the quantity of each active ingredient must be stated, along with the percentage of the recommended daily amount (RDA) for an adult, maximum doses are rarely shown. This may be of little importance where the water-soluble vitamins are concerned but may be relevant for the fat-soluble vitamins due to the potential build up in the body. Vitamins A and D can be harmful in overdose, but many products, including those available from 'health food' shops and other outlets, contain large amounts of these substances.

The dangers of excessive use have been highlighted by reports into the side effects associated with pyridoxine. Women have been encouraged to take this vitamin for a variety of menstrual and menopausal problems, but some individuals have exhibited peripheral neuropathy. The Department of Health issued a warning about the adverse effects, and high dosage products were put under direct supervision of the pharmacist in registered pharmacies. No controls can be exerted on products sold in other retail outlets, so purchasers will not get the advice necessary to prevent potential damage.

The restriction on prescribing of vitamins for specific deficiency states may explain the burgeoning market for 'tonics' and 'pick-me-ups'. Advice on diet and lifestyle should be sufficient for a healthy adult to improve their well-being. Even if listened to, the public still perceives that vitamins will be good for them and may purchase them anyway.

Folic acid is one of the few vitamins to have a product licence. The products are now licensed for the prevention of first occurrence of neural tube defects, including spina bifida, in all women. Any woman planning a pregnancy should take them and they should be taken up to the end of the first trimester of any pregnancy that occurs. Publicity campaigns have been used to raise awareness of their availability, and advice on this and many other aspects of pre-conception care is available from pharmacies. Referral to a GP or practice nurse is made if appropriate.

Summary

This chapter briefly reviews the background to the availability of OTC medicines in the UK today. The legal and ethical implications of such availability are considered, with reference to the role of pharmacists and other health care professionals in promoting effective and appropriate use of such products. The remainder of the chapter deals with some of the categories of drugs found in OTC medication. The legal category and uses are given, along with the more common side effects, interactions and complications of use. Full details of the latter aspects can be found in product literature or obtained from the relevant pharmaceutical company.

Over the counter medication is a great tradition in this country and its benefits are many. There are far more products and therapeutic groups on the market than have been mentioned here. Easy access to certain drugs means that the health service is not terminally overloaded, as GPs do not have to deal, in the main, with the treatment of minor conditions. Time and money are saved, both by the NHS and the patient, and the health care budget can be spent on serious illness.

The very nature of the practice of selling medicines means that there will always be drawbacks. Drug misuse will always occur and overdoses and side effects will cause difficulties for some. The problems highlighted here can be overcome by a commitment to public education about drugs and medicines, and the role of pharmacists, doctors and nurses in the prevention of harm and the giving of advice on health care matters.

It seems likely that more potent preparations will be deregulated in the future and the conditions for which they are used may need careful consideration before sales are made. The ethos of protection of the public by the relevant professionals warrants wide discussion to ensure that the public good is being served. Despite the fact that this will probably not take place, individual professional responsibility and the duty of care towards patients and customers should ensure that standards of service are improved wherever possible, and the consumer allowed to make an informed choice as to their self medication.

References

Doran, T.F., De-Angelis, C., Baumgardner, R.A. & Mellits, E.D. (1989) Acetaminoplen: more harm than good for chickenpox? *J. Paediatr.* **114**, 1045–8.

Joint Working Group of the Research Unit of the Royal College of Physicians & the British Paediatric Association (1991) Guidelines for the management of convulsions with fever. *Br. Med. J.* **303**, 634–6.

Kramer, M.S. Naimark, L.E., Roberts-Bräuer, R., McDougall, A. & Leduc, D.G. (1991) Risks and benefits of paracetamol antipyresis in young children with fever of presumed viral origin. *Lancet* **337**, 591–4.

White, W.H. (1898a) *Materia Medica*, J. & A. Churchill, London, pp. 369–71.
White, W.H. (1898b) *Materia Medica*, J. & A. Churchill, London, pp. 329–30.

Further reading

Harding, G., Nettleton, S. & Taylor, K. (1994) *Social Pharmacy*. Pharmaceutical Press, London.
Mehta, D.K. (1997) *British National Formulary No. 34*. British Medical Association and Royal Pharmaceutical Society of Great Britain, London.
Reynolds, J.E.F. (1996) *Martindale. The Extra Pharmacopeia*, 31st edn. Royal Pharmaceutical Society of Great Britain, London.
Royal Pharmaceutical Society of Great Britain (1997) *Medicines, Ethics and Practice*, Vol. 18. RPSGB, London.
Walker, R. & Edwards, C. (1994) *Clinical Pharmacy and Therapeutics*, Churchill Livingstone, Edinburgh.

Chapter 8

The Nurse's Role in Prescribing

Lynn Austin, Barbara Dicks and Tracey Thornton

Introduction

This chapter presents the background to the nurse's new role in prescribing including protocol prescribing, and the necessary legislative and administrative changes to enable initial prescribing for community nurses. The preparation of nurses for prescribing is discussed, and findings are highlighted from the evaluation at the original community nurse prescribing demonstration sites. The chapter provides information regarding items commonly prescribed by nurses and contained in the *Nurse Prescribers' Formulary* (NPF). This includes details on the indications for use, mode of action, contra-indications and side effects. The concluding section provides an overview of the likely developments in relation to nurse prescribing.

Background

The demand for nurse prescribing rights, particularly for nurses working in the community, has been voiced since the early 1980s (RCN, 1980). This prescribing lobby gained momentum following the publication of the Cumberlege Report (DHSS, 1986) which strongly advocated prescribing rights for community nurses and placed the prescribing debate firmly on the policy agenda.

The Department of Health's (DH's) response to pressure for prescribing rights for nurses was an exploration of the potential benefits of community nurses' prescribing, the findings of which were published in the Crown Report (DH, 1989). The report focused on three types of prescribing: initial prescribing from a nurses' formulary; supplying within a group protocol, for example for immunization programmes; and altering the timing and dosage of a GP prescribed medication, for example in the management of analgesia for patients who are terminally ill.

Ultimately, the legislative changes, enacted in October 1994 (The Medicinal Products Act 1992) permitted one of the three types of prescribing advocated in the Crown Report, namely initial prescribing by community nurses with a recognized qualification (i.e. a district nurse or health visiting qualification) who had undertaken the English National Board approved course (ENB, 1992). This is perhaps because in many respects custom and practice, arising from delegated medical responsibility, had resulted in nurses already taking on roles with regard to the administration of medicines, usually in accordance with specifically devised local protocols. This practice is widely used and is discussed in more detail below.

Nurse prescribing by protocol

There has been considerable debate about the appropriateness or otherwise of the term protocol prescribing. It is frequently stated that nurses who purport to prescribe by protocol are in actual fact not prescribing as such, but administering or supplying medicines. This section will not attempt to comment further on this debate, but will focus on the clinical benefits to patients, nurses and doctors, that have arisen from the now established practice of protocol prescribing. The direction prescribing by protocol may take in the future is discussed in the concluding section of this chapter.

Rationale for protocol prescribing

The last 10 years have seen a proliferation of specialist nursing activities whereby clinical nurse specialists or nurse practitioners have been involved in a growing range of nurse led initiatives, and it has been in response to such developments that prescribing by protocol arrangements have proliferated.

It has already been noted that nurses in hospital are not able to prescribe medicines but, by acting within clear criteria which have been agreed with the relevant medical staff, they can on the strength of the following section (58b) of the Medicines Act 1968 be said to be effectively administering medicines:

> No person shall administer (otherwise than to himself) any such medicinal product unless he is an appropriate practitioner or a person acting in accordance with the directions of an appropriate practitioner.

It has been the wording of this section of the Medicines Act, that has provided the initiative for the development of nurse prescribing by protocol.

Furthermore, the United Kingdom Central Council for Nursing, Midwifery and Health Visiting (UKCC), through the Code of Professional Conduct and Scope of Practice, enables practitioners to understand more clearly professional accountability, and in so doing provides a framework for nurses to practice in a more autonomous way. Whilst the UKCC (1997) clearly views prescribing separately from the supply and administration of medicines, it supports in principle protocol prescribing for individuals and groups that has become in many areas custom and practice.

Protocol development

It is important to see the development of protocols as distinct from the established system whereby nurses make adjustments to prescribed medications to suit the individual requirements of the patient. In the case of protocol prescribing the nurse, working to an agreed protocol (which has been signed by a doctor), following nursing assessment and using her own clinical judgement, initiates the prescription of a drug. Until recently there were no nationally agreed guidelines for protocols and their development was dependent on local arrangements (DH, 1998). The Medicinal Products Act 1992, which permits nurses to prescribe a limited range of drugs, and the associated legislation which provides a framework within which qualified community nurses can prescribe, have emphasised the importance of nurses being appropriately prepared. Community nurses wishing to be put forward as initial nurse prescribers must have successfully completed a nurse prescribing course programme (Courtenay & Butler, 1998). In contrast it is the case that for protocol prescribing, there is as yet no formal programme of preparation: it is therefore imperative that only nurses who are proven experts in a specific area prescribe using protocols.

In our experience this has meant that only designated clinical nurse specialists or nurses with equivalent expertise can prescribe using protocols. These nurses are experts in the care concerned and have been educated in the actions, contra-indications and side effects of the drugs they are prescribing, and work to an agreed patient focused protocol for the management of a specific symptom (Mallett, 1997).

The protocols in use at the Royal Marsden Hospital comprise two parts. The first part details the symptom to be alleviated, the aims of the treatment and the strategy for evaluating its effectiveness (Fig. 8.1) and the second part focuses specifically on the medication to be used as part of the overall management of the symptom (Fig. 8.2)

Clinical benefits

It is the case that the division of labour in medicine and nursing remains intrinsically unchanged. It is usual for doctors to assess and diagnose the patient's condition and to choose the treatment strategy, whilst nurses implement the medical plan. However, the development of a variety of nursing roles has led to considerable blurring of boundaries between medicine and nursing. During recent years nurses have become involved in an increasing number of nurse led initiatives. Prescribing by protocol has developed almost out of necessity to ensure that care is delivered in a patient focused manner. One of the reasons for developing protocol prescribing at the Royal Marsden Hospital was to support nurse led clinics. It soon became apparent that the time patients

Nurse specialist: ....

Designation: ....

Supervising physician: ....

Symptom(s): Acute radiation toxicity, proctitis from pelvic radiotherapy

Aims of **treatment** or **care**:

- Reduce anal soreness
- Decrease pruritis
- Reduce anal bleeding

Methods:

- Assess severity of, and distress associated with, symptoms
- To apply Scheriproct ointment (topical steroid drug)
- 2 x daily (3–4 times daily on first day and take for a few days after symptoms have cleared
- Provide verbal instruction and written support

Evaluation:

- Assess patient weekly either in outpatient clinic or by telephone
- Review two weekly in clinic
- Assess degree of comfort and symptoms

If bleeding persists or symptoms become worse review and administer Scheriproct suppositories

Fig. 8.1   Plan for symptom management.

attending nurse clinics waited for their prescription was reduced (Mallett, 1997). It is frequently noted that one of the major advantages for patients of nurse led services is that nurses are perceived to be more approachable than doctors. This fact was particularly apparent in a study which examined patients' views of prescribing in the community (Luker *et al.*, 1997c).

It is true to say that the proliferation of prescribing by protocol has arisen because arrangements for nurse prescribing in general have been so slow in coming on stream. Although it has to be acknowledged that prescribing by protocol is a back door approach and caution is required whilst waiting for wider legislation to become a reality, practitioners have adopted this practice as it is so obviously in the patients' best interests.

Initial prescribing by community nurses

Before the introduction of initial prescribing by community nurses the potential benefits of this new role were frequently noted in the popular nursing press

Nurse prescriber: . . . .

Designation: . . . .

Responsible physician: . . . .

Medication	Action	Contraindications, interactions and side effects
Scheriproct ointment	Topical steroid + Local anaesthetic	See BNF No. 34 Sept. (1997) pages 53–55

Indications for treatment	Range within which medication can be prescribed and altered (i.e. timing and dose)	Clinical information and dose measurements required	Indications for review of treatment and time allowed	Rationale for referral to physicians
Anal soreness, pruritus, pain or discomfort	5–7 days, 2 × daily (3–4 times daily on first day)	Use of symptom assessment and distress tool	Symptom reviewed weekly or if discomfort increased or bleeding occurred	If patient experiences no improvement. If bleeding is more than occasional spotting

Signature of Nurse prescriber: . . . .

Signature of Physician: . . . .

Signature of Director of Patient Services/CNO: . . . .

Date protocol agreed: . . . .

Rationale for review: Initial assessment of protocol

Frequency of review: 3 months

Date protocol to be reviewed: . . . .

Fig. 8.2   Protocol for patients with acute radiation toxicity; proctitis from pelvic radiotherapy.

(Fawcett-Henesy, 1988; Nursing Standard, 1990; Poulton, 1994). Anticipated benefits included increased convenience to patients and their carers due to a reduction in the number of journeys required to obtain prescribed items; this was also expected to lead to the earlier commencement of treatment. Patients expected to benefit were elderly people, people with a disability, those living in rural areas, families with a low income, travelling families, homeless people and patients newly discharged from hospital. Nurses were also expected to save time. Additionally, it was thought that relationships between themselves and their colleagues would be enhanced, and nurses' job satisfaction and status would increase once they were seen to be accountable for prescribing decisions. In many respects nurse prescribing was seen to be legitimizing everyday practice with regard to items such as wound care products, as nurses commonly selected products which the GPs simply endorsed by writing a prescription.

Nurse prescribing evaluation

Following the enactment of legislation which permitted suitably qualified nurses to prescribe from a specifically devised formulary (BMA *et al.*, 1994), an evaluation was undertaken in eight demonstration sites in England. This looked at nurses' prescribing behaviour, the impact of nurse prescribing on patients and health care professionals, and the economic implications associated with this new role.

The formulary included items commonly employed by nurses in their day-to-day work. Items included were wound management products, topical applications, antipyretics/analgesics, laxatives, antifungal agents, and treatments for infestations. Details on the properties of the more commonly used products are outlined in a later section.

Community nurses at the prescribing sites undertook specific training in their new role in accordance with the ENB guidelines (1992). This included an open learning pack with approximately 15 hours' worth of study material followed by an intensive 2 day course. These covered various aspects of prescribing including pharmacology, accountability and the legal and ethical aspects of prescribing.

Items prescribed by nurses in the study varied by type of nurse and reflected the different aspects of work undertaken. Whilst health visitors tended to prescribe items for skin conditions, candidiasis and pyrexia, district nurses predominantly prescribed wound care items. Practice nurses also commonly prescribed wound and skin care products, and additionally were the group of nurses most likely to prescribe appliances and reagents for diabetes. Although nurses did prescribe items such as analgesics and aperients, these were initially treated more cautiously; concern expressed was based on a fear of not identifying an underlying pathology or the potential side effects of the medication (Luker *et al.*, 1998a).

Many of the benefits anticipated in the literature were found to occur in practice at the eight demonstration sites (Luker *et al.*, 1997a–d). Nurses were viewed as competent to prescribe items included in the *NPF*. Because most items in the *NPF* are available over the counter and many patients opt to obtain items in this way (Luker *et al.*, 1997f), some respondents indicated that the *NPF* should be extended to include other items such as antibiotics, immunization products and treatments for asthma (Luker *et al.*, 1997d,e, 1998b).

In addition to the professional success of nurse prescribing, initial fears that prescribing costs would escalate as a result of this change were quelled to some extent by the findings from the economic analysis of the evaluation (Luker *et al.*, 1997a), which found no evidence to suggest the prescribing costs in the eight demonstration sites had increased more than they would have done in the absence of nurse prescribing.

The Nurse Prescribers' Formulary

The NPF is published in the *British National Formulary* (Mehta, 1997) and is reproduced in Appendix 1. This section presents details of some of the items included in the *NPF* for situations commonly encountered by community nurses namely, constipation, pain relief, candidiasis, infestations and wound and skin conditions.

Laxatives

Constipation can be described as the infrequent and difficult passage of dry and hard faeces. The accompanying symptoms may include straining and abdominal discomfort, a sensation of incomplete evacuation and mild abdominal distension. Most forms of constipation are easily treated by increasing the amount of fibre in the diet, having an adequate fluid intake and taking regular exercise. Laxatives should generally be reserved for:

- Post myocardial infarction patients who, when straining at stool, may exacerbate angina.
- Patients with heart failure, where fluid intake may be restricted.
- Cases where straining may increase the risk of bleeding, e.g. haemorrhoids.
- Drug induced constipation.
- Bowel evacuation prior to diagnostic and surgical procedures.
- Constipation related to illness or surgery.
- Constipation in pregnancy when above measures have failed (but as with all drugs in pregnancy it would be wise to consult the relevant literature before prescribing or refer to a doctor).
- Elderly people with inadequate muscle tone.

(Luscombe, 1994)

Table 8.1 Different classes of laxatives in Nurse Prescribers' Formulary.

Bulking agents	Ispaghula husk
	Sterculia
Stimulant laxatives	Bisacodyl
	Docusate sodium
	Senna
	Danthron (dantron)
	Glycerol
Faecal softeners	Docusate sodium
	Arachis oil
Osmotic laxatives	Lactulose
	Magnesium hydroxide
	Phosphates (rectal)
	Sodium citrate (rectal)

Overuse of laxatives may lead to dehydration and electrolyte disturbance. Laxatives can be divided into four main categories: (Wynne & Edwards, 1992; Edwards & Stillman 1993; Medicines Resource Centre, 1994). Table 8.1 shows the classes of laxatives in the *NPF*.

Bulk forming laxatives

Bulk laxatives are polysaccharide or cellulose derivatives. They soften and increase stool bulk by absorbing water in the colon. This produces distension of the intestines and stimulates peristalsis. To avoid intestinal obstruction and faecal impaction they should be taken with plenty of fluid (approximately $\frac{1}{4}$ pint or 130 ml of cold water) and administration should be avoided immediately before retiring to bed.

Bulk laxatives take several days to achieve full effect and are therefore unsuitable for acute relief. They are more appropriate for long term use in those who have uncomplicated constipation and a normal gut motility, e.g. pregnancy, haemorrhoids, and anal fissures.

The main side effects are flatulence and abdominal distension. Gastrointestinal (GI) obstruction and faecal impaction have also been reported.

Stimulant laxatives

Stimulant laxatives increase intestinal motility by an irritant effect on the bowel wall. This stimulates sensory nerve endings and produces colonic contraction. The onset of action is 6–12 hours. They may therefore be given at night to produce a bowel movement the following morning. Their use should preferably be restricted to short term as chronic use may lead to tolerance, bowel atony and hypokalaemia.

Side effects include abdominal cramps and local irritation. Preparations containing danthron (dantron), (Co-danthramer and Co-danthrusate), are particularly useful in the elderly and terminally ill as they combine a stimulant laxative with a faecal softener. Patients should be counselled that these preparations may colour the urine red.

Faecal softeners

Faecal softeners are surfactants which lubricate and soften hard faeces in the bowel by reducing the surface tension and facilitating the absorption of water.

Docusate sodium, as well as being a stimulant laxative, acts as a faecal softener. It acts within 1–2 days when given orally. It is useful in patients where bulk laxatives have been ineffective and straining should be avoided. It may also be considered in patients where bulking agents are unsuitable or in combination with a stimulant laxative to promote peristalsis.

Arachis oil is a faecal softener often given as an enema. It lubricates and softens impacted faeces and promotes a bowel movement. The enema should be warmed before use. Arachis oil is produced from peanuts and should not be given to patients who have nut allergy.

Osmotic laxatives

Osmotic agents retain fluid in the bowel by osmosis; this stimulates peristalsis and produces a soft stool. The most common agents are magnesium salts and lactulose.

Magnesium has a very rapid effect producing a bowel movement 1–2 hours after administration. Magnesium containing laxatives should be reserved for use when a rapid action is required, as magnesium may be absorbed leading to hypermagnesaemia, especially in renal failure.

Lactulose is a semi-synthetic disaccharide which is not absorbed from the GI tract. As well as having an osmotic action it is metabolised by colonic bacteria to lactic and acetic acid which stimulate peristalsis in the large bowel. Lactulose needs to be taken regularly and produces an effect within 2–3 days. It is not suitable for rapid relief of constipation. Side effects of lactulose include flatulence, abdominal cramps and discomfort. Lactulose should be avoided in intestinal obstruction and galactosaemia.

Phosphate is used as an enema and is of value for bowel clearance before surgery or diagnostic procedures, and for the acute treatment of severe constipation. Information on the different laxatives available is shown in Table 8.2.

Analgesics

Analgesics can be classed as opioid or non-opioid. Opioid analgesics are used for the treatment of severe pain of visceral origin, whereas non-opioid analgesics are preferred to treat mild to moderate pain. Non-opioid analgesics

Table 8.2   Information on the different laxatives available.

Drug	Adult dose	Notes
Bulk forming agents		
Ispaghula husk granules (3.5 g per sachet), powder (3.4 g, or 6 g per sachet)	1 sachet in water twice daily	Preferably taken after meals More palatable if made as a jelly Ensure adequate fluid intake to prevent intestinal obstruction
Sterculia granules (100 g or 7 g per sachet)	1–2 heaped 5 ml spoonfuls or 1–2 sachets once or twice daily	Wash down with plenty of liquid without chewing, preferably after meals
Stimulant laxatives		
Bisacodyl 5 mg tablets 10 mg suppositories	1–2 tablets at night 1 suppository in the morning	Tablets act in 10–12 hours; suppositories act in 20–60 minutes. Can cause local irritation and stomach cramps. May also be used before radiological procedures. Paediatric suppository also available, contains 5 mg bisacodyl
Senna 7.5 mg tablets granules (15 mg/5 ml spoonful) 7.5 mg/5 ml solution	15–30 mg taken at night Initial dose should be low, then gradually increased	Act in 8–12 hours Preparations on sale to public recommend a lower dose
Senna and ispaghula husk granules	1–2 5 ml spoonfuls with water once or twice daily for 1–3 days	Ensure adequate fluid intake and do not take immediately before retiring to bed Take after food
Stimulant/faecal softener		
Glycerol suppositories Docusate sodium 100 mg capsules 50 mg/5 ml solution	1 when required Up to 500 mg daily in divided doses Up to 50 ml daily in divided doses	Moisten with water before use. Mild irritant Acts within 1–2 days. Useful following stroke or myocardial infarction, haemorrhoids or anal fissure when straining may be hazardous. Avoid rectal preparations if haemorrhoids/anal fissure
Enemas	One when required	Paediatric solution also available
Danthron (dantron)	Initially 5–10 ml or 1 capsule at night	Available as co-danthramer or co-danthrusate. Acts in 6–12 hours. Colours urine red/pink and causes skin irritation, especially in incontinent patients. Restricted indications after consultation with doctor
Faecal softeners		
Arachis oil	One enema when required	Warm before use. Avoid in patients with nut allergy
Osmotic laxatives		
Lactulose	Initially 15 ml twice daily	Takes up to 48 hours to act
Magnesium hydroxide	25–50 ml when required	Avoid prolonged use especially in renal impairment
Phosphate	Given as an enema when required	Contra-indicated in inflammatory bowel disease Sodium absorption may occur
Sodium citrate	Give when required	Small volume microenema

Table 8.3   Characteristics of aspirin and paracetamol.

	Aspirin	Paracetamol
Indications	Mild to moderate pain, pyrexia	Mild to moderate pain, pyrexia
Adult dose	300–600 mg every 4–6 hours **MAXIMUM** 2.4 g in 24 hours without doctor's advice	0.5–1 g every 4–6 hours **MAXIMUM** of 4 g in 24 hours
Contra-indications	Children under 12 years Breastfeeding Gastro-intestinal ulceration Haemophilia Gout Hypersensitivity to aspirin or other NSAIDs	None but should be used with caution in hepatic and renal disorders
Side effects	Gastro-intestinal irritation causing dyspepsia and occult blood loss Bronchospasm Skin reactions Angioedema Increased bleeding time	These are rare Rashes Blood disorders Acute pancreatitis Liver damage in acute overdosage
Drug interactions	Oral anticoagulants Methotrexate Mifepristone Probenecid Sulphinpyrazone Other NSAIDs	Possibly warfarin with prolonged use

can be further divided into non-steroidal anti-inflammatory drugs (NSAIDs) and paracetamol. The characteristics of asprin and paracetamol are shown in Table 8.3.

Aspirin

Aspirin, the first NSAID to be discovered, has antipyretic, analgesic and anti-inflammatory properties. Its mechanism of action is to prevent the synthesis of prostaglandins from arachidonic acid by inhibiting the enzyme cyclo-oxygenase (Bowman & Rand, 1984; Foster, 1986).

Antipyretic effects. Aspirin has no effect on normal body temperature, or elevated temperature due to excessive physical exercise. During fever, endogenous pyrogen is released from leucocytes which activates the synthesis of prostaglandins in the hypothalamus. These prostaglandins then act on the temperature controlling centres to produce fever. Aspirin inhibits the formation of prostaglandins and prevents the rise in body temperature.

Analgesic effect. Prostaglandins themselves do not produce pain but potentiate the pain caused by other mediators of inflammation (e.g. bradykinin, histamine). Aspirin exerts its analgesic effect by inhibiting prostaglandin formation in inflamed tissue.

Anti-inflammatory effect. Prostaglandins are potent inflammatory mediators, and aspirin relieves inflammation by inhibiting prostaglandin production. The prescribing of aspirin by nurses is restricted to the treatment of mild to moderate pain and relief of pyrexia. It should not be prescribed by nurses to decrease platelet aggregation following stroke or myocardial infarction, or for the treatment of rheumatoid arthritis.

Paracetamol

Paracetamol has analgesic and antipyretic properties. The mechanism of action is similar to aspirin and involves the inhibition of prostaglandin synthesis. Unlike aspirin, paracetamol has no anti-inflammatory properties (Foster, 1986). Paracetamol is widely available to the general public and is an ingredient of many over the counter analgesic preparations. Since it is extremely toxic in overdosage, it is important to check that patients are not already taking over the counter products or combination analgesics containing paracetamol.

Local anaesthetics

Local anaesthetic drugs reversibly block the conduction of impulses along nerve fibres resulting in the loss of sensation only to a specific area which is served by the affected neurones. The most commonly used drug is lignocaine (lidocaine) (Foster, 1986).

Lignocaine (lidocaine) is effective in all forms of local anaesthesia. It is particularly useful for surface anaesthesia as it is readily absorbed through mucous membranes. It is available in various forms for use in catheterisation (see Table 8.4). A 5% ointment may also be used for topical administration. Since lignocaine (lidocaine) is readily absorbed, care should be taken in those patients with epilepsy, anal disorders, cardiac disease and hepatic impairment. It should not be used in the mouth as it may lead to choking. Side effects include convulsions, cardiac depressant effects and allergic reactions. Lignocaine (lidocaine) gel preparations included in the *NPF* are shown in Table 8.4.

Drugs for the mouth

Stomatitis and oral thrush may be caused by ill fitting dentures, the use of broad spectrum antibiotics, cytotoxic agents or inhaled corticosteroids. In many cases treatment with topical antifungal agents may be required. Removal of the causative agent, if possible, and strict oral hygiene may help alleviate symp-

Table 8.4 Different preparations of lignocaine gel in *Nurse Prescribers' Formulary.*

Preparation	Proprietary name
Lignocaine (lidocanine) gel 2%	Xylocaine gel (20 g) Xylocaine accordion gel (single use syringe 20 g)
Lignocaine (lidocaine) 2% and chlorhexidine 0.25% gel	Xylogaine antiseptic gel (20 g) Instillagel (disposable syringe 6 ml, 11 ml) Xylocaine antiseptic accordion (single use syringe 20 g)

toms and prevent recurrence. Patients on inhaled corticosteroids should be advised to use a spacer device and rinse their mouth with water after use.

Patients with unexplained mouth ulcers of greater than 3 weeks' duration require urgent referral to exclude oral cancer. Various preparations are available for the relief of stomatitis and oral thrush.

Miconazole

Miconazole is an imidazole antifungal with a broad spectrum of activity against pathogenic fungi and some Gram positive bacteria. Its mode of action is to inhibit the synthesis of ergosterol which is an important component of the cytoplasmic membrane in fungi but not mammalian cells (Pedler, 1994). It is available as an oral gel which should be smeared around the infected area using a swab or clean finger. Some absorption may occur following topical administration. It should therefore be used with caution in pregnancy and patients taking warfarin. It should be avoided in patients with porphyria.

Nystatin

Nystatin is a polyene antifungal with a broad spectrum of activity. It is not absorbed following topical administration. It is available as pastilles or an oral solution. The usual dose is 100 000 units, four times a day after food. The pastilles should be sucked and the oral solution rinsed around the mouth before being swallowed. Patients with diabetes should use a sugar-free preparation. Treatment is usually for 7 days and should be continued for 48 hours after symptoms have resolved (Pedler, 1994).

Compound thymol glycerin

This preparation has no antifungal activity, but may be used to cleanse the mouth and relieve the pain of oral ulceration. It should be used as a mouthwash three or four times daily when necessary, either undiluted or diluted with 3 volumes of warm water.

Drugs for threadworms

Mebendazole

Mebendazole, a benzimidazole carbamate derivative, is the drug of choice for treating threadworms in patients over 2 years old. It acts by irreversibly inhibiting glucose uptake by the worms, resulting in depletion of the worms' energy sources, glycogen and adenosine triphosphate and their slow death (Reynolds 1996). It is given by mouth but is poorly absorbed from the GI tract. The usual dose is 100 mg as a single dose. If reinfection occurs, this dose may be repeated after 2–3 weeks. Side effects include abdominal pain, diarrhoea and allergic reactions. It should not be used in pregnancy. Further information on doses is depicted in Table 8.5.

Table 8.5   Doses of mebendazole and piperazine.

Drug	Patient group	Dose
Mebendazole: 100 mg tablets oral suspension 100 mg per 5 ml	Adult & child >2 years	1 tablet sucked or chewed 5 ml **May be repeated if necessary after 2–3 weeks**
Piperazine citrate elixir 750 mg per 5 ml	Adult 7–12 years 4–6 years 2–3 years	15 ml daily for 7 days 10 ml daily for 7 days 7.5 ml daily for 7 days 5 ml daily for 7 days **7 day course may be repeated after 1 week if necessary**
Piperazine and senna powder (dissolve in water before taking)	Adult & child >6 years 1–6 years 3 months–1 year	1 Sachet stat Two-thirds sachet stat One-third sachet stat **Repeat dose after 14 days**

Piperazine

Piperazine is thought to act as an inhibitory agonist on the musculature of worms leading to relaxation. The living paralysed worms are then easily dislodged from their position by peristalsis and are expelled in the faeces (Reynolds, 1996). The dose depends on the preparation prescribed and the age of the patient (see Table 8.5) Side effects include nausea, vomiting, colic, diarrhoea, dizziness and muscle incoordination. In patients with neurological or renal impairment, drowsiness, confusion and clonic contractions have been reported. It should therefore be used with caution in patients with epilepsy or severe liver or renal disease. It should only be used in pregnancy when advised by a doctor.

The use of anthelmintics should be used in conjunction with strict hygiene measures to break the cycle of autoinfection. Patients should be informed of the following points:

- Treat the whole family.
- Wash hands and scrub nails before eating, drinking and after each visit to the toilet.
- Keep nails short during infection.
- Bathe on rising to remove eggs laid during the night.
- Wash bed clothes and underclothes when diagnosis is made and regularly over the next 2–3 weeks.

Drugs for scabies and headlice

Carbaryl and malathion

Carbaryl is a reversible cholinesterase inhibitor belonging to the carbamate group of pesticides. It is used clinically to treat headlice. Malathion is a prodrug which is activated to the organophosphorus anticholinesterase, maloxon, by insects. It is used clinically to treat headlice and scabies. These drugs exert their effects by preventing the breakdown of acetylcholine and interfering with neuromuscular transmission in headlice causing paralysis and preventing them from feeding (Nathan, 1997). Both are available as a lotion or shampoo. In the treatment of headlice the lotion should be applied to the dry hair and scalp and any other infected areas, and allowed to dry naturally. The hair should be combed and the lotion removed after 12 hours by washing.

The shampoo is applied to wet hair and left for 5 minutes; the hair is rinsed and then the application is repeated. The hair should be towel dried and combed. This procedure should be repeated twice at 3 day intervals.

Important points to note when treating headlice are:

- The lotion is preferred to the shampoo because it remains in contact with the hair for longer and is thought to be more effective.
- Treatment should be repeated after 7 days to kill any lice emerging from any eggs that have survived the first application.
- Alcoholic lotions should be avoided in asthmatics and young children.
- Most Health Authorities have a rotational policy to prevent resistance. It is important to find out from the local pharmacy which preparation is currently recommended.

Malathion may also be used to treat scabies. The aqueous lotion should be applied to the whole body, omitting the head and neck, and washed off after 24 hours.

Permethrin and phenothrin

Permethrin and phenothrin are pyrethroid insecticides with low mammalian toxicity. They are rapidly absorbed across the insect cuticle and exert their action on the sodium channels of nerve axons causing excitation and then paralysis. Phenothrin is recommended for the treatment of headlice and should be applied to dry hair and allowed to dry naturally. The hair should be shampooed after 2 hours and combed while still wet. Permethrin can be used in both headlice and scabies. The cream rinse is used to treat headlice. This is applied to clean damp hair and rinsed off after 10 minutes. In scabies the cream is applied to the whole body (excluding the head in adults) and washed off after 8–24 hours. When treating scabies patients should be advised:

- to treat the whole family
- to use only aqueous preparations
- to pay particular attention to webs of fingers and toes when applying lotion
- not to apply preparations after a hot bath as this may increase absorption into the blood, removing it from its site of action on the skin
- that itching may persist for some days after treatment and can be relieved with calamine lotion. However, this is only a short term effect. Other anti-pruritic preparations, such as crotamiton cream, are available over the counter.

Skin preparations

Emollients

Emollients are agents which have a soothing effect on the skin by hydrating the epidermis. They should be applied frequently as their effects are short lived. Preparations in the *NPF* are aqueous cream, hydrous ointment (oily cream) and emulsifying ointment. The latter is usually used as an alternative to soap.

Barrier preparations

These contain a water repellent agent and are used to protect against irritation or repeated moistening, particularly around stoma sites and for nappy rash. Zinc and castor oil ointment is probably the most effective, but preparations containing dimethicone are also available (e.g. Vasogen, Siopel and Conotrane cream).

Pruritus

Pruritus can be due to systemic disease such as drug allergy, jaundice and malignancy, as well as skin diseases like eczema, scabies and urticaria. It is preferable to treat the cause where possible, but agents such as calamine lotion can be soothing.

Fungal infections

Fungal infections thrive in a moist environment. Susceptible areas should be kept clean and dry if possible. Established fungal infections can be treated with clotrimazole cream (Canesten). This is an imidazole antifungal which should be applied 2–3 times daily and continued for 14 days after the infection has cleared.

Boils

Boils are usually treated with systemic antibiotics. Magnesium sulphate paste is sometimes used as an adjuvant to treatment. It should be applied under a dressing. Boils may be associated with diabetes.

Wound management products

Film dressings

Film dressings allow the evaporation of water and are suitable to reduce friction on pressure points or for relatively shallow wounds. They should not be used on fragile skin as they are adhesive and can cause damage when removed.

Hydrocolloids

All hydrocolloids contain methylcellulose and some contain pectin and gelatin. When they come into contact with the wound exudate they liquefy, hydrating the surface and promoting wound healing. They also promote the formation of granulation tissue and provide pain relief by covering nerve endings with gel and exudate. Over-granulation can sometimes occur. Initially they may need to be changed daily but once the exudate decreases, they can be left in place for up to 7 days.

Hydrogels

These compounds are hydrophilic polymers in an aqueous base. They encourage wound healing by hydrating the wound surface, lifting slough and necrotic tissue. They are usually changed daily and require a secondary dressing.

Alginates

These contain sodium alginate or a mixture of calcium and sodium alginate and are derived from seaweed. When they come into contact with wound exudate, they form a moist gel over the surface and promote wound healing. They also have haemostatic properties and are useful to control bleeding. In heavily exuding wounds they are changed daily, but as the exudate reduces, this can be done less frequently. They are unsuitable for dry or necrotic wounds and usually require a secondary dressing. Rope is available for cavities and sinuses.

Foams

Foam dressings absorb exudate laterally and create a moist environment for wound healing. In heavily exuding wounds they should be changed daily, but in those with less exudate, they can be left in place for up to 7 days. No secondary dressing is required. Cavity dressings are also available, but cannot be obtained in the community. (Anderson, 1994).

Dressings listed in the Drug Tariff are shown in Table 8.6.

Nurse prescribing: the future

The developing role of nurses working in the community, for example practice nurses and nurse practitioners, has ensured that the debate surrounding pre-scribing rights for nurses has not abated as a result of introducing limited prescribing rights for some nurses. Many believe that prescribing rights should be extended to other groups. Additionally, it is argued that the current for-mulary is too restrictive as nurses influence doctors' prescribing behaviour and are already making prescribing decisions in areas such as asthma, diabetes, contraception, antibiotics and immunizations, commonly in conjunction with the use of protocols. For this reason it is argued that the formulary should be extended to accommodate the role nurses play in these areas (Mayes, 1996; RCN, 1980, 1995; Wedgewood, 1995). This was acknowledged to some extent by the Crown Report (DH, 1989) which noted that treatment decisions made by nurses are authorized without question by GPs. The concerns regarding the current limitations of nurse prescribing were resolved to some extent by the publication of *Primary Care: Delivering the Future* (DH, 1996) which outlined plans for a staged roll-out of nurse prescribing with a view to national roll-out by 1998. Whilst the change in government has led to a delay, commitment to a full roll-out has been expressed by the Secretary of State for Health and there are indications that prescribing may be extended to other specialist nurses. In addition, the concern surrounding group protocol prescribing and the limita-tions of the formulary has prompted a further review of the prescribing, supply and administration of medicines (DH, 1997). The full findings of the review team are awaited, although an interim report on prescribing by protocol has been published (DH, 1998). The review team notes that, in general, patients should receive medicines on an individual basis, but acknowledges that there is likely to be some need for the supply and administration of medicines under group protocol in certain limited situations. In the absence of a clear legal position it is suggested that group protocols for the supply and administration of medicines should comply with set criteria; these include the clinical con-

Table 8.6 Dressings available in the *Drug Tariff*.

	Size	Type of wound
Low adherent dressings		
NA Dressing	Both 9.5 cm × 9.5 cm	Dry or lightly exuding wounds
Tricotrex		
Vapour permeable films		
Opsite	10 cm × 12 cm	Post-operative dressing
Tegaderm	10 cm × 12 cm	Donor sites
Bioclusive	10.2 cm × 12.7 cm	Decubitus ulcers
Cutifilm	7.5 cm × 10 cm	Amputation stumps
	10 cm × 14 cm	Stoma care
Hydrogels and desloughing agents		
Intrasite gel	15 g sachet	Desloughing
Dextranomer (Debrisan)	4 g beads	Light or medium exuding wounds
	4 × 10 g sachet of paste	Necrotic wounds (Avoid if anaerobic infection)
Alginates		
Kaltogel	5 cm × 5 cm	Moderately exuding wounds
	10 cm × 10 cm	Pressure sores
		Leg ulcers
Kaltostat	5 cm × 5 cm	Haemostatic
	7.5 cm × 12 cm	
	2 g packing	Rope useful for cavities
		Heavily exuding wounds
Sorbsan	5 cm × 5 cm	
	10 cm × 10 cm	
	Packing 30 cm	
	Ribbon with probe 40 cm	
Tegagen	5 cm × 5 cm	
	10 cm × 10cm	
Hydrocolloids		
Comfeel/Comfeel Plus	10 cm × 10 cm	Desloughing agents
	15 cm × 15 cm	Necrotic wounds
	20 cm × 20 cm	Light and medium exuding wounds (not if infected)
Comfeel Alginate	4 cm × 6 cm	
	10 cm × 10 cm	
Granuflex	10 cm × 10 cm	
	15 cm × 15 cm	
	15 cm × 20 cm	
	20 cm × 20 cm	
Tegasorb	10 cm × 12 cm (oval)	
	13 cm × 15 cm (oval)	
Foam dressings		
Lyofoam	7.5 cm × 7.5 cm	Exuding wounds
	10 cm × 10 cm	Burns
	10 cm × 17.5 cm	Decubitus ulcers
Allevyn/Allevyn adhesive	15 cm × 20 cm	Donor sites
	5 cm × 5 cm	Granulation
	10 cm × 10 cm	
	10 cm × 20 cm	
	20 cm × 20 cm	

dition or situation to which the protocol applies, the staff authorised to take responsibility for the supply or administration of medicines under a group protocol, a description of the treatment available under the protocol, and details of the management and monitoring of the protocol.

Summary

There is no doubt that nurses do have a key role to play in the management and administration of medicines, and this is discussed in detail in Chapters 11 and 12. Historically, prescribing has been the prerogative of doctors. Despite the fact that some nurses can administer controlled drugs, sometimes on a *pro re nata* (PRN) basis, nurses in general are not legally entitled to prescribe mild analgesics such as paracetamol or aspirin. However the Medicines Act 1968 does permit doctors to delegate responsibility to nurses to administer medicines in accordance with their instructions. This delegated responsibility can be observed in a hospital setting where nurses often assume responsibility for the selection of wound and skin care products. In some instances, the administration of medicines in a hospital setting has been formalized by the production of local protocols (Mallet, 1997; Marshall, 1997).

However, the legality of prescribing items in accordance with locally devised protocols is an area of debate at present (Naish, 1996). This should be resolved following the publication of findings from the DH consultative document (DH, 1997) which will be used to establish the circumstances in which health professionals can undertake new roles with regard to the prescribing or supply of medicines, and the associated implications for legislation and training.

References

Anderson, R. (1994) Pressure sores and leg ulcers. In: *Clinical Pharmacy and Therapeutics* (eds R. Walker & C. Edwards), pp. 769–81. Churchill Livingstone, Edinburgh.

Bowman, W.C. & Rand, M.J. (1984) *Textbook of Pharmacology*, 2nd edn. Blackwell, Oxford.

British Medical Association & Royal Pharmaceutical Society of Great Britain in association with the Health Visitors' Association & Royal College of Nursing (1994) *Nurse Prescribers' Formulary 1994* (pilot edition). British Medical Association and Pharmaceutical Association, London.

Courtenay, M. & Butler, M. (1998) Nurse prescribing – the knowledge base. *Nursing Times* **94**(1), 40–2.

Department of Health and Social Security (1986) Neighbourhood nursing – a focus for care. *Report of the Community Nursing Service Review (Cumberlege Report)*. HMSO, London.

Department of Health (1989) *Report of the Advisory Group on Nurse Prescribing* (Crown Report). HMSO, London.

Department of Health (1996) *Primary Care: Delivering the Future*. HMSO, London.

Department of Health (1997) *Review of Prescribing. Supply and Administration of Medicines.* NHS Executive, Leeds.

Department of Health (1998) *Review of Prescribing, Supply and Administration of Medicines. Report on Supply and Administration of Medicines under Group Protocol.* HSC, 1998/051, NHS Executive, Leeds.

Edwards, C. & Stillman, P. (1993) Constipation. *Pharm. J.* **251**, 53–5.

English National Board (1992) Nurse prescribing: guidelines for the preparation of district nurses and health visitors. *Circular 1992/30/MB.* English National Board for Nursing, Midwifery and Health Visiting, London.

Fawcett-Henesy, A. (1988) Tools of the trade. *Community Outlook* (supplement to the *Nursing Times*). February.

Foster, R.W. (ed) (1986) *Basic Pharmacology,* 2nd edn. Butterworths, London.

Luker, K.A., Ferguson, B., Austin, L., Hogg, C., Jenkins-Clark, S., Willock, J., Smith, K. & Wright, K. (1997a) *Evaluating Nurse Prescribing.* Department of Health, London (unpublished report).

Luker, K.A, Austin, L., Hogg, C., Ferguson, B. & Smith, K. (1997b) Nurse prescribing: the views of nurses and other health care professionals. *Br. J. Community Health Nursing* **2**, 69–74.

Luker, K.A., Austin, L., Hogg, C., Ferguson, B. & Smith, K. (1997c) Patients' views of nurse prescribing. *Nursing Times* **23**(17), 51–54.

Luker, K.A. & Austin, L. (1997d) Nurse prescribing: study findings and GP views. *Prescriber* **8** (9), 31–34.

Luker, K.A., Austin, L., Willock, J., Ferguson, B. & Smith, K. (1997e) Nurses' and GPs' views of the nurse prescribers' formulary. *Nursing Standard* **22**(11), 33–8.

Luker, K.A., Hogg, C., Austin, L., Ferguson, B. & Smith, K. (1997f) Over-the-counter items bought by a sample of community nurse patients. *Br. J. Community Health Nursing* **2**(2), 75–82.

Luker, K.A., Hogg, C., Austin, L., Ferguson, B. & Smith, K. (1998a) Decision making: the context of nurse prescribing, *J. Adv Nursing* **27**, 657–5.

Luker, K.A., Austin, L., Hogg, C., Ferguson, B. & Smith, K. (1998b) Nurse patient relationships: the context of nurse prescribing. *J. Adv. Nursing* **28**, 235–42.

Luscombe, D.K. (1994) Constipation and diarrhoea. In: *Clinical Pharmacy and Therapeutics* (eds R. Walker & C. Edwards), pp. 153–66. Churchill Livingstone, Edinburgh.

Mallett, J. (1997) Nurse prescribing by protocol. *Nursing Times* **93**(8), 50–2.

Marshall, J. (1997) Protocols and emergency nurse practitioners. *Nursing Times* **93**(19), 58–9.

Mayes, M. (1996) A study of prescribing patterns in the community. *Nursing Standard* **5**(8), 4–5.

Medicines Resource Centre (1994) The treatment of constipation. *MeReC Bull.* **5**, 21–4.

Mehta, D.K. (1997) *British National Formulary No 34.* British Medical Association and Royal Pharmaceutical Society of Great Britain, London.

Naish, J. (1996) Prescribed confusion. *Nursing Times* **92**(49), 56.

Nathan, A. (1997) Products for hair and scalp problems. *Pharm. J.* **258**, 629–32.

Nursing Standard (1990) Nurses demand the right to prescribe. *Nursing Standard (suppl.)* **4**(44), 13–14.

Pedler, S.J. (1994) Fungal infections. In: *Clinical Pharmacy and Therapeutics* (eds R. Walker & C. Edwards), pp. 587–99. Churchill Livingstone, Edinburgh.

Poulton, B.C. (1994) Nurse prescribing broadening the scope of nursing practice. *Int. Nursing Rev* **41**(3), 81–4.

Reynolds, J.E.F. (1996) *The Extra Pharmacopoeia*, 31st edn. Royal Pharmaceutical Society of Great Britain, London.

Royal College of Nursing (1980) *Nurse Prescribers of Oral Contraceptives for the Well Woman*. RCN, London.

Royal College of Nursing (1995) *Whose Prescription?* RCN, London.

United Kingdom Central Council for Nursing, Midwifery and Health Visiting (1997) *Response to the Review of Prescribing, Supply and Administration of Medicines*. UKCC, London.

Wedgewood, A. (1995) The case for prescribing the pill. *Nursing Times* **91**(50), 25–7.

Wynne, H.A. & Edwards, C. (1992) Which Drug? Laxatives. *Pharm. J.* **248**, 17–19.

Chapter 9
Prescribed Medicines in Primary Care (General Practice)

Nicholas W. Hough

Controversies in therapeutics

This chapter is intended to give a flavour of some of the 'controversies' which surround the use of medicines in primary care. Three specific therapeutic areas or categories of drugs are discussed, but a different three could equally have been chosen in order to highlight the same difficulties and types of issues that GPs have in deciding which drugs to prescribe. In the space available, what follows is not meant to be an exhaustive review of each subject but represents, from the author's point of view, some important factors which influence prescribing practice and drug choice. Readers who want to follow up any of the topics in more detail should consult the reading list at the end of the chapter, and also refer to the *British National Formulary (BNF)* (Mehta, 1997) for detailed prescribing information about individual drugs mentioned. Following the discussion on the three therapeutic areas, information is given on repeat prescribing, bulk prescribing and prescribing for addicts.

'Controversy' is not meant to convey the image of doctors arguing about what constitutes best prescribing practice; the word is used here because there are often valid reasons, either substantiated in the medical literature or born out of clinical experience, for accepting different positions on treatment preferences. These may involve the choice between one class of drugs or another, or the selection of one particular drug within the same category. Further debate may arise from a consideration of patient factors which determine different approaches to treatment; for example, is treatment being given where lifestyle changes might be more appropriate and equally effective, or is it out of convenience that something is prescribed long-term rather than attempting to eliminate the source of the problem in the first place?

There is much debate about the use of new drugs in place of older more established ones. Undoubtedly, many new medicines bring much wanted benefits, especially in conditions and diseases where previous treatments have been relatively ineffective. However, many new drugs represent only minor modifications of existing agents, or are reformulations of older drugs, such as modified-release tablets/capsules, which do not really herald major advances in therapy. Some new drugs with novel modes of action, such as interacting with a different receptor site or inhibiting a different enzyme, are often heavily promoted to doctors with the emphasis on this fact, but this does not necessarily mean that they are more likely to be effective in the long or even the short term.

There is also a price to pay for innovation, and particularly in days of increasing budgetary awareness, new treatments have to show evidence of cost-effectiveness. Even this does not always carry the case for a new drug if, whilst the total costs of treatment are reduced as a result of savings made elsewhere in the health service (e.g. through reduced hospitalisation), the size and rate of rise of the drugs bill increases.

Finally, there is the debate around implementing evidence-based practice. In theory, the field of medicines use and prescribing should be particularly suited to this approach, since drugs are subject to the most intense research and investigation through clinical trials in order to gain a product licence. Reports of the results of such clinical trials with both new and established drugs abound in the medical literature, and this should provide a sufficient evidence-base for those involved in undertaking meta-analyses and systematic reviews of the literature. However, there remains the major problem that, when taking part in clinical trials, what happens to patients and how they respond to treatment do not often reflect the real life situation. The gap between the real world where patients initially present with undifferentiated symptoms, and the research environment where patients are 'worked up' and full diagnostic procedures are available, means that practitioners cannot always apply to their everyday practice the results of well controlled and properly conducted clinical trials.

Some of the preceding issues are illustrated in the following three discussions which focus on the use of acid suppressants, the treatment of hypertension, and the use of non-steroidal anti-inflammatory drugs (NSAIDs). The discussion is kept relatively brief here, while some of the issues are quite complex if the medical literature on these subjects is reviewed in greater depth.

Use of acid suppressants (drugs for healing peptic ulcers)

The treatment of acid-related gastro-intestinal (GI) disorders is worthy of close scrutiny because the two main groups of drugs – the histamine type-2 receptor antagonists (H_2RAs) and the proton pump inhibitors (PPIs) – currently account for just over 10% of the total NHS primary care drugs bill! Considering that these two types of drugs were only first widely available about 20 years ago and 5 years ago, respectively, it is not difficult to appreciate the massive impact they must have had on clinical practice in recent years. However, one might also reasonably conclude that we either have an 'epidemic' of acid-related GI disorders on our hands, or that these types of drugs are far too readily prescribed instead of doing something else to eliminate the need for them in the first place.

The following is a list of the H$_2$RAs and PPIs presently available in the UK.

H$_2$RAs	PPIs
• Cimetidine	• Omeprazole
• Ranitidine	• Lansoprazole
• Famotidine	• Pantoprazole
• Nizatidine	

Background to the use of H$_2$RAs and PPIs

Both groups of drugs have been shown to be remarkably safe when used for relatively long periods, and that they are also very effective in relieving symptoms and preventing serious complications. These are the probable reasons for their widespread popularity amongst doctors and patients alike; there are few people who have not heard of Zantac (and even Losec), even though they may not have been prescribed it for themselves.

It has long been appreciated that these types of drugs do not bring about a complete cure in those conditions which respond to lowering the acidity (increasing the pH) of gastric secretions. Rather, these drugs allow the normal mucosal repair processes to take place in the stomach and duodenum, thereby 'healing' erosions and ulcers which would persist in more acidic conditions. Consequently many patients with proven ulcer disease require long term treatment, perhaps lifelong, with H$_2$RAs and PPIs in order to prevent relapse and the potentially serious complications thereof.

Since discontinuing therapy often leads to ulcer recurrence, the decision has to be taken whether to use a daily maintenance dose, or to treat each recurrence with a separate course of healing therapy. Those with more frequently relapsing disease (e.g. more than once a year), frail and elderly people would be more suitable for the former, whereas more healthy patients with infrequent symptoms might be offered the latter.

Economic as well as clinical considerations also come into play, since long term maintenance therapy, albeit using lower doses than those used for healing ulcers, is expensive. However, this has to be seen against the total costs of ulcer relapse which may well include more expensive hospitalisation. It has been argued many times that the high costs associated with the use of modern acid suppressants have been more than offset by savings in hospital care, not too mention relief of patient suffering and reduced loss of earnings due to ill health.

Recent developments with ulcer healing drugs

In the specific area of acid suppression therapy, most attention over the last 10–15 years has been paid to optimising the dosing regimen of H$_2$RAs, e.g. moving from divided daily doses to once daily therapy. Also, attention has been focused on reassuring doctors of the safety of using drugs which profoundly suppress acid secretion for long periods of time. Concerns were particularly expressed when PPIs were first introduced, but gradually these fears have subsided and patients have been maintained on therapy for several years without obvious dangers coming to light.

However, over much the same time period as this was happening some researchers were beginning to question the role of a bacterium present in the stomachs of ulcer patients. Whilst it was known that certain other factors besides gastric acid were involved in predisposing patients to ulcer development (e.g. smoking, excessive alcohol intake, lifestyle), few gastroenterologists were inclined to believe that there was a causative infectious link.

The bacterium *Campylobacter pylori*, now called *Helicobacter pylori*, had actually been known about for some time, but it was an Australian doctor who was one of the first to demonstrate the potential for 'curing' ulcer disease completely. He deliberately 'infected' himself by swallowing a suspension of the above organism, developing the tell-tale signs of ulcer disease, and then took an antibiotic which 'cured' the problem (Marshall *et al.*, 1985). Others were also working along the same lines, so it is difficult to say precisely at what stage widespread opinion on the treatment of peptic ulcers began to change in a new direction.

Another strand in this story was the knowledge that ulcers 'healed' with a different type of drug from the acid suppressants, namely a bismuth-based preparation, tended to relapse less frequently 'off treatment' (i.e. when it was discontinued after ulcer healing had occurred) than those in people who had previously received H$_2$RAs and PPIs to heal their ulcers. However, compared to H$_2$RAs and PPIs, bismuth was not very popular because preparations of it were, and still are, not very palatable and there were also some fears about toxicity. Thus, a great deal of attention was focused on long term maintenance therapies with acid suppressants.

The current situation

It is now recognised, however, that 'curing' peptic ulcer disease is a realistic therapeutic goal in many patients. It is very common to see the phrase 'eradication therapy' to describe the use of a combination of drugs to eliminate *H. pylori* from the stomach, and patients are categorised, if they have been appropriately tested, as *H. pylori* positive or negative. However, there are still many problems to overcome, so acid suppressants have by no means had their day. Some of the issues to be resolved are discussed below and more details can be found in the references in the further reading list under Acid Suppressants.

- Which patients have ulcers caused by *H. pylori* and how can they be identified in general practice?
- Is it appropriate to treat patients 'blind', i.e. without undertaking, or whilst awaiting the results of, *H. pylori* screening?

- Should attention be focused on new patients, or those already on long term maintenance with acid suppresssants, or both?
- Which is the best 'eradication' regimen – finding the balance between effectiveness and compliance?
- How should eradication be confirmed – follow-up testing or observing symptoms?
- Will resistance emerge with the more widespread use of antibiotics?

In many ways, the fact that peptic ulcer disease can be cured should be a significant advantage to those who look after patients in primary care. In theory, there should be fewer repeat prescriptions for relatively expensive drugs like PPIs and H_2RAs, which will help reduce the size of the drugs bill. On the other hand, there are patients with ulcers and/or symptoms who will not benefit from eradication therapy, including those with gastro-intestinal problems due to the use of NSAIDs and those with gastro-oesophageal reflux disease (GORD). Neither of these groups is suitable for eradication therapy, and GORD seems to be the major reason for the particularly widespread use of PPIs. If there were space here, the latter would lend itself to a discussion of whether patients should pay more attention to lifestyle changes rather than relying on medication for relief of their symptoms.

Near patient testing kits are now available which can be used in general practice to detect the presence of *H. pylori* antibodies in a drop of blood. Previously, the only methods available were a breath test and endoscopic biopsy, both requiring attendance at hospital. Not enough is known about the reliability of testing patients in the surgery for it to be widely recommended, but some GPs are taking a more positive approach and are managing an increasing number of ulcer patients with eradication therapy.

There are those who feel that pre-treatment testing is not required because the prevalence of *H. pylori* associated ulcers is so high that a course of eradication therapy is as good a first step as any. If the patient is *H. pylori* positive and complies with an effective eradication regimen, a positive outcome will confirm the diagnosis for the doctor, the patient's symptoms will be relieved and a potentially serious problem cured, and the expense and inconvenience of long term therapy will be avoided. If the patient's symptoms continue after completing a proven treatment, then another cause for the problem can be sought, probably necessitating specialist investigation.

Patients who have been shown to require long term maintenance therapy (because they relapse 'off treatment') may also be suitable for eradication therapy without first confirming the presence of *H. pylori*. The fact that they are in this 'therapeutic state' strongly suggests that there is some precipitating factor that has not been dealt with adequately. Many patients might accept the short term inconvenience associated with many of the eradication regimens in the knowledge that this might eliminate the need for the alternative of lifelong tablet taking.

H. pylori *eradication regimens*

Table 9.1 lists only a few of the possible *H. pylori* eradication regimens; there now appear to be well over 100 different combinations available, each with its own merits. Particular efforts have been made to reduce both the number of drugs in the combination and the duration of therapy, whilst at the same time maintaining efficacy. The 'gold standard' against which all options are compared is 'triple therapy' for 2 weeks, as shown in Table 9.1. The first attempts at 'dual therapy' tended to have slightly lower eradication rates, but more patients may be able to adhere to treatment, perhaps making them nearly as effective in practice as 'triple therapy' because of its inevitable compliance problems. One H_2RA, ranitidine, has now been chemically linked to the bismuth molecule in the same tablet in a further attempt to simplify treatment.

Table 9.1 *Helicobacter pylori* eradication regimens[a]

One week regimens (acid supressant plus two antibiotics)
Omeprazole 20 mg b.d./40 mg o.d. OR lansoprazole 30 mg b.d.
with either
metronidazole 400 mg t.d.s. AND amoxycillin (amoxicillin) 500 mg t.d.s.
  OR
Tinidazole 500 mg b.d. OR metronidazole 400 mg b.d. AND clarithromycin 500 mg b.d./
250 mg b.d.
  OR
Amoxycillin (amoxicillin) 1 g b.d. AND clarithromycin 500 mg b.d.

Two week regimens (bismuth compound plus two antibiotics):
Tripotassium dicitratobismuthate 120 mg q.d.s. AND oxytetracycline 500 mg q.d.s. AND
metronidazole 400 mg t.d.s.

---

[a] Based on British Society of Gastroenterology – Dyspepsia Management Guidelines, September 1996; see Medicines Resource Centre (1997) which provides further details, and also Mehta (1997) for more examples of regimens and some advisory notes.

Management of gastro-intestinal disorders in general practice

As stated, the 'eradication' approach is not suitable for NSAID related problems or GORD. It is possible to enquire about the use of NSAIDs and take appropriate action, but it may be impossible to differentiate between the symptoms of GORD and peptic ulcer. This is one of the main problems facing GPs in this therapeutic area because without being able to determine precisely what is responsible for a patient's symptoms, many prescriptions are written presumptively. It is, of course, impractical to endoscope every patient before doing something to relieve their immediate symptoms.

One approach is to use a 'step-wise' progression through the range of acid suppressant drugs available: first a trial of simple antacids that can be bought in a pharmacy plus lifestyle advice, followed if necessary by a course of H_2RAs, and finally referral and/or a course of PPIs. However, this can be very time consuming for the GP and patient, perhaps requiring several visits to the surgery. Since dyspepsia is one of the commonest presenting symptoms in general practice, it is not too surprising that PPIs appear to be used increasingly frequently as a first line therapy. Thus the patient gains access to a potent and very effective treatment, though not a cure, and the GP saves a lot of valuable time.

Guidelines and protocols, covering treatment and referral, have been produced by many health authorities and specialist groups based on these types of approach, as seen in the British Society of Gastroenterology Guidelines on Dyspepsia (Medicines Resource Centre, 1997). They take into account the fact that the nature and severity of the symptoms do not always help in establishing a diagnosis; mild symptoms can be associated with more severe ulceration, and patients with few physical symptoms can suddenly present with a bleeding peptic ulcer. There are also some symptoms which require immediate specialist investigation, such as weight loss, anaemia or other signs of blood loss. Age is another important factor since gastric cancer is less common under the age of about 45 years.

It may be that eradication therapy will replace the need for so many prescriptions of long term H_2RAs and PPIs in peptic ulcer disease. Even so, there still seems to be a problem with the prevalence of GORD, a condition that responds very well to PPIs but not so well to H_2RAs. Lifestyle changes would probably do much to lessen the burden of suffering for patients and expense to the NHS, especially in the areas of smoking cessation, curbing excessive alcohol intake, and improving poor dietary habits. The next few years will see whether the initial promise of eradication therapy can bring real benefits to a wide range of patients and also reduce 'therapeutic dependence' on long-term maintenance therapy with acid suppressants.

Hypertension

Hypertension is one of the commonest cardiovascular disorders managed by GPs, although it is widely thought that it is still undertreated and could be targeted more effectively as a cardiovascular risk factor. There is a wide variety of effective drugs available in several different pharmacological categories, the main ones being thiazide diuretics, beta-adrenoceptor blocking drugs (beta-blockers), calcium channel blockers (calcium antagonists), and angiotensin-converting enzyme inhibitors (ACE inhibitors). Other less popular established drugs include the alpha-antagonists, methyldopa, and ganglion blockers.

Hypertension is still a very popular area for the pharmaceutical industry in terms of introducing new drugs, both variations within an existing class, and drugs with a completely novel mode of action; recent new categories include the angiotensin-II receptor antagonists and the potassium channel blockers. Consequently there is much debate about the relative merits of the different treatments available. This debate is also fuelled by the fact that the older drugs, which still have a definite place in therapy, cost only a few pence per month per patient, whereas the newer classes of agents may be between £10–20 per month.

It is difficult to put an exact figure on how much the NHS spends in treating hypertension, since many of the drugs are also used for other cardiovascular disorders and it is impossible to dissect out the relevant proportions from national prescribing analysis and cost (PACT) data. It is likely that the total costs of anti-hypertensives run into tens of millions of pounds, but this must be seen in the context of savings to the rest of the health service through the prevention of major complications, such as heart failure, stroke and renal failure, which may require expensive hospital treatment.

Which drugs should be used?

Treating hypertension is an effective intervention because it has been shown to prevent long-term complications such as stroke and· more serious cardio-vascular disease. It is the basis of the evidence for this which, for many cardiovascular specialists, determines a rational approach to drug selection from the many alternatives available. There are only two groups of drugs which have been shown to reduce long-term mortality from the complications of hypertension and these are the thiazide diuretics, for example bendro-fluazide (bendroflumethiazide), and the beta-adrenoceptor blocking drugs (beta-blockers), for example propranolol.

There is widespread support for the use of these types of drugs as first line treatment, and some concern that the newer, more expensive drugs should not replace them before they are proved to produce the same overall benefits. However, there is also the argument that since all classes of antihypertensives reduce blood pressure to approximately the same extent, then the same longterm benefits might reasonably be expected regardless of which class of drug is used at the outset (Medicines Resource Centre, 1995).

The costs of abandoning thiazides and beta-blockers entirely in favour of newer agents might run into tens or even hundreds of millions of pounds, and would not represent an evidence-based medicine approach to treatment. Given the current emphasis in the NHS for selecting medical interventions on the basis of proven evidence of effectiveness, it would seem only logical to select those antihypertensive agents which have actually been shown to prevent long-term complications.

There are two further points to consider, however, before finally arriving at a rational approach to the selection of antihypertensive medication. The first is that not all patients with hypertension can tolerate or be safely prescribed thiazides or beta-blockers. For example, asthmatic patients should not be given beta-blockers because these drugs might precipitate bronchospasm, and thia-zide diuretics should be avoided in patients with gout since they may elevate uric acid levels. There are a number of other adverse effects associated with these two groups of drugs which may preclude their use as first line treatment in patients with certain other medical conditions. Secondly, there are patients with additional cardiovascular problems for whom one of the newer drugs might bring dual benefits. For example, hypertensive patients with symptoms of coronary heart disease (angina) or poor peripheral circulation may usefully be treated with a calcium antagonist, and ACE inhibitors may be preferred in the diabetic hypertensive because of their potentially protective effects on the kidney. Recent data have cast doubt over the safety of, particularly, short-acting calcium antogonists; for example, an increased risk of cardiovascular events such as myocardial infarction has been observed in a number of studies when compared to other forms of antihypertensive medication. The evidence in the medical literature is sometimes controversial on this topic and the issues have not been completely resolved.

Current approaches to antihypertensive therapy

As a result of all of this, recently published guidelines for the treatment of hypertension have tended to promote an approach based on tailoring the drug to the individual patient, taking into account factors such as those outlined above. Previously, guidelines were based on the 'stepped care' approach, where the first step meant a thiazide diuretic or beta-blocker, followed by a combination of drugs if single drug therapy failed to bring about a sufficient decrease in blood pressure. The newer drugs, such as ACE inhibitors and calcium antagonists, were reserved for those patients failing to respond to this type of approach, or for those intolerant to the more established drugs, or where the latter were specifically contra-indicated.

There is still some emphasis on the fact that the only positive data on long-term outcomes is derived from clinical trial experience with thiazides and beta-blockers, but there is now also more recognition of the differing needs of specific types of patients and the need to take a more pragmatic approach to treatment.

A list of the types of drugs which may be used to lower blood pressure is given in Table 9.2. Some older drugs are no longer routinely used to treat new patients with hypertension, but they may be continued in some patients who have remained stable on them for many years, and for whom a change in therapy might be an unnecessary inconvenience. Thus drugs such as methyl-dopa, or vasodilators (in combination with beta-blockers to prevent reflex tachycardia), and even adrenergic neurone blockers may rarely be seen.

Practical advice for prescribers

There are currently in excess of 60 different 'active ingredients' available in a much larger number of formulations. There are some which are combination tablets containing two different drugs, and some which are modified-release in order to prolong their duration of action. Although there are some advantages in having so many alternatives to choose from, by and large most GPs could

Table 9.2   Antihypertensive agents – examples from each major therapeutic class.

Beta-adrenoceptor blocking drugs (beta-blockers):	Atenolol Propranolol Oxprenolol Metoprolol Labetalol
Thiazide diuretics:	Bendrofluazide (bendroflumethiazide) Chlorthalidone (chlortalidone) Hydrochlorothiazide Indapamide
Angiotensin-converting enzyme inhibitors (ACE inhibitors):	Captopril Enalapril Lisinopril
Calcium channel blockers (calcium antagonists):	Nifedipine Verapamil Amlodipine Diltiazem
Other examples of antihypertensive agents:	Prazosin (alpha-adrenoceptor blocker) Methyldopa (centrally acting) Losartan (angiotensin II receptor antagonist)

probably manage with a reasonably small selection. Bearing in mind all the points mentioned previously about relative merits of the different classes of antihypertensive drugs available, it would be a rational prescriber who became familiar with, maybe, a dozen or so drugs selected from the wide range available across the different therapeutic classes.

New types of drugs should be critically examined to determine whether they really add anything new to the already overcrowded antihypertensive market. Recent examples may offer some advantages in specific groups of patients, but on the whole there is no overwhelming evidence to support their use ahead of more tried and tested effective treatments.

The treatment of hypertension is not just a matter of choosing the right drug for the right patient, however, or even having the most evidence-based cardiovascular drug formulary. One of the most important factors is how to identify those patients who need treatment, how to manage their ongoing therapy, and how to avoid treating those patients who do not really have hypertension. This all comes down to how the practice operates and whether an agreed protocol has been developed with input from all those who are likely to be involved in its implementation.

It has often been emphasised that patients should have their blood pressure recorded on three separate occasions before instituting antihypertensive therapy. This is to ensure that a true reading has been obtained and that patients are not 'labelled' as hypertensive when they are not. 'White coat' hypertension describes the effect that some patients experience when they undergo examination, namely that their blood pressure rises as a consequence of the 'stress' involved in visiting the doctor. After repeated measurements over a period of several months these patients are found to have normal blood pressure, and are therefore spared the consequences of embarking on lifelong therapy for a condition they do not have.

This last point highlights the need for patients who really do have hypertension to understand that their treatment is likely to be lifelong. Compliance, or as it is now known 'adherence to medication' or 'concordance', is probably more of a problem in a condition like hypertension which is generally symptomless, but for which there is the hope of fewer complications later in life if treatment is adhered to. The rationale behind 'tailoring the drug to the patient' becomes even more important if it ensures that the patient experiences the minimum of adverse effects and finds the treatment easy to take.

Non-steroidal anti-inflammatory drugs (NSAIDs)

These drugs attract a lot of attention because many can be bought and they are so frequently prescribed, particularly in those patients who are amongst the most susceptible to the adverse effects of this type of therapy. Furthermore, this is a therapeutic area where there have been many new drugs over the years, often introduced by their manufacturers with the promise of reduced gastrointestinal toxicity. In practice, however, this has not generally been shown to be the case, and prescribers still need to exercise caution in their use of NSAIDs, and to consider whether prescribing them for some patients is necessarily the most appropriate course of action to take.

For what are NSAIDs prescribed?

NSAIDs are used in conditions for which their anti-inflammatory properties are required, such as rheumatoid arthritis, and in many situations where their analgesic effects are considered to be beneficial, for example soft tissue injuries and back pain. It is in these latter situations that many have questioned whether NSAIDs are the most appropriate choice of therapy, and also whether enough steps have been taken to try other forms of therapy before moving on to NSAIDs.

It is generally considered that in single doses there is not much to choose between the simple analgesic paracetamol and an NSAID in terms of analgesic properties. The difference between them is found when they are used chronically, because when used in this way, as their name suggests, the NSAIDs also have anti-inflammatory properties. Thus they are particularly useful in those conditions associated with an inflammatory component such as rheumatoid arthritis, but there is some debate as to their relative benefits in non-inflammatory conditions such as osteoarthritis.

Choosing between NSAIDs

One of the main difficulties in determining the most appropriate place in therapy for the various NSAIDs which are available is the nature of the vast amount of clinical trial data that has been generated to support their use. Although there is a considerable mass of documented evidence of their effectiveness, several important questions remain unanswered. Given that there are in excess of 20 different NSAIDs available, that is different chemical entities as opposed to dosage forms, it is extremely difficult to rank them in terms of their potency or risk–benefit ratio. In terms of their safety profiles, and generally what most doctors are concerned about is gastro-intestinal toxicity, it is similarly difficult to determine with absolute certainty which NSAIDs should be preferred.

Furthermore, in some conditions in which NSAIDs are very widely prescribed, there are not enough data comparing them with the simple analgesic paracetamol or paracetamol/low-dose opiate combinations (e.g. co-dydramol). The paucity of data in this respect was commented on fairly recently (Dieppe *et al.*, 1993) and only three or four randomised double-blind clinical trials with a few representatives of the NSAID group were identified, which compared their efficacy with that of paracetamol in the treatment of osteoarthritis.

Differences in efficacy and safety

What has emerged from the widespread clinical experience gained with the use of NSAIDs is that there is some variability in the degree to which different patients respond to the same or different drugs. It is generally thought that about 60% of patients can be expected to respond to any one NSAID; those that do not will probably respond to another. The problem is that it is impossible to predict in advance which patients will do well, both in terms of gaining the benefits of therapy and avoiding side effects (Medicines Resource Centre, 1994).

Several attempts have been made to identify which of the NSAIDs are likely to be the safest and which should be avoided as first line treatments. There are some specific problems associated with certain individual members of this group, but the general problem is one that has already been referred to – namely gastro-intestinal toxicity. NSAIDs are known to cause damage to the gastro-intestinal tract and in extreme cases this can be severe enough to cause haemorrhage leading to death.

Using records of prescription numbers, i.e. the number of prescriptions of a particular NSAID issued over a given period of time, and combining this with the number and type of adverse effects reported to the Committee on Safety of Medicines (CSM) in association with various NSAIDs, some attempts have been made to express the incidence of gastrointestinal adverse effects across the group as a whole. This type of work has been supplemented by other retrospective case control studies and there has been some consistency in the results obtained.

For seven oral NSAIDs the CSM has issued advice on the relative risks of serious gastro-intestinal effects associated with their use; of those NSAIDs considered, azapropazone is associated with the highest risk, and ibuprofen the lowest. Five others are associated with intermediate risks – piroxicam, keto-profen, indomethacin, naproxen and diclofenac (in piroxicam's case the risk may possibly be higher). The CSM advised that there were not enough data to draw any conclusions about all the other available oral NSAIDs.

Practical prescribing advice for GPs

The fact that ibuprofen and certain other NSAIDs have been identified as being associated with a relatively lower risk of gastro-intestinal toxicity should not lead prescribers into a false sense of security regarding how these drugs should be used. The CSM also recommends that in addition to generally preferring one of the NSAIDs associated with low risk, treatment should be started at the lowest recommended dose, and no more than one NSAID should be used for the same patient at the same time.

Obviously, these drugs should be avoided in patients with peptic ulcer disease, and in patients with a history of this condition they should only be used after other forms of treatment have been carefully considered. Elderly people are another group for whom particularly special care should be taken when prescribing NSAIDs, and the *BNF* (Mehta, 1997) contains further advice in this respect. In summary it states that:

- for *osteoarthritis, soft tissue lesions* and *back pain*, weight reduction, warmth, exercise and the use of a walking stick should be tried first;
- for these same conditions and *rheumatoid arthritis*, NSAIDs should be avoided unless paracetamol (alone or in a combination product containing a low-dose opiate, for example co-codamol or co-dydramol) fails to relieve the pain
- if the latter is the case then a very low dose of a NSAID should be added to the paracetamol (ibuprofen should be tried first), and
- if an NSAID is considered necessary, the patient should be monitored for signs of gastro-intestinal bleeding for 4 weeks

(Combination products containing paracetamol with a low dose opiate may not provide significant additional pain relief compared to paracetamol alone. The low dose opioid may also be enough to cause side effects such as constipation and can complicate the treatment of overdose.)

One approach that has been widely recommended is that doctors should prescribe from a range of just three or four of the 'safer' NSAIDs. and thereby gain through clinical experience a better understanding of how well they work and are tolerated in the types of patients seen in their practices. In addition to adopting this approach, it should be remembered that whereas the analgesic effects of these drugs usually become apparent after only a few days, their anti-inflammatory effects may take up to 2–3 weeks to be recognised. Therefore, before switching to another NSAID within the selected range, an appropriate length of time should be allowed for the initial treatment to take full effect.

Some commentators regard the spread of prescribing across the NSAID group as a measure of prescribing quality. Thus, those who rely on a relatively small range of drugs might be considered to be more rational prescribers than those who seem to use a wide variety with no obvious preference for two or three drugs over all the others. The latter approach may reflect a desire to keep trying something new in the hope of getting a little extra therapeutic benefit. However, as mentioned previously, there is not a great deal of evidence to separate these drugs in terms of efficacy, and it seems only logical that the best approach may be to restrict oneself to a few well tried and trusted drugs so that a better understanding of how to get the best out of them is obtained.

New NSAID molecules and new formulations

One of the features of this group of drugs which keeps them in the headlines is the introduction of new formulations and even new chemical varieties of NSAIDs. In many cases there is little to be gained from reformulating oral NSAIDs, and many would regard this as purely a marketing ploy in order to maintain brand loyalty amongst doctors. However, certain products seem to have gained widespread popularity amongst patients and prescribers, and these may be the ones that provide a simpler dosage regimen or which smooth out fluctuations in plasma levels, thereby reducing the risk of adverse effects associated with high peak concentrations.

The costs of some of these products may be significantly higher than that of the 'standard' or original formulation, particularly if a generic version is available. Given the widespread prescribing of NSAIDs, this is an important point to take into account along with the risk–benefit assessment which should be undertaken when prescribing any NSAID.

A few years ago there was a move to produce topical formulations of NSAIDs, offering the promise of more targeted drug delivery over the surface of the affected joint(s), thereby eliminating the need to expose the gut to the direct presence of the NSAID molecules. Whilst attractive in principle, there has been a lot of controversy as to whether these formulations really improve the delivery of drug to the site of action, or whether they achieve anything more than a traditional rubefacient. Furthermore, they are not necessarily free of systemic side effects, although they probably carry a reduced risk. Some of them are now available over the counter in pharmacies, and those which are prescribable on the NHS have seen their prices reduced as a result of the Selected List Scheme (see Chapter 1).

One approach to reducing the problem of gastro-intestinal toxicity with NSAIDs has been the use of misoprostol. This is a synthetic prostaglandin analogue with antisecretory and mucosal protective properties which can be used to promote gastric and duodenal ulcer healing. It can also prevent ulcers associated with NSAIDs when co-prescribed with them, and both a combination tablet (with diclofenac) and a combination pack (with naproxen) are available to make this a convenient option.

However, misoprostol is not necessarily thought to be the complete solution to the problem of gastro-intestinal toxicity with NSAIDs, and it is probably most appropriate for frail or very elderly people. For other patients, more attention should be paid to avoiding the use of NSAIDs in the first place, for example by using paracetamol, or minimising the risk by selecting one of the safer agents at the lowest possible effective dose. The misoprostol–diclofenac combination is widely promoted to prescribers, and so it is important that they understand its appropriate place in therapy and do not prescribe it indiscriminately for everyone who needs an NSAID.

The latest in the line of new chemical varieties of NSAIDs are the selective COX-2 inhibitors, meloxicam being the first example of such a drug to become available in the UK. NSAIDs work mainly by preventing the production of prostaglandins through the inhibition of cyclo-oxygenase (COX), an enzyme which exists in two forms. COX-1 is involved in protecting the gastric mucosa, whereas COX-2 is involved in producing inflammatory mediators (chemicals produced locally at the site of inflammation).

Theoretically, preferential blocking of COX-2 should result in an anti-inflammatory effect, and there is some evidence that NSAIDs with selectivity in this respect may have less risk of causing gastro-intestinal toxicity. However, there are probably other factors which determine gastro-intestinal toxicity, and the risk associated with different NSAIDs is not necessarily proportional to their relative COX-2 selectivity. Although it has been demonstrated in the short term to cause less gastro-intestinal toxicity than some other NSAIDs, meloxicam needs to be shown to be safer than ibuprofen before it can be considered to be a drug of first choice.

Repeat prescribing

Repeat prescribing has attracted a great deal of attention recently. This is because of increasing pressure to improve the arrangements whereby 'repeats' are issued, and recognition of the potential of computerised patient record systems (in general practices) to enable this to happen. There are both clinical and financial reasons for this particular prescribing activity to come under close scrutiny.

It has long been recognised that whilst repeat prescribing is often convenient and time-saving for doctors and patients alike, there is sometimes much waste of medicines. This may occur because patients no longer need them (on clinical grounds) or, for a variety of reasons, do not fully comply with treatment(s) that may have been initiated some time in the past.

Adequate supervision and regular review at appropriate intervals is, therefore, vital in ensuring that patients continue to benefit from repeat prescriptions for long-term medication. This also helps to minimise the risks of patients being exposed to unnecessary adverse effects. It is also important to ensure that large quantities of unused medicines are not accumulated which may subsequently be discarded, thereby wasting scarce NHS resources. Various estimates suggest that over half of all prescribed items are issued on 'repeats' and so the financial implications of uncontrolled repeat prescribing are obvious.

Repeat prescribing is an activity which is well suited to the processes of medical audit, and many practices have now put into place well defined policies for the issuing and monitoring of 'repeats'. These include checking systems on the practice database which remind the doctor of the need to review individual patients at appropriate intervals.

Improved information systems should also help eliminate the problems which occur when patients are seen by different doctors who may then change the treatment without communicating this information to others involved in caring for the same individual. This situation can arise on discharge from hospital or referral to an out-patient clinic. Patients may be unable to remember which treatment they are supposed to be receiving and which has been discontinued. It is particularly in these circumstances that improvements in patient care can be realised through accurate record keeping and proper arrangements for the continuance of long-term therapies.

Computerised systems are not in themselves the whole answer, and may actually lead to prescriptions being automatically issued when they are not needed – it is just as important to delete items from the list of 'repeats' as it is to ensure that the patient is reviewed at appropriate intervals. A potential development that has been discussed to help with these problems is the increased involvement of community pharmacists in managing the issue of 'repeats'. This may be through a system of 'instalment dispensing', authorised at the outset by the doctor, but involving the pharmacist in a more proactive way so that patients do not accumulate medicines that they do not need.

This is only a very brief outline of some of the issues which arise when discussing repeat prescribing and the interested reader is referred to more detailed accounts elsewhere (Harris, 1996; Audit Commission, 1994; National Audit Office, 1993).

Bulk prescriptions

The *Drug Tariff* defines a 'bulk' prescription as an order for two or more patients, bearing the name of a school or institution in which at least 20 persons reside, where the doctor is responsible for the treatment of at least 10 of those patients (National Health Service, 1997). This is the only exception where the doctor can issue one prescription form for more than one individual patient, and, as stated, the prescription form is headed with the name of the institution and not the name of the patients.

The bulk prescription can only be for a drug which is prescribable under the NHS, and this must not be a prescription only medicine (POM) as defined in the Medicines Act 1968; it may also be for a prescribable dressing as long as it does not contain a product which is a designated POM.

Prescribing for addicts

The Misuse of Drugs Regulations 1973 permit only medical practitioners who hold a special licence issued by the Home Secretary to prescribe diamorphine ('heroin'), dipipanone (Diconal) or cocaine for addicts. Other doctors must refer any addict who needs these drugs to a treatment centre.

In the first instance, doctors must notify the Chief Medical Officer at the Drugs Branch of the Home Office, in writing, of any person who is addicted to any one of 14 'notifiable drugs', these being listed in the relevant section of the *BNF* which covers controlled drugs and drug dependence. This notification must be confirmed annually if the patient is still being treated by the particular doctor concerned. An index of registered addicts in maintained in the Home Office and it is necessary to check this in order to prevent persons trying to obtain supplies of controlled drugs from more than one doctor.

Addicts who are to obtain prescriptions for their drug supplies are usually introduced to a convenient pharmacy where agreement exists to make such supplies. There are two types of prescription form which may be used: the form FP10(MDA), or in Scotland GP10, issued by general practitioners, and the form FP10(HP)(ad), or in Scotland HBP(A), issued mainly by special drug dependency units.

Special requirements exist for the actual writing of prescriptions for controlled drugs. These are beyond the scope of this chapter, but they are also described in the *BNF* section on prescribing controlled drugs and drug dependence.

In the NHS, it is possible to arrange for supplies to be made to addicts by 'instalments'. A weekly prescription is sent to the pharmacy by post for dispensing in daily instalments. No alterations are permitted to the arrangements covered by the existing prescription and any changes requested by the addict must be made by represcribing the amount to be supplied by instalments.

It is a criminal offence for a pharmacist to dispense an instalment out of turn, i.e. to make the next day's supply a day early. Neither can pharmacists make 'emergency supplies' of controlled drugs nor take orders over the telephone.

The system of supplying instalments is intended to help prevent overdose and to bring some routine into the daily life of the addict. Pharmacists have to maintain careful records of supplies of controlled drugs and be familiar with the arrangements made under the Misuse of Drugs Act for all transactions involving controlled drugs.

Many community pharmacists exchange clean syringes and needles for contaminated equipment used by injecting substance and drug misusers. Clients requesting syringes and needles are encouraged to return any used equipment to the pharmacy. Used contaminated material should ideally be brought to the pharmacy by clients in a sealed 'sharps' container (RPSGB, 1997).

Summary

There are many factors which influence prescribing decisions – whether to prescribe at all, for how long, and what class of drug will be most suitable. This chapter highlights some of the issues involved with reference to three very common therapeutic topics in general practice. These are the use of acid suppressant drugs, the treatment of hypertension and the use of non-steroidal anti-inflammatory drugs. The chapter does not set out to cover these areas in great depth, but mentions those clinical and pharmacological aspects which are immediately relevant to the present discussion, and the views expressed represent the author's interpretation of the most familiar known features of the drugs and indications for which they are prescribed. There are enough facts to make the chapter informative to those who do not regularly read around the topic of prescribing in general practice, and additional reference sources are suggested for those who have had their appetite stimulated for further information.

General practice prescribing is an important topic, not least because of the proportion of the NHS drugs bill (approximately 80%) which is accounted for compared to that which is spent in the hospital sector. It represents a very interesting field because GPs now have to pay more attention to the costs of their prescribing whilst meeting the clinical needs of all their patients. Without the luxury of the more sophisticated diagnostic technologies available to their hospital counterparts, GPs still have to make important therapeutic decisions which can have a major bearing on the well-being of their patients. It is the balance of doing something for their patients without the time and resources necessary for a complete diagnostic work-up that makes prescribing in general practice such a fascinating and challenging area.

References

Audit Commission (1994) *A Prescription for Improvement – Towards More Rational Prescribing in General Practice.* HMSO, London.

Dieppe, P.A., Frankel, S.J., & Toth, B. (1993) Is research into the treatment of osteoarthritis with non-steroidal anti-inflammatory drugs misdirected? *Lancet* **341**, 353–4.

Harris, C. (1996) *Prescribing in General Practice.* Radcliffe Medical Press, Oxford.

Marshall, B.J., Armstrong, J.A., McGechie, D.B. & Glancy, R.J. (1985) Attempt to fulfil Koch's postulates for pyloric campylobacter, *Med. J. Austr.* **142**, 436–9.

Medicines Resource Centre (1994) Choosing a non-steroidal anti-inflammatory drug. *MeReC Bulletin 5*, No. 12.

Medicines Resource Centre (1995) Hypertension – which drugs for which patient? *MeReC Bulletin 6*, No. 2.

Medicines Resource Centre (1997) Dyspepsia, peptic ulcer and *Helicobacter pylori. MeReC Bulletin 8*, No. 2.

Mehta, D.K. (1997) *British National Formulary No. 34.* British Medical Association and Royal Pharmaceutical Society of Great Britain, London.

National Audit Office (1993) *Repeat Prescribing by General Practitioners*. HMSO, London.
National Health Service (1997) *Drug Tariff*. HMSO, London.
Royal Pharmaceutical Society of Great Britain (1997) *Medicines, Ethics and Practice 18*. RPSGB, London.

Further reading

For all three topics (acid suppressants, anti-hypertensives and NSAIDs)

The *British National Formulary* (*BNF*) (Mehta, 1997), contains detailed information about *all* the different individual drugs in these therapeutic categories and also useful prescribing notes at the beginning of each relevant chapter or section.

Individual topic headings

Acid suppressants

Medicines Resource Centre (1993a) Gastro-oesophageal reflux disease, *MeReC Bulletin 4*, No. 5.
Medicines Resource Centre (1993b) Peptic ulcer disease. *MeReC Bulletin 4*, No. 10.
Medicines Resource Centre (1994) Update on proton-pump inhibitors. *MeReC Bulletin 5*, No. 7.
Medicines Resource Centre (1997) Dyspepsia, peptic ulcer and *Helicobacter pylori*. *MeReC Bulletin 8*, No. 2.

Hypertension

Medicines Resource Centre (1993a) Essential hypertension – management guidelines. *MeReC Bulletin 4*, No. 7.
Medicines Resource Centre (1993b) The treatment of hypertension in the elderly. *MeReC Bulletin 4*, No. 9.
Medicines Resource Centre (1995a) Hypertension – which drugs for which patients? *MeReC Bulletin 6*, No. 2.
Medicines Resource Centre (1995b) Losartan, a new type of antihypertensive. *MeReC Bulletin 6*, No. 6.

NSAIDs

Medicines Resource Centre (1992) Misoprostol. *MeReC Bulletin 3*, No. 6.
Medicines Resource Centre (1993) Athrotec. *MeReC Bulletin 4*, No. 3.
Medicines Resource Centre (1994) Choosing a non-steroidal anti-inflammatory drug. *MeReC Bulletin 5*, No. 12.
Medicines Resource Centre (1996) Two new NSAIDs: meloxicam and aceclofenac. *MeReC Bulletin 7*, No. 12.

Chapter 10
Prescribed Medicines in Secondary Care

Adrian Brown

Introduction

This chapter will focus on some of the principles and practice of prescribing in specific therapeutic areas. It is beyond the scope of the chapter to discuss the pharmacology of individual agents in detail, and the reader is referred to standard texts on the subjects in question. Instead, emphasis will be placed on general principles and practical elements of hospital prescribing.

Anti-infective agents

Most hospitals operate an 'antibiotic policy' which needs to be regularly amended on the basis of local patterns of disease prevalence and the presence of individual pathogens isolated from infected patients over time. The major problem regarding antibiotic use within hospitals relates to the development of resistance of organisms to specific drugs. There are many mechanisms by which antibiotic resistance can occur: for instance an organism may develop changes in cell membranes structure to limit entry of the antibiotic (e.g. aminoglycosides, tetracyclines), or it may develop the capacity to produce a specific enzyme which inactivates the antibiotic (e.g. staphylococci which produce beta-lactamases against penicillins). It is well recognised that antibiotics used inappropriately may increase the likelihood of resistant organisms resulting. Antibiotic policies are therefore aimed at maximising the chances of successful eradication of the infective agent from the patient, and minimising the risks of resistance developing (Lind, 1995). The principles of appropriate antibiotic use apply to both patients in hospital and in the community, although it may be argued that the imperative to minimise resistance in hospital is stronger, as hospitalised patients are more likely to be critically ill (Jones *et al.*, 1997).

Broad principles of antibiotic use in hospital may be summarised as follows:

(a) Antibiotics should only be used where there is clear evidence that the therapeutic outcome will be improved.

The above principle is self-evident. Nonetheless, there are many instances both in hospital and community prescribing when this does not apply. For example, an antibiotic may be prescribed for an infection which is most likely to be viral (e.g. pharyngitis, acute bronchitis) or for a self-limiting condition (most forms of gastroenteritis) where the drug is most unlikely to alter the course of the illness, and may actually be counter-productive. Antibiotics are frequently used short-term to prevent infection during particular surgical procedures (surgical prophylaxis).

(b) A narrow spectrum agent should be chosen in preference to a broad-spectrum agent when the pathogen is identified.

Treatment should be specific and aimed at eradication of the causal organism. An agent with broader action is likely to kill endogenous bacteria in the gut and elsewhere (the 'bacterial flora'), and cause adverse effects (diarrhoea). In contrast, a broad spectrum agent should be reserved for treating infections when pathogens are unknown (e.g in emergency admissions before culture and sensitivities can be carried out) and in infections caused by more than one pathogen. Over-use of broad spectrum agents will increase the likelihood of resistance developing.

(c) The agent chosen should have adequate activity against the pathogen.

In practice, choosing the appropriate drug is sometimes difficult. Antibacterial activity is usually inferred from *in vitro* data, either published data relating to the drug from standard sources (e.g. the *British National Formulary (BNF)* (Mehta, 1997) or the maufacturer's data-sheet) or results of sensitivity testing from the hospital laboratory.

In bacterial sensitivity-testing, a sample of pathogen obtained from the patient (e.g. from a urine or sputum sample) is incorporated into a semi-solid culture medium able to sustain the growth of the organism in question. On the surface of this medium is placed a series of small disks of paper each impregnated with a different antibiotic. A lid is then placed on the dish and the closed unit is allowed to incubate at an optimal temperature for several hours, enabling growth of the organism to take place. After this time, the lid is removed and the bacterial culture examined. If any of the antibiotics contained within the paper disks are active against the organism, this will be reflected in an absence of bacterial growth around the particular disk (a 'zone of inhibition'). If however, the organism is able to exist in close proximity to a disk, then it is clearly resistant to that particular agent.

Bacterial sensitivity testing in this way has the clear advantage that it relates to the actual organism which is currently infecting the patient, and not to theoretical data gleaned from a previous clinical trial, which may or may not apply to specific patients. There are two main drawbacks: firstly, it takes several hours to achieve a result, which may be costly to a critically ill patient, and secondly because the result is obtained *in vitro*, it takes no account of the patient's host defence mechanisms.

(d) The agent chosen should have the lowest risk of toxicity.
All antibiotics may cause adverse effects; in some cases these may be life-threatening. Some toxicity may be dose-related (e.g. penicillins in very high dose may cause neurotoxicity), and occasionally may correlate to circulating plasma concentrations of the agent (e.g. ototoxity from gentamicin). In the latter case, it is appropriate to measure concentrations of antibiotic on a regular basis, and to adjust the dose accordingly during the course of treatment. Usually, however, toxic effects are not predictable on the basis of dosage, and may only be identified by careful monitoring of the patient. Some drugs, such as penicillins and cephalosporins, have a low incidence of toxicity and, unless patients are known to be hypersensitive to them, can be used safely at a relatively wide range of dosages. Other drugs (e.g. rifampicin, clindamycin and chloramphenicol) have a much higher incidence of adverse effects and require careful observation of the patient whilst they are receiving them. As in all therapeutic decisions, the difficult balance of risk and benefit applies in the selection of the most appropriate antibiotic for a particular patient.

(e) The agent should be used at the most appropriate dose for the shortest time required for successful treatment.
Choosing the most appropriate dose and length of treatment may be a difficult balance to strike. It is clear that patients should not be overdosed, as this will increase the risk of adverse effects. Underdosing the patient however will lead to sub-optimal therapy and the risk of antibiotic resistance developing and treatment failure.

(f) The oral route should be used unless there are clear reasons for parenteral therapy.
Many antibiotics can be given orally, by injection and perhaps by other routes (rectally, topically, intrathecally, etc). Some agents, however, cannot be given orally, either because they are broken down rapidly in the stomach (e.g. some penicillins) or because they are simply not absorbed from the gastro-intestinal tract (e.g. aminoglycosides). In the latter case, the drug must be given parenterally, but in many cases there is a choice whether to give oral therapy or not. An intravenous injection achieves an immediate 'peak' plasma level which may be an advantage for a patient who is critically ill, for whom even the delay of a few hours in starting effective therapy may represent a serious risk. In practice, however, most patients requiring antibiotic therapy are not so critically ill, and the time taken to absorb the antibiotic after oral administration is unlikely to compromise the outcome of therapy. Intravenous injections are clearly invasive, carry some risk of introducing further pathogens into the patient and are more likely to result in adverse effects, particularly local reactions (thrombophlebitis, tissue necrosis from extravasation, etc.). Injectable forms of an antibiotic are almost always more expensive than the same dose given orally, and often require reconstitution and perhaps special giving sets and consum-

ables. Unless there are compelling reasons for intravenous administration (e.g. no oral form of the drug exists; the patient cannot swallow; unconsciousness; severe nausea and vomiting) oral therapy is preferred.

Anticancer drugs

Traditionally there have been three treatment modalities aimed at eradication of malignant disease: surgery, radiotherapy and chemotherapy. Sometimes two or three of these approaches are used in the same patient, depending on the condition and clinical features. It is arguably in chemotherapy that the most significant advances have been observed in recent years, a trend which seems set to continue into the future.

A wide variety of drugs is used in the treatment of malignant disease. In general these comprise: cytotoxic agents (toxic to all body cells, but exhibiting some selectivity to tumour cells if used appropriately); hormonal agents (natural or synthetic agents which inhibit the growth of hormone-dependant tumours such as breast, ovary and prostate), and adjuvant/investigational agents (e.g. interferons, cytokines). This section focuses on the use of cytotoxic agents.

Cytotoxic agents

These comprise a heterogeneous group of drugs with several sub-groups of related compounds. As the description suggests, they are toxic to all human cells (normal cells as well as cancer cells) and most exert maximal toxicity on cells which are actively dividing, rather than those which are 'resting'. As many tumours have a large proportion of actively dividing cells (i.e. a high 'growth fraction') cytotoxic drugs will display some selectivity for damaging tumour cells to a greater extent than normal 'host' cells. The chemical groupings mentioned do not imply particular clinical specificity. Thus chlorambucil (an alkylating agent) is used mainly in the treatment of leukaemias; cyclophosphamide (another alkylating agent) may also be used against a variety of solid tumours. Some examples of commonly used cytotoxic drug sub-groups are:

- *Alkylating agents* These irreversibly damage DNA by forming cross-links between the two strands of the DNA molecule and thereby stop DNA replication. Examples of specific drugs include cyclophosphamide and chlorambucil.

- *Antimetabolites* These interrupt synthesis of DNA or other vital metabolic processes involved in cell division. Generally these agents are chemically similar to substances normally involved in these pathways, thereby blocking the action of the active substance. Examples include methotrexate and 5-fluorouracil.

- *Anthracyclines* These agents bind to DNA in a similar manner to the alkylating agents. Examples include doxorubicin (Adriamycin) and mitozantrone (mitoxantrone).

- *Vinca alkaloids* These are agents isolated from plants of the genus *Vinca* (periwinkle). They affect the cell division process by interrupting the production of proteins comprising the 'spindle' structure which allows alignment of chromosomes immediately before cell division. Examples are vincristine and vindesine.

- *Platinum compounds* These again inhibit DNA replication in a manner not completely understood, but which is likely to involve binding to DNA. An example is cisplatin.

Several other sub-groups of cytotoxic agents exist, and several completely new agents are likely to be released onto the market in the next couple of years.

Toxicity of cytotoxic agents

As has been suggested, cytotoxic drugs are also toxic to normal cells, especially those cell types with a high growth fraction. All the above drugs share some common toxicities therefore, reflecting their action on these cells and tissues. Typical normal cells with high growth fractions are found in the bone marrow, in the cells of the hair follicles and in the mucosal cells throughout the gastro-intestinal tract. Most cytotoxic agents can therefore cause bone marrow aplasia (leading usually to underproduction of white blood cells and platelets), alopecia, and gastro-intestinal irritation (leading to nausea, vomiting and ulceration). Some drugs are particularly prone to produce a certain type of toxicity (e.g. cyclophosphamide – alopecia; cisplatin – nausea). In addition, some have toxic effects peculiar to the individual drug or class: vinca alkaloids, for example, are neurotoxic and may produce peripheral neuropathies, whereas doxorubicin may cause a life-threatening cardiomyopathy. The rational use of cytotoxic chemotherapy requires that the patient gains maximum benefit (i.e. high level of damage to tumour cells) with the minimum risk of toxicity. This is frequently difficult to achieve, but careful adherence to prescribing protocols increases the chances of a successful outcome. Some specific measures which may be employed to counteract common adverse effects of cytotoxic chemotherapy are outlined below.

Management of nausea and vomiting

Although virtually all cytotoxic drugs may cause nausea, those which have provided the greatest problems of management are the platinum compounds, particularly cisplatin. The nausea associated with this substance may be so profound as to deter patients from completing their therapy course unless it can be controlled. Nausea caused by cisplatin is frequently resistant to conventional antinausea agents such as prochlorperazine and cyclizine. Patients may respond to metoclopramide parenterally, but only when the latter is given as a high-dose regimen (in doses up to 10 mg/kg over 24 hours) when there is a strong likelihood of extrapyramidal side effects to the drug. The first-line agents used to counter cisplatin induced nausea are the 5HT-3 antagonists ondansetron, granisetron and tropisetron. These drugs are usually very effective in preventing symptoms arising if given before and during chemotherapy. Side effects to these drugs are usually mild and include constipation and headaches but are occasionally associated with adverse cardiovascular reactions (arrythmias, chest pain) involuntary movements, disturbed vision and transient changes in liver enzymes. Some patients may also benefit from the addition of dexamethasone, which seems to increase the effectiveness of the antinausea agent, although it has no antinausea action of its own. A benzodiazepine (e.g. lorazepam) may also be beneficial, as it possesses amnesic properties, and reduces the patient's recollection of the experience.

Reducing the effects of cytotoxic drugs on the bone marrow

In general terms there is little that can be done to achieve a reduction in the effect of cytotoxic drugs on the bone marrow. Amifostine is one of a small group of drugs developed as a 'bone marrow protectant'. It seems to act as a free-radical scavenger and offers some protection to the bone marrow against cisplatin and alkylating agents used in the treatment of solid tumours. It has been shown to reduce the fall in white blood cells and platelets which accompany treatment with these agents. Interestingly, it also offers protection against these effects in patients receiving radiotherapy.

In leukaemias, however, malignant cells are present in the bone marrow, and it is there that the maximum drug activity is sought. Most effort has been made in deriving measures to enhance bone marrow recovery after exposure to the cytotoxic agent, either by the use of a specific antidote to the drug, or more recently by the use of bone marrow growth factors. An example of the use of an antidote would be the so-called 'leucovorin rescue' following high dose methotrexate therapy. Here, calcium folinate (leucovorin) is given for several doses as a specific antagonist to methotrexate which otherwise would give rise to profound bone marrow suppression at doses of above $1 g/m^2$, given for maximal effects on malignant cells. Human granulocyte colony stimulating factors (G-CSF) are sometimes used to assist recovery of bone marrow function following cytotoxic chemotherapy. These agents must be used with caution, however, as they may also aid tumour recovery in some cases (e.g. in myeloid leukaemias).

Extravasation of cytotoxic agents

Most cytotoxic agents are intensely vesicant, and when given parenterally must be injected into the line of a fast flowing infusion to facilitate rapid distribution in the circulation. A venflon may become displaced from its site, particularly if the needle punctures the vein wall; this will cause the tip to protrude outside the vein into the surrounding tissue (extravasation). It is advantageous where possible to administer highly vesicant drugs, such as platinum agents, via a control line which minimises local irritation and avoids risk of extravasation. Continued administration of cytotoxic agents will cause tissue necrosis around the vein which may be of sufficient extent to require surgery, possibly amputation. Care must be taken to repeatedly examine the cannula site to ensure the needle is appropriately located, and that there is no local irritation evident. Most units operate an extravasation policy which involves the use of a 'kit' containing certain materials to minimise the extent of damage following an extravasation incident. Often included in such a kit are two agents. The first is hyaluronidase, an enzyme which can break down connective tissue: local injection of this agent into the area enhances dissipation of the cytotoxic agent from the site of deposition, and reduces its local concentration. Secondly, sodium thiosulphate is a reducing agent and is particularly effective in neutralising the action of platinum drugs (cisplatin and carboplatin), both of which are extremely damaging to surrounding tissues if extravasated.

Alopecia

Most patients are aware that cytotoxic agents cause hair loss, and this may be the single most distressing feature of their treatment, particularly for women. Drugs given at high dose in a pulsatile fashion (e.g. one injection every 2 weeks for several treatments) will cause a weakening of the hair shaft each time the drug is given. The hair will then tend to break at the area of weakness. It must be stressed to the patient that the hair follicles have not been irreversibly damaged, and that the hair will grow back after the course of therapy is completed. When lower dose cytotoxic agents are given for a long period, perhaps for palliation maintenance, such as the use of busulphan for chronic myeloma, hair loss may be more long-lasting. General measures to maintain hair and scalp condition are particularly important during and after cytotoxic therapy, and may enhance the patient's sense of well being. If hair loss is long term and/or becomes cosmetically unacceptable, specialist advice on the provision of wigs is available in most centres. Attempts have been made to limit the exposure of the hair follicle cells to the drug. For example, ice compresses have been designed to be applied to the scalp, to cause local vasoconstriction during the time the individual is exposed to the cytotoxic drug. Local vasoconstrictor agents (e.g. noradrenaline (norepinephrine)) have been administered subcutaneously for the same purpose. These measures have largely met with minimal success in reducing hair loss, and may actually have been counter-productive in that they run the risk of reducing drug exposure to secondary tumours below the scalp.

Environmental exposure of cytotoxic agents to staff

It has long been recognised that cytotoxic drugs may cause chromosomal changes (i.e. are mutagens) in individuals exposed to them. A Finnish case controlled study in 1985 investigated the risks to pregnant nurses of occupation exposure to cytotoxics (Selevan *et al.*, 1985). The authors found that exposure to cyclophosphamide, doxorubicin and vincristine conferred a significant increase in the risk of foetal loss to that of control. The increased risk ranged from $\times 3.96$ for doxorubicin to $\times 2.46$ for vincristine. The mechanism of this effect was unknown. In health care staff involved in the reconstitution and administration of cytotoxics, the exposure is likely to be long-term, but of low intensity. Although much research has been carried out in this area, the increased risk to such individuals is unknown. Most units carry out periodic checks of blood counts in staff regularly involved in cytotoxic reconstitution, with some units performing more sophisticated testing (e.g. looking for chromosome abnormalities). The Calman report into the future of cancer services (DH & Welsh Office, 1995) recommended that all cytotoxic agents should be reconstituted or otherwise assembled into a 'ready to use' product in a dedicated facility within the hospital pharmacy. Cytotoxic agents should not be manipulated on the open ward environment by nursing staff. This is now generally the case. Most hospital pharmacies have access to an isolator, a completely enclosed unit where the product is protected from contamination by the operator and *vice versa*. The infusion containing the required amount of drug for the particular patient is conveyed to the ward and merely requires connection to an infusion giving set by the nurse or doctor attending the patient.

Prescribing of cytotoxic drugs

Most prescribing for cancer treatment is carried out in accordance with standard protocols. These may be nationally or locally agreed, depending on the condition, and other factors may apply. For example, most patients with leukaemias and certain other malignancies are effectively entered into one of the national clinical trials which are ongoing to establish the optimum treatment for the condition. Protocols may be very specific and run for a particular time schedule. There are specific inclusion and exclusion criteria, and patients not eligible for one particular protocol will be included in another. The individual drugs are often prescribed on a dedicated prescription sheet which is separate from other hospital prescriptions. In some hospitals, prescriptions are generated by the pharmacy department having been written on a standard computer spreadsheet package.

Doses are calculated according to patient's weight and other factors (e.g. renal function, fluid balance, etc.) and a computerised facility reduces the risks of error inherent in manual calculation. Chemotherapy prescriptions will also include the provision of adjuvant drugs (e.g. antinauseants, steroids, antidotes) where applicable.

For conditions where the role of drug therapy is less clear (e.g. non-small-cell lung cancer; adjuvant chemotherapy of bowel cancer after surgery) chemo-therapeutic regimens may be decided locally and are unlikely to be as complex as those for leukaemias and lymphomas.

Cardiovascular agents

There is a wide range of cardiovascular drugs prescribed both within hospitals and in the community. This section concentrates on two major developments in therapy in conditions regularly encountered within hospitals .

Thrombolytic agents for myocardial infarction

The advent of streptokinase in the acute management of myocardial infarction has dramatically improved the prognosis of patients presenting with this condition. Streptokinase is a fibrinolytic enzyme derived from a streptococcal bacterium which can dissolve the thrombus which has given rise to the infarct, if administered within 12 hours of the onset of symptoms. Recent trials have shown mortality to improve still further if oral aspirin is combined with streptokinase. Streptokinase (1.5 million units) is administered intravenously over 60 minutes; oral aspirin is continued daily for at least 4 weeks. As strep-tokinase is a foreign protein, it is antigenic and may provoke antibody pro-duction for an indefinite time in an individual. The result of this phenomenon is that if that individual has a further myocardial infarct, a subsequent injection of streptokinase would be inactivated by their circulating antibodies and thus the treatment would be ineffective. More recently, recombinant human tissue plasminogen activator (r-TPA) has become available as an alternative throm-bolytic to streptokinase for patients who have received the latter drug in the past. r-TPA is not antigenic; hence can be given if the patient suffers a second infarct in the future. The main drawback of r-TPA is the cost: at around £700 per dose it is around ten times as expensive as the £70 cost of streptokinase. It is likely that other similar agents will become available in the near future. The main clinical problems of thrombolytics relate to their tendency to produce bleeding in susceptible individuals, and that they may produce re-perfusion arrhythmias after the initial thrombus has dispersed (Rogers, 1995).

ACE inhibitors in congestive heart failure

Angiotensin converting enzyme (ACE) inhibitors have been demonstrated in several trials to enhance life expectancy and quality of life in patients with congestive heart failure. ACE inhibitors act by blocking the enzyme responsible for activation of the endogenous vasoconstrictor agent angiotensin and hence lowering peripheral resistance to cardiac output. They also effectively decrease circulating aldosterone levels, thereby increasing sodium loss and causing potassium retention within the renal tubules.

There is some debate about which ACE inhibitors may be the most effective in the management of heart failure, with some members of the group not yet licensed for this indication. However, it seems most likely that this is a class effect, with most experience having been gained from the more established agents such as captopril, enalapril, lisinopril, ramipril and perindopril (Baker *et al.*, 1994).

The major problem associated with ACE inhibitors relates to initiation of therapy: if the starting dose is too high, blockade of the renin/angiotensin/aldosterone system may cause a precipitant reduction in renal perfusion, acute renal failure and catastrophic hypertension. This problem has led to fatalities, with an increased risk in elderly patients receiving diuretics. For this reason it is usual to start therapy with a 'test' dose (6.25 mg captopril, or 2.5 mg enalapril) whilst the patient is hospitalised, and to monitor blood pressure closely over the next few hours. If this dose is tolerated, a subsequent dose may be increased to a provisional maintenance dose (e.g. captopril 12.5 mg b.d.) which can then be titrated upward against the patient response over the next few days. ACE inhibitors should not be used in patients with renal artery stenosis or with aortic stenosis, as these conditions predispose to acute renal failure. ACE inhibitors may occasionally cause angio-oedema which may be life threatening. They cause a troublesome cough in a significant minority of patients. These problems have been documented with all members of the group, but there is some evidence to suggest that they may be expected to be less frequent with the newer drugs than the older agents.

Renal function and electrolyte balance (especially potassium, which may rise) should be monitored regularly in all patients receiving ACE inhibitors for heart failure.

Drugs used in respiratory conditions

Respiratory illness accounts for a large proportion of acute hospital admissions in the UK. Many of these patients have an acute exacerbation of asthma, or of chronic obstructive airways disease arising from a chest infection. In the latter case, common pathogens may include *Streptococcus* spp., *Moraxella catarrhalis* and *Haemophilus influenzae*. Initial treatment is normally with a broad-spectrum antibiotic (e.g. amoxycillin (amoxicillin)) until sputum can be tested for culture and sensitivity.

In addition to eradication of the infection, most patients have poor respiratory function which requires appropriate management. This section will briefly discuss the role of bronchodilators and corticosteroids in the management of acute respiratory disease in hospitalised patients.

Beta-2 adrenoceptor agonists

The hormone adrenaline (epinephrine) acts on beta-2 receptors in the bronchial smooth muscle to produce relaxation and hence bronchodilation. However, adrenaline (epinephrine) also acts on beta-1 receptors elsewhere in the body to produce stimulation of the heart muscle and may predispose to cardiotoxicity such as arrhythmias. Attempts have been made to produce drugs which mimic the beta-2 effects of adrenaline, but have little or no beta-1 action. These 'selective' beta-2 agonist drugs include salbutamol, terbutaline and fenoterol. More recently, longer acting beta-2 agonists have been developed such as salmeterol and bambuterol.

Beta-2 agonists delivered by inhaler have been the mainstay of management of airways obstruction for many years until recently, when their regular use in asthma management was questioned. According to the current British Thoracic Society Guidelines (British Asthma Guidelines Co-ordinating Committee, 1997) they should not be used more than three times per week as sole therapy for the management of chronic asthma. If they are needed more frequently than this, the patient should be given regular inhaled corticosteroid as first line management. However, beta-2 agonists continue to have an important role in the management of acute asthma where they are administered by nebuliser, and often produce remarkable resolution of symptoms and improvement of respiratory function.

In theory, the use of beta-2 agonists should be supported by objective tests of an improvement in airways obstruction. The most practical test to demonstrate reversibility in airways obstruction is measurement of the peak expiratory flow rate (PEFR or peak flow) which can be readily carried out at the bedside. Normally a 'pre' and 'post' nebuliser reading is taken, the difference between the two being the 'reversibility' of bronchoconstriction, which in turn justifies the continued use of the bronchodilator. In practice, however, little reversibility may be seen, although patients will often claim a significant subjective improvement in their breathlessness. This is especially so in patients with chronic obstructive airways disease. It may be that beta-2 agonists have a secondary effect (perhaps local anti-inflammatory) which is distinct from their effects on relaxing bronchial smooth muscle. This has tentatively been suggested to occur with salmeterol.

Beta-2 agonists, although 'selective' to beta-2 receptors, are not 'specific', and will produce beta-1 effects on the myocardium if given in sufficient dosage. When the drugs are administered by nebuliser, the dose is often large enough to produce tachycardia. Patients also experience tremor of the hands and fingers from nebulised beta-2 agents. When given in a portable inhaler device, the dose of beta-2 agonist is usually much smaller than that given by nebuliser. Few patients are likely to suffer side effects from a standard inhaler if they maintain their correct dosage.

A major factor deciding success of use is inhaler technique. With a standard pressurised inhaler (metered dose inhaler, MDI), the patient is obliged to inspire just as they press the body of the canister into its holder to release a dose. This technique, even in a person who is not breathless, takes time to learn adequately; some patients simply cannot cope with the device and most of the administered dose becomes deposited in the mouth rather than reaching the bronchioles. When attached to the inhaler, a 'spacer' chamber (e.g. Volumatic or Nebuhaler) removes the need to coordinate breathing with the release of drug and improves the efficiency of drug supply in most patients. A range of alternatives exists, each with its own strengths and weaknesses. A breath-actuated inhaler, for instance, is a modified MDI such that there is no need to press the canister to release the dose of drug; release is stimulated by the patient sucking on the mouthpiece, i.e. during inspiration. Most other alternatives are 'dry powder' devices and contain no propellant (e.g. Rotacaps, Diskhaler, Turbohaler, Accuhaler). These are often more efficient than the pressurised MDI devices in terms of drug delivery to the bronchioles, but some patients dislike the sensation of inhaling dry powder. Again, there is no need to coordinate breathing with drug release; this occurs automatically.

Corticosteroids

Systemic steroids, either by injection or given orally, continue to have an important role in the management of acute asthma in hospitals. The most significant change in the management of chronic asthma has been in the increased use of maintenance inhaled steroids given regularly. Regular inhaled steroid is now part of Stage II of the British Thoracic Society's guidelines on asthma management (British Asthma Guidelines Co-ordinating Committee, 1997). The agents used include beclomethasone (beclometasone) (Becotide, Beclazone), budesonide (Pulmicort) and fluticasone (Flixotide). The main problems of long term steroid inhalation include candidal infection of the mouth and throat, and the possibility of systemic absorption and eventual side effects. With the former, the risk of candida increases with the proportion of steroid deposited within the oral cavity, rather than being delivered to the bronchioles as intended. The risk is higher with 'less efficient' systems such as a standard metered dose inhaler (MDI) and reduces if a spacer attachment is used, or if a dry powder system is preferred. The risk can also be minimised if the patient is advised to rinse out their mouth with water after each use of the inhaler. In relation to systemic side effects from steroid inhalation, these can occur and have been most widely described with beclomethasone (beclometasone) when given at its highest dosage (e.g. 500 μg b.d. or more). The consequences are most marked for children, in whom long term steroid administration may cause suppression of the hypothalamic/pituitary/adrenal axis and ultimately a reduction in growth. Both children and adults experience an addisonian crisis if the steroid is stopped abruptly. Fluticasone appears to have very low systemic absorption when given by inhalation and hence has been associated with a lower incidence of systemic side effects, even at high dose. This agent would be preferred in children, and may become the drug of choice in all age groups as more data are collated (Whitaker, 1996).

Gastro-intestinal agents

The most frequently encountered gastro-intestinal conditions in hospital practice include peptic ulcer (Rauws & Van Der Hulst, 1995), gastro-oesophageal reflux disease (GORD) and inflammatory bowel disease. Hospital prescribing tends to relate to the acute phases of these conditions; follow up and long term care normally take place within primary care.

Drugs used in the management of gastro-oesophageal reflux disease (GORD)

This is a common presentation both within hospital out-patients departments and via accident and emergency units where it may be confused with cardiac pain. It has been estimated that up to 20% of patients admitted to a coronary care unit later turn out not to have had cardiac pain; most of them were suffering from the pain of gastro-oesophageal reflux.

The majority of patients with GORD are cared for by their GP and in many cases the condition is mild and sporadic, requiring simple antacids or an alginate suspension (e.g. Gaviscon) for resolution of symptoms when they occur.

A proportion of patients develop severe symptoms, however, which may mimic angina or myocardial infarct. In severe GORD there is an increased risk of the development of oesophageal ulceration, leading to stricture and difficulty in swallowing (dysphagia). Moreover, there is an increased risk of oesophageal cancer in poorly controlled patients. Some patients may be amenable to surgery; those with a hiatus hernia, for example, may be cured by surgical resection. The majority of patients have no apparent anatomical defect, and must therefore be managed medically. The drugs available are essentially the anti-secretory agents used for peptic ulcer healing (De Vault & Castell, 1995). In severe GORD, however, these agents often need to be given at a high dose for long-term (perhaps lifelong) management. Typical doses used are cimetidine 800 mg b.d. or omeprazole 20 mg b.d. Another approach is to use a prokinetic agent such as cisapride. This drug promotes peristalsis and hence inhibits reflux of stomach contents into the oesophagus. It has no effect on gastric acid secretion. Cisapride is as effective as omeprazole in resolving the symptoms of GORD, and may be given together with omeprazole when the latter has only been partially effective. Cisapride should not be given with certain drugs which reduce its metabolism and cause it to accumulate (e.g. erythromycin, ketoconazole), as it has been associated with cardiac arrhythmias under these circumstances.

Management of inflammatory bowel disease (IBD)

Ulcerative colitis and Crohn's disease are conditions usually requiring hospital admission for investigation, diagnosis and initial management. Drugs are used to induce a remission (normally whilst the patient is in hospital) and to maintain remission after discharge. Initial management is similar for the two conditions.

Corticosteroids

Corticosteroids (especially prednisolone) are the most effective agents in inducing a remission of the acute phase of the disease. Prednisolone may be given orally, by injection, or topically (as an enema or rectal foam) depending on the extent and location of the disease. The main limitations of corticosteroids are their toxic effects, especially on long-term use. Moreover, the drugs appear to be only partially effective in maintaining a remission in many patients. Much research has been carried out to develop an orally active agent which is as effective as prednisolone but does not possess its adverse safety profile. Efforts have focused on producing a drug which has low systemic absorption together with high topical activity, being carried to the inflamed areas of intestinal wall. The agent fluticasone has these characteristics and is presently being investigated in this therapeutic area. An alternative approach is to use a drug which, although absorbed, is rapidly metabolised by the liver, and is thus largely unavailable to produce serious systemic effects. The drug would require to be in a form which would allow deposition at the inflamed sites of intestine, so it could exert a local effect before being absorbed and eliminated. Budesonide falls into this category; it has recently become available as Entocort and appears to be as effective as oral prednisolone in inducing a remission in many patients with Crohn's disease of the small bowel. It would be expected not to produce the typical long-term side effects of prednisolone.

Aminosalicylic acid derivatives

The mainstay of long-term treatment of ulcerative colitis is sulphasalazine (sulfasalazine). This drug is not significantly absorbed orally. It passes to the colon where it is broken down by bacteria into sulphapyridine (a sulphonamide) and mesalazine (5-aminosalicylic acid). The latter agent is active as a locally acting anti-inflammatory. The sulphapyridine is partially absorbed via the intestinal mucosa and may produce adverse effects systemically. Sulphasalazine (via sulphapyridine) may therefore produce any of the side effects of sulphonamides, such as sensitisation and blood dyscrasias. It also causes a reversible reduction in sperm count which may be sufficient to produce male infertility. The mesalazine, however, is not absorbed and is not thought to produce any systemic effects. Despite the possibility of the side effects listed above, sulphasalazine is generally well tolerated (by 90% of patients) and remains a first choice treatment of ulcerative colitis. The drug is of more limited value in Crohn's disease, however, as this condition may affect any portion of the GI tract, and not only the colon where sulphasalazine is activated. These limitations have led to a search for an alternative means of delivering mesalazine to areas of inflammation within the GI tract.

Mesalazine itself has become available as particles with a pH-dependant coating, which facilitates the release of drug in the small intestine and colon, and has been effective in the control of both ulcerative colitis and Crohn's disease in these areas (Brogden & Sorkin, 1989). Olsalazine, which comprises two mesalazine molecules bonded together, is an alternative agent to sulpha-salazine which, like the latter, is cleaved in the colon to release mesalazine into the colonic lumen.

Summary

This chapter concentrates on the principles of prescribing medicines within a hospital environment, using specific drugs and clinical situations as examples. Many of these principles also pertain within primary care.

Although the expenditure on drugs within the NHS amounts to only a small proportion of total NHS resources, it represents a considerable outlay which can be accurately measured, and on which NHS management may exert some degree of control. However, the past decade has seen a vast increase in the therapies available to treat many conditions, and an increase in patients' expectations of the treatments they will receive. Most newer therapies are more expensive than existing drugs, making control of drug expenditure difficult. However, more expensive therapies may actually be cost effective if they are significantly better (i.e. more effective, or with lower toxicity) than older drugs. Treatment with a new antibiotic, for example, may eradicate an infection more quickly than an older drug, and lead to a patient spending less time in hospital; hence there is a cost-saving overall. It has recently been realised that there may be differences in perceived quality of life measurements in comparing one treatment with another in particular patients. Both a new and an existing treatment may heal a duodenal ulcer in a patient within 4 weeks, but the new treatment eradicates the patient's symptoms within the first 3 days, whereas the older treatment takes 2 weeks for this to occur. Evaluation of these factors to establish overall advantages of new treatments over existing ones has led to the development of 'evidence-based practice' and the discipline of pharmaco-economics.

Many of the innovations in therapy have aimed at hospital patients initially, as a novel therapy often requires more intensive patient monitoring. As pre-scribers' familiarity with a new treatment grows, however, there is a tendency for it to be used increasingly within a primary care setting. A typical example of this would be the use of ACE inhibitors to manage heart failure. Until recently, patients needed to be hospitalised for initiation of this treatment due to the risk of precipitating dramatic drops in blood pressure on the first dose. Several of these agents are now licensed for initiation of treatment in the community as optimum 'safe' starting doses are now better understood. The next 10 years are likely to see many patients being effectively managed at home whilst on increasingly complex drug treatments.

Finally, as hospital prescribing becomes increasingly 'protocol driven', professionals such as clinical nurse specialists, pharmacists and others will be increasingly involved in the prescribing process. These personnel will be responsible for much of the assessment of the effectiveness of a given treatment, and will need to possess a clear understanding of pharmacological principles in order to discharge that responsibility effectively and safely.

References

Baker, D.W., Konstam, M.A., Bottorff, M. & Pitt, B. (1994) Management of Heart Failure I. Pharmacologic treatment. *J. Am. Med. Assoc.* **272**(17), 1361–6.

British Asthma Guidelines Co-ordinating Committee (1997) British guidelines on asthma management; 1995 review and position statement. *Thorax* **52** (suppl), s1–s21.

Brogden, R.N. & Sorkin, E.M. (1989) Mesalazine: A review of its pharmacodynamic and pharmacokinetic properties and therapeutic potential in inflammatory bowel disease. *Drugs* **38**, 500–23.

DeVault, K.R. & Castell M.O. (1995) Guidelines for the diagnosis and treatment of gastroesophageal reflux disease. *Arch Int. Med.* **155**, 2165.

Department of Health & Welsh Office (1995) *A Policy Framework for Commissioning Cancer Services.* HMSO, London.

Jones, R.N., Pfaller, M.A. & Cormican, M.G. (1997) Infectious diseases (bacterial and fungal): principles and practice in antimicrobial therapy. In: *Avery's Drug Treatment* (eds T.M. Speight & N.H.G. Holford), 4th edn. Adis International, Auckland, New Zealand.

Lind, M.J. (1995) Chemotherapy. *Med. Int.* **23**, 422–5.

Mehta, D.K. (1997) *British National Formulary No. 34.* British Medical Association and Royal Pharmaceutical Society of Great Britain, London.

Rauws, E.A.J. & Van Der Hulst, R.W.M. (1995) Current guidelines for the eradication of *Helicobacter pylori* in peptic ulcer disease. *Drugs* **50**, 984–90.

Rogers, W.J. (1995) Contemporary management of acute myocardial infarction. *Am. J. Med.* **99**, 195–206.

Selevan, G.G., Lindbohm, M.L., Horning, R.W. & Hemminki, K. (1985) A study of occupational exposure to antineoplastic drugs and feotal loss in nurses. *N. Engl. J. Med.* **313**, 1173–8.

Whitaker, K. (1996) Effect of Fluticasone on growth in children with asthma. *Lancet* **348**, 63–4.

Chapter 11

The Nurse's Role in Medicines Administration – Legal and Procedural Framework

John A. Sexton

Introduction

The responsibilities of nurses, as well as doctors and pharmacists, in relation to the handling and administration of medicines are derived from a complex mix of statute law, convention and historical practice. Figure 11.1 illustrates examples of some of the sources of these responsibilities. In the UK the two most important pieces of primary legislation controlling medicines use are the Medicines Act 1968 and the Misuse of Drugs Act 1971.

As might be expected, these acts of parliament contain paragraphs outlining various responsibilities of the professions, and restrictions placed on them. However, they were primarily designed as enabling acts. That is, they give power to Ministers of the Crown to implement further regulations through instructions known as *Orders* or *Statutory Instruments* (*SI*). The great advantage of this type of legislation is that laws about medicines use can be constantly updated to meet changing circumstances or to implement European directives without the need for new acts of parliament. As a result, the regulations often become more relevant than the original legislation. For example, the Misuse of Drugs Act 1971, as will be seen, is the major statute restricting the possession and supply of *controlled drugs*. However, it was only given effect by the Misuse of Drugs Regulations 1973 (SI 1973 No. 799) and subsequent regulations. These were consolidated in new Misuse of Drugs Regulations in 1985 (SI 1985 No. 2066) though there have been further revisions since, such as the classification of temazepam as a controlled drug in the light of escalating abuse problems. In a similar way, orders made under the Medicines Act enabled small packs of ibuprofen to be offered for general sale in supermarkets and other outlets. On the other hand, some parts of acts of parliament are never brought into force. An example of this is Chapter 66 of the Medicines Act 1968, which gives the Secretary of State power to make regulations concerning the appearance and

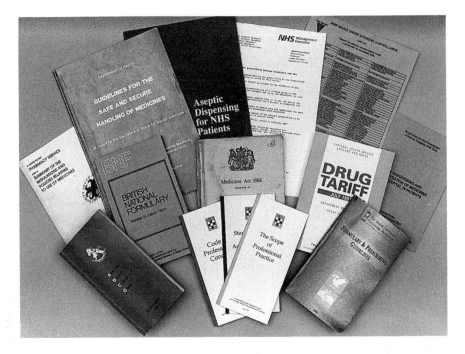

Fig. 11.1 Examples of documents imposing the legal and procedural framework in relation to medicines administration by nurses.

standards of community pharmacies. Despite repeated lobbying by the Royal Pharmaceutical Society, no regulations have ever been made and the Society continues to deal with the issue as a professional matter.

Other legislation governs the operation of the National Health Service (NHS) and conduct of the health professions. Professional bodies such as the United Kingdom Central Council (UKCC) are given wide powers to regulate their professions and set and enforce codes of ethics and practice. In addition, within the NHS, a variety of non-statutory guidance has been issued by the Department of Health (DH), and more recently by the National Health Service Executive (NHSE) and its counterparts in Scotland and Northern Ireland. In recent years a series of multidisciplinary reports has upheld a standard of practice to be adhered to throughout the NHS. While it is not generally a criminal offence in itself to break these codes, staff disregarding them may find themselves removed from their professional registers and/or facing disciplinary action from their employers for unprofessional conduct. Most NHS hospital trusts have standard procedures, usually derived from this mass of legislation and professional and cultural practice, which are printed and available for reference by all relevant staff. Figure 2 shows the various influences on the practice of individual nurses that have been discussed.

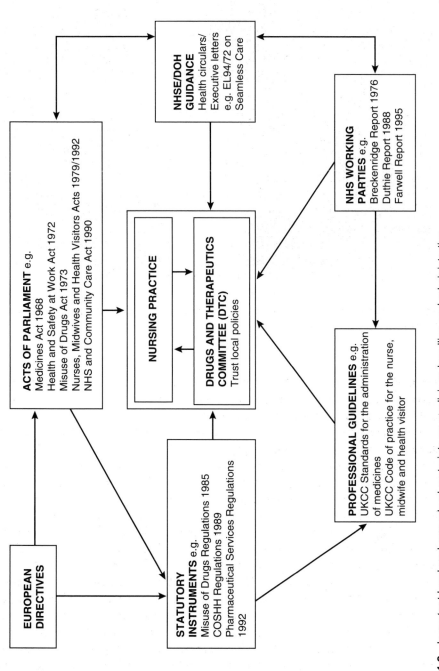

The Medicines Act 1968

Absurd as it seems to us now, before 1968 there was no comprehensive medicines legislation in the UK. A whole range of laws passed during the first part of the twentieth century controlled the manufacture and supply of different types of medicines. As the patent and herbal medicines were replaced by more potent medicines during the therapeutic explosion of the 1960s, it became clear that this legislation was woefully inadequate. This fact was highlighted in the thalidomide tragedy following the prescription of what had been heralded as a safe medicine in pregnancy. Following this disaster, the Medicines Act 1968 was passed to put into place a completely new structure for the marketing and use of medicines. This act remains in force, functioning effectively through a long series of regulations made thereunder. Some of these regulations, as mentioned earlier, have been issued to comply with European directives. Others have been intended to meet changing circumstances in the patterns of supply, for example community nurse prescribing, and the development of new products.

The Medicines Act 1968 established a licensing system for medicines for human use. (Other parts of the act relate to veterinary use of medicines.) The licensing authority is the *Medicines Control Agency*, acting for the government ministers responsible. The only statutory body established by the act is the *Medicines Commission*, which oversees the whole licensing process. Two other well known subsidiary bodies are the *Committee on Safety of Medicines*, described in Chapter 13, and the *British Pharmacopoeia Commission*. Before a medicine is marketed, evidence must be produced of safety and efficacy following which a *Product Licence* is granted. This allows the company concerned to manufacture and market a medicine for specific indications with the dose, side effects, interactions and similar information for health professionals clearly agreed. This licence can be revoked or amended by regulations issued on the advice of the Medicines Commission, if further safety or efficacy data is obtained after marketing. When the Medicines Act 1968 was first implemented, some 39 035 *product licences of right* were granted to products on the market at that time, pending review by the *Committee on the Review of Medicines*. The majority of these preparations were voluntarily withdrawn by their manufacturers before their review took place due to a sales volume too low to justify the work needed to get a Product Licence, or because of anticipated difficulty in satisfying the regulatory authorities about the safety or efficacy of a product (Anon., 1986). As a result, health professionals and patients can be satisfied that licensed products in the UK have been shown to perform as well and as safely as can be expected.

The Product Licence also restricts the availability of products by defining the legal category of the medicine under the Medicines Act 1968: prescription only medicine (POM), pharmacy medicine (P), or general sale list medicine (GSL). All proprietary medicines should bear a *Product Licence Number* (or *European Marketing Authorisation Number*) and legal status code.

Legal categories of medicines in the Medicines Act 1968

Prescription only medicine

Prescription only medicines (POMs) may only be supplied to a patient on the instruction of an appropriate practitioner, that is a doctor or dentist. In a similar manner, the Medicines Act 1968 declares that no person may administer (otherwise than to himself) any such medicine unless he is an appropriate practitioner or a person acting in accordance with the directions of an appropriate practitioner (Applebe and Wingfield, 1993). It will be seen that doctors, including general practitioners, may personally administer POMs to their patients without a prescription, though some record should be kept as part of good practice. NHS regulations specify payments to GPs for drugs personally administered. Possession of a POM without a prescription does not in itself constitute an offence unless that product is also a controlled drug. Nurses should avoid being placed in the position of having to administer a POM without a valid prescription or clear protocol which removes the need for one.

All injections except insulin preparations are POMs. Often, when medicines have been safely used on prescription for a time with good safety data, regulations are amended to move them to a lower category, and well known recent examples of this include ibuprofen, loperamide, clotrimazole vaginal preparations and topical hydrocortisone. Occasionally it may become necessary to reclassify medicines back to POM status; terfenadine has been reclassified as a POM due to increasing evidence of toxicity and interactions.

General Sale List medicine

At the other end of the scale of restriction of supply, medicines on the General Sale List (GSL) can be freely sold in outlets such as supermarkets, garages and drugstores. Small packs of analgesics, simple cough mixtures and vitamin preparations are the most commonly available items.

Pharmacy only medicine

All licensed medicines not the subject of a prescription-only order or on the General Sale List are, by default, pharmacy medicines. These can be freely purchased at any registered community pharmacy providing the pharmacist is present and in a position to personally supervise the sale. Pharmacists have a responsibility under professional codes to refuse the sale if they feel the patient might come to harm by purchasing the medicine or is abusing it. To facilitate this intervention, sales protocols are in place in all community pharmacies to enable sales assistants to direct particular patients, for example those pregnant or taking other medicines, to the pharmacist for further investigation.

Interestingly, the same medicine, for instance ibuprofen, might be a POM, a GSL, or a pharmacy medicine, depending on the indication, pack size, and dose instructions. In the USA, no Pharmacy Only category exists and all medicines are either prescription only or available for open sale, often in very large quantities. Conversely, in most European countries, no GSL category exists and community pharmacists have a total (and lucrative) monopoly on the sale of medicines.

Hospitals and the Medicines Act 1968

It should be noted that all medicines for in-patients in hospitals are *de facto* POMs, except in special circumstances such as officially approved nurse-prescribing schemes. It can be argued that in most nurse-prescribing schemes nurses are not prescribing so much as following a protocol for which a medical practitioner or group with medical practitioners on it (e.g. drugs and therapeutics committee) has taken ultimate responsibility. This is not as a result of the Medicines Act 1968 but rather the multidisciplinary reports referred to later. Hospital pharmacy departments are not registered pharmacies and therefore cannot sell medicines to staff or the public unless they are GSL medicines. However, many have sought registration with the Royal Pharmaceutical Society and sell medicines in small hospital pharmacy shops.

Medicines manufacturing and preparation

Under the Medicines Act 1968, the Medicines Commission not only licenses the products through the previously mentioned Product Licence, but also the manufacturing and preparation of these products. However, while hospital pharmacies do indeed need to obtain Manufacturing Licences to prepare batches of products, exemptions exist for actions taken to meet the immediate needs of particular patients. Under Section 10 of the Medicines Act 1968, pharmacists may prepare products to dispense against prescriptions for patients. In a similar way, Section 11 allows nurses and midwives to assemble medicinal products in the course of their profession without needing a Manufacturing Licence.

The Misuse of Drugs Act 1971

Unlike the Medicines Act 1968, the Misuse of Drugs Act 1971 (MDA) is not concerned with the efficacy and promotion of medicines. Instead, for reasons of public safety, it prohibits the possession, supply and manufacture of certain medicinal and other products, except where such possession, supply or manufacture has been made legal under the regulations. These regulations made under the act are known as the Misuse of Drugs Regulations 1985 and divide these so called *controlled drugs* into various schedules subject to different levels of restriction. Most substances controlled under the MDA are either POMs or totally banned substances, but some strengths and preparations might even be pharmacy medicines, for example kaolin and morphine mixture BP.

Originally the MDA covered mainly opioids and amphetamines (amfetamines), but lately new schedules have been created to restrict aspects of the possession and supply of drugs such as benzodiazepines (and especially temazepam) and anabolic steroids, much beloved by body-builders. Possession of controlled drugs is restricted to the patient or those with legitimate grounds (e.g. community midwives, pharmacists, nurses in charge of a ward or nursing home, etc.). The Schedules of the Misuse of Drugs Regulations (1985) are listed below and summarised in Table 11.1.

Schedule 1 controlled drugs (licence needed)

These are substances with no orthodox therapeutic uses and include poppy straw, lysergic acid diethylamide (LSD) and cannabis. Possession is only legal if the person involved has a licence from the Home Office, for purposes such as research. As a result, if patients are admitted to hospital with a substance such as cannabis in their possession, the ward or the pharmacy may not legally accept and store this. Local protocols exist for this type of situation and generally involve informing the duty manager and police. Of course, staff are under no obligation to inform the police which patient had the cannabis since patient confidentiality must be considered. If the quantities involved are large it may be appropriate to divulge the source to the police, but hospital managers and legal advisers and the consultant would need to be advised first (Appelbe and Wingfield, 1993).

Schedule 2 controlled drugs ('full controlled drugs')

These drugs are the full controlled drugs such as morphine, diamorphine, pethidine and amphetamines. Regulations specify the required information on prescriptions, and other restrictions, and these are detailed below. Exemptions from some of these requirements apply for certain drugs, as shown in Table 11.1. Stocks of Schedule 2 controlled drugs may only be destroyed by a pharmacist if a witness such as a police officer is present, but pharmacists and nurses may destroy patients' own drugs which are no longer needed, preferably as soon as possible after receipt. However, nurses should be careful that in destroying patients' non controlled drugs, they are not breaking local guidelines.

Schedule 3 controlled drugs (CD with no register entry)

Products considered less likely to abuse than Schedule 2 controlled drugs are restricted under Schedule 3. Most commonly these include temazepam and buprenorphine (Temgesic Sublingual), as well as most barbiturates. Like full controlled drugs, regulations on storage, prescription writing and emergency supply apply unless exempted. However, no register entries are needed and supervision of stock destruction is not necessary. It should be observed that

Table 11.1 Some of the Restrictions of the Controlled Drugs Regulations 1985 as Subsequently Amended.[a]

	Schedule of registrations				
	Schedule 1: CDs (Home Office licence)	Schedule 2: CDs subject to full controls	Schedule 3: CDs with no register entry	Schedule 4: CDs anabolic steroids/ benzodiazepines	Schedule 5: CDs needing invoice retention
Example of drugs	Cannabis resin, LSD	Morphine, diamorphine, pethidine, dexamphetamine (dexamfetamine)	Temazepam, buprenorphine, most barbiturates	Chlordiazepoxide, diazepam, nitrazepam, testosterone	Pholcodine linctus, co-dydramol, kaolin and morphine mixture
Drug locked in a CD cupboard	Yes	Yes (except quinalbarbitone (secobarbital))	No (except temazepam, diethylpropion, buprenorphine)	No	No
CD register needed	Yes	Yes	No	No	No
Written requisition	Yes	Yes	Yes	No	No
Prescription in doctor's own handwriting	Yes (need a Home Office Licence)	Yes	Yes (except temazepam and phenobarbitone)	No	No
Detailed prescription needed	Yes	Yes	Yes (except temazepam)	No	No
Emergency supplied permitted by pharmacists	No	No	No (except phenobarbitone for epilepsy)	Yes	Yes

[a] Some Hospital Trusts may treat certain preparations as if they belong in a more restricted category, or apply additional restrictions to preparations. Consult your own nursing procedures for local practice.

many hospitals treat these drugs as fully restricted Schedule 2 controlled drugs.

Schedule 4 controlled drugs (CD anabolics and benzodiazepines)

Most nurses should not even notice that medicines in this category are now controlled drugs. The restrictions in this category apply mainly to those wishing to import, export, manufacture or destroy at a commercial level. However, in the light of continuing abuse, it may be that further restrictions will be applied in the future by government or at a local level by individual hospitals.

Schedule 5 controlled drugs (CD invoices retention)

These are preparations which contain controlled drugs in quantities too low to be a problem. The only requirement is that invoices are kept for 2 years. Typical examples include codeine linctus, and kaolin and morphine mixture BP, which are pharmacy medicines. Interestingly, morphine sulphate mixture 10 mg/5 ml is a Schedule 5 Controlled Drug which is a POM, but it is treated as a full Schedule 2 controlled drug in many hospitals.

Prescriptions for Schedule 2 and 3 controlled drugs

The *British National Formulary* (BNF) (Mehta, 1997) denotes Schedule 2 and 3 controlled drugs with the symbol CD. As seen above, and in Table 11.1, these are the categories to which restrictions apply. The prescription must:

- Be written by a doctor resident in the UK and whose signature is known to the pharmacist
- Be written in ink
- Specify the name and address of the patient
- Have all details written in the doctor's own hand (except for temazepam or preparations containing only phenobarbitone (phenobarbital)
- Be signed and dated by the doctor, not more than 13 weeks before the date presented for dispensing. (A date-stamp is acceptable but not computer-generated dates)
- Contain the name, dose, form and strength (where appropriate) of the preparation (not for temazepam)
- Specify the total quantity or number of doses of the preparation in *both words and figures* (not for temazepam)

In general a pharmacist may not dispense a prescription unless these conditions are met and the doctor's signature is known. In addition, diamorphine, dipipanone and cocaine may not be prescribed *to addicts* in the absence of a Home Office licence. Breach of these regulations by a pharmacist is a criminal offence. In practice, the need to comply with the law often creates inconvenience and delays for nurses and patients when prescribers fail to adhere to the regulations. Hospital nurses in charge of wards and departments may requisition controlled drugs from the pharmacy department, specifying the quantity of drug required. Operating department assistants and practitioners may not requisition, but may hold the keys to the controlled drug cupboard under the supervision of the nurse in charge. Midwives are additionally allowed to possess and administer pethidine, obtained on a requisition from the 'appropriate medical officer' or other appointed supervisor. Midwives must record supplies and use of the pethidine they hold, and may not destroy unwanted or expired stock themselves but should return it to their supervisor.

The Poisons Act 1972

Only products containing a substance on the *Poisons List* made under the Poisons Act 1972 are considered to be 'non-medicinal poisons' or 'poisons'. An example is strychnine. In addition, if the substance is being used for a medicinal purpose, its use is regulated by the Medicines Act 1968. The Poisons List contains two parts. Part I poisons are similar to POM in that they must be sold from a community pharmacy under the supervision of a pharmacist. Part II poisons, may, in addition, be sold by *Listed Sellers* and their nominated deputies, whose names appear in lists maintained by local authorities. In addition to the Poisons List, the Poisons Act 1972 also has regulations made under it called the *Poisons Rules* which modify the provisions of the Act. These rules contain eight schedules but it is most unlikely that nursing staff will be asked to use listed poisons.

The Health and Safety at Work Act 1974: Control of Substances Hazardous to Health (COSHH) Regulations

It is far more likely that nurses will be aware of the regulations made under the Health and Safety at Work Act 1974 on the control of substances hazardous to health (SI 1988 No. 1657). These regulations exist to protect staff from hazards resulting from exposure to substances in the workplace, such as chemicals, micro-organisms, medicines and so forth. Other risks, such as those from radiation and asbestos are covered by other legislation and so excluded (Appelbe & Wingfield, 1993).

Employers are required to assess the risk that substances carry, which will depend on the substance, the form it is being used in, how long staff will be exposed to it, and what precautions can be taken. Manufacturers of potentially hazardous substances must provide full details of the risks, on labels, leaflets and other information, as appropriate, and in hospitals there will be a health and safety manager deputed to maintain files of this information where appropriate. Employers are required to:

- Train and inform staff of the dangers from the substance
- Prevent or minimise exposure to the substance
- Monitor exposure and staff

The following steps are advised in the regulations to reduce risk:

- Avoiding the use of the substance altogether
- Using a safer substance or a safer form
- By enclosing the process and extracting the by-products
- By improving ventilation and hygiene facilities
- By instituting safer handling procedures
- By introducing protective equipment

Most substances that nurses handle will carry fairly small risks but these should not lead to complacency. Passive smoking is a similar occupational hazard in other employment areas but one recognised as an increasing problem. Many nurses are women of childbearing age and this group is especially vulnerable to exposure to many of the hazards. In many hospitals, it is still the practice for medical and nursing staff to prepare cytotoxic infusions. The risks associated with this practice can never be as low as in pharmacy preparation by trained staff with full protective clothing and accessories working in a laminar flow cabinet.

Other products have risks, though. The risk of contact allergy is well known with medicines such as chlorpromazine and antibiotics, and, even though many of these preparations are now film- or sugar-coated tablets or sealed capsules, staff should avoid touching them during medicines administration. Nurses using nebulised pentamidine will be aware that the premixed nebuliser solution will produce less atmospheric risk than mixing the dry powder originally intended for injection. In addition, during nebulisation of pentamidine, various steps are taken (using an exhaust filter/venting the exhaust line/ patient education) to avoid staff exposure to the vapour.

NHS and Community Care Act 1990

This Act was passed to enable the creation of NHS Trusts, fundholding general practices, and in general, the whole concept and practice of the 'purchaser– provider' split in British health care delivery. Originally the Medicines Act 1968 did not apply to NHS hospitals because of the principle of crown immunity, though in practice its provisions were always followed in the NHS. However, since the passing of the NHS and Community Care Act 1990, crown immunity has ceased to exist in NHS hospitals, and the Medicines Act 1968 applies

(Merrills & Fisher, 1995). Other regulations made under the NHS and Community Care Act 1990 (The Pharmaceutical Services Regulations 1992: SI 1992 No. 662) empower the Secretary of State for Health to issue the *Drug Tariff* as described below. Amendments to these regulations allowed a community nurse-prescribing 'demonstration' in eight areas (discussed further in Chapter 8).

The Drug Tariff

While the Medicines Act 1968 and Misuse of Drugs Act 1971 are concerned with restricting the manufacture, marketing and availability of medicines, the *Drug Tariff* is issued each month to identify the availability of medicines within the NHS through community pharmacies. Most nurses will be familiar with the principle that some dressings and surgical sundries are not available to patients following discharge. The reason for this is that in the *Drug Tariff*, there is an assumption that all required medicines will be made available to patients needing them. (This principle has been slightly weakened by those sections of the *Drug Tariff* that blacklist the prescribing of, for example, common cough and cold remedies and many branded benzodiazepines). However, the cost of dressings, appliances, wound management materials, and foods and toiletries (borderline substances) will only be reimbursed to community pharmacists if the product is specifically listed in the *Drug Tariff*. Many products are only allowed for specific indications or in certain sizes. The *Drug Tariff* does not apply in hospitals, but various guidance letters mean that with respect to medicines it is generally followed. However, hospitals often purchase dressings and devices which GPs cannot prescribe, hence these items will need to be supplied to the patient from the ward or department if continuity of supply is to be maintained following discharge. This will incur costs to the NHS Trust which are really the responsibility of the primary care purchasers, and local guidance should be sought before hospital property is given away. (In a similar way, community prescription forms (FP10s) should not be used for GPs to order stock drugs for their practice.)

Community nurse prescribing

The primary legislation to enable nurses to prescribe (The Medicinal Products: Prescription by Nurses etc. Act 1992) was passed on 16 March 1992. In October 1994 the necessary commencement order and secondary legislation amending the Medicines Act 1968 came into force. Additionally, at this time, an amendment to the Pharmaceutical Services and Charges for Drugs and Appliances Regulations came into force; this permitted pharmacists to dispense nurse prescribed items.

A *Nurse Prescribers' Formulary* (NPF) was produced which includes items covering a number of treatment areas associated with nurses' day-to-day practice, for example wound and skin care items, laxatives, minor analgesics and treatments for candidiasis. The preparations are listed in Appendix 1. The majority of these items are available over the counter, although six categories of POMs are included.

In addition to the production of an *NPF*, coloured FP10s (green for district nurses and health visitors and lilac for practice nurses) were issued to prescribing nurses: this was for ease of identification by the Prescription Pricing Authority (PPA). Full details of NHS prescription forms used in England and Wales are given in Table 11.2.

Table 11.2 NHS prescription forms which can be dispensed by community pharmacists.[a]

Form	Colour	Description
FP10	White	Standard NHS prescription form used by general practitioners for items allowed by the *Drug Tariff*.
FP14	Yellow	NHS prescription form used by dental practitioners. Only valid for items listed in the *Dental Practitioners' Formulary*
FP10 (D)	Blue or green	NHS prescription form used by dispensing doctors to order an item they do not carry
FP10 (PN)	Lilac	NHS prescription form for use by approved practice nurses. Only valid for items listed in the *Nurse Prescribers' Formulary*
FP10 (CN)	Green	NHS prescription form for use by approved health visitors and community nurses. Only valid for items listed in the *Nurse Prescribers' Formulary*
FP10 (HP)	Orange/red	NHS prescription form issued by hospital clinics for dispensing in community pharmacies (used when hospital dispensing is not possible)
FP10 (MDA)	Light blue	NHS prescription form used by general practitioners to prescribe any Schedule 2 Controlled Drug[b] in instalments (and water for injections) for addicts
FP10 (HP)Ad	Pink	NHS prescription form used by Drugs Treatment Centres to prescribe in instalments for addicts. Only valid for six controlled drugs: cocaine, dextromoramide, diamorphine, dipipanone, methadone and pethidine[b]

[a] These are the forms used in England and Wales. The forms used in Scotland and Northern Ireland differ slightly in range, purpose, and title.
[b] **Under the Misuse of Drugs Act 1971 diamorphine, dipipanone, and cocaine may only be prescribed for addicts by doctors who hold a Home Office licence.**

Nurse prescribing was originally restricted to eight demonstration sites, one in each region of England. The evaluation of nurse prescribing at each of these sites has now been completed (Luker *et al.*, 1997). Nurse prescribing was subsequently extended to other sites since the publication of DH Report *Primary Care: Delivering the Future* (Department of Health, 1996) with a view to full implementation of nurse prescribing in England by April 1998.

Multidisciplinary reports concerning NHS hospitals

The Aitken Report (1958), Gillie Report (1970), and Roxburgh Report (1972) were major multidisciplinary reports prepared to provide guidance to the NHS on the control of medicines in hospitals. The first two were commended to the NHS by Department of Health and Social Security (DHSS) circulars, and the latter by the Scottish Home and Health Department. These reports operationalise the legal requirements of the Medicines and Misuse of Drugs Acts and are responsible for everyday practices recognised in hospitals today. For example, all these reports recommended that medicines should be stored in locked cupboards, the keys of which were the responsibility of the sister in charge, and that sisters should maintain a controlled drug register, which is not a provision of the Misuse of Drugs Act 1971 (Applebe & Wingfield, 1993).

However, changes in hospital practice led to the setting up of a new Joint Sub-Committee of the DHSS Standing Medical, Nursing and Midwifery, and Pharmaceutical Advisory Committees, chaired by Professor R.B. Duthie. The so called Duthie Report (1988) provides the current guidance for NHS hospitals that consolidates and revises the guidance to Health Authorities and Boards on medicines handling and storage in hospitals, community clinics, and the ambulance services. The report remains in force despite the health-service reforms of the 1980s and 1990s which created the provider NHS Trusts. Although the Duthie Report's recommendations have no legal force, they should be the basis of all NHS Trusts' medicines handling policies, and breach of these by staff will usually be considered a disciplinary matter. The Duthie Report is out of print, and original copies are difficult to obtain. Although the report is over 80 pages long, it is split into sections intended for different situations, (the ward, the pharmacy, and so forth) and copies should be held by all senior nursing managers and chief pharmacists. At intervals, the health departments of the government, or, lately, the NHS Executive, have also issued lesser guidance documents called *Health Circulars* or *Executive Letters* which revise guidance on such issues as the use of child resistant containers or discharge medication policy.

The Duthie Report 1988

The Duthie Report required Health Authorities (and therefore the more recently created Trusts) to establish, document and maintain procedures to *ensure and demonstrate that medicines are stored and handled in a safe and secure manner,* and to designate a senior pharmacist to ensure this. The report considered there to be a *medicines trail* in hospitals, which began with formulary, contracting and quality control work in the pharmacy, proceeded through ordering, distribution, storage and dispensing, and ended up with the patients actually receiving the dose intended by the prescriber. Under the Duthie Report, all procurement of medicines, including that for investigational and trial use, should occur through the pharmacy department. At every stage of the medicines trail when medicines change hands, the report required the procedures to state clearly the required:

- Responsibility
- Record-keeping
- Reconciliation.

The medicines trail described in the Duthie Report is shown in Fig. 11.3.

Storage and handling of medicines at ward level

The appointed nurse in charge of a ward has the responsibility under the Duthie Report for ensuring that the written hospital and ward procedures are followed, and that the security of the medicines held on the ward is maintained. She or he may delegate some of the required duties, for example reconciliation of controlled drugs stocks, or administration or ordering of medicines, but retains the ultimate responsibility. Other sections of the Duthie Report contain slight variations concerning medicines use in areas such as theatres, casualty departments, intensive care units, and clinics. Major issues required to be considered in all these areas are listed below.

- Patients' own drugs are often brought in on admission and a local policy will exist for their handling. They are the property of the patient and should neither be disposed of without the patient's consent, nor used for other patients. They may be used for the patient in question following identification by a doctor or pharmacist, and some hospitals encourage this, especially for non-formulary items and partially used calendar packs. Items not destroyed or disposed of must be stored securely on the ward for return to the patient, or sent home with an identified adult as determined by local policy and practice and the wishes of the patient. (A difficult conflict of professional responsibilities arises if the medicines are unfit for use or if the item has been discontinued by the medical staff, but the above principles generally apply.)

- Stock and non-stock medicines held on wards are ordered and received from the pharmacy department under the responsibility of the appointed nurse in charge. Samples and clinical trial materials must not be accepted on wards, and if found there they should be sent to a pharmacist. The appointed nurse

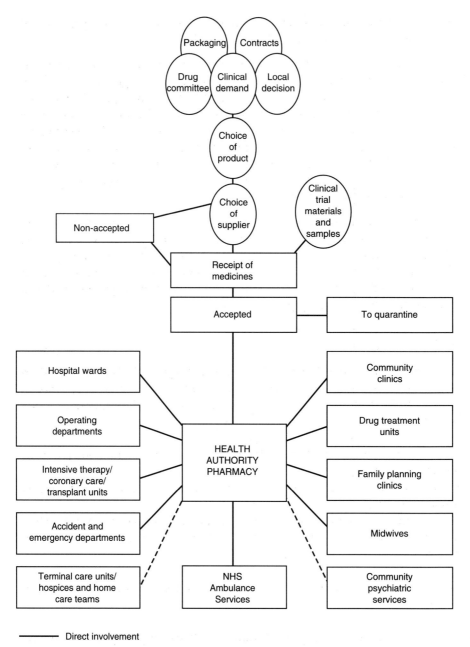

Fig. 11.3 The medicines trail in hospitals (Duthie, 1988). (Crown copyright: reproduced with the permission of the Controller of Her Majesty's Stationery Office.)

must ensure that all receipts of medicines are documented appropriately and stored securely as soon as possible after receipt.

- In a similar way the storage of and access to medicines at ward level is always the responsibility of the appointed nurse in charge, though parts of this duty are usually delegated. There should be separate, locked cupboards for internal medicines, external medicines, controlled drugs, and medicines needing refrigeration or storage in a freezer. There should also be separate storage for diagnostic reagents, intravenous and topical fluids, and flammable products. Pharmacy will check the storage of medicines every 3 months, but nursing staff should reconcile controlled drugs, ideally every day unless local policy varies this.

- Unwanted and expired medicines should be returned to pharmacy. They should only be destroyed on the ward if it is felt they might be diverted, and of course, controlled drugs should not be destroyed or disposed of. (Under the Misuse of Drugs Act 1971 patients' own controlled drugs may be destroyed on the ward, but Duthie does not encourage the practice and as a result local policies usually prohibit this.)

Administration

According to the Duthie Report (1988), all medicines use in hospitals must be considered prescription-only except where specifically exempted. This is because administration, whether by a nurse or nurses, or the patient, may take place only where:

- An instruction is recorded in writing by a medical practitioner on an official prescription chart
- In accordance with local policy (for example nurses' discretionary medicines lists, local 'nurse prescribing schemes')
- In exceptional circumstances, following an oral request from a medical practitioner, but this must not be for a controlled drug and the prescription must be written within 24 hours

Administration of the dose to the patient could take place in a variety of ways, stated to be:

- Self-administration by the patient following dispensing of an out-patient or take-home prescription
- Administration by a suitably qualified practitioner
- Administration by an authorised nurse or nurses following authorisation by an appropriate (usually medical) practitioner, or on their own responsibility within local guidelines. Where single-nurse administration is allowed locally, this should not apply to controlled drugs, weight-related doses, or administration to children under 12 or involving calculations

- Self-administration by in-patients as part of a locally approved scheme. Self-administration schemes are not covered in great detail in the Duthie Report, except that each patient should have a locked non-portable cupboard or drawer for their medicines.

The Farwell and Breckenridge Reports

One particular area of pharmacy practice that has seen major expansion in recent years has been the growth of aseptic dispensing of a whole range of products. As long ago as 1976 the Breckenridge Report advised that all additions of drugs to fluids for intravenous administration should be carried out in the hospital pharmacy department (Breckenridge, 1976). However, due to resource limitations, even as recently as 1995 less than half of acute NHS Trusts were offering even a partial centralised intravenous additive service (CIVAS) for antibiotic reconstitution (Needle, 1995). However, many hospitals do provide aseptic dispensing facilities for antibiotics and/or for products such as total parenteral nutrition solutions, patient-controlled analgesia sets, ophthalmic products such as drops and intra-ocular injections, cytotoxics, and dialysis fluids. For most of these products final sterilisation is not possible and so the products are very vulnerable to the effects of any contamination, which may be especially important in seriously ill patients. As a result of two children's deaths after receiving infected parenteral nutrition solution (Cousins & Upton, 1995) a report primarily written by Dr. John Farwell with specialist pharmaceutical input was published in 1995 (Farwell, 1995): the report *Aseptic Dispensing for NHS Patients* aimed to ensure that aseptic preparation continued to be carried out to the highest standards. To maintain an audit trail from assembly of ingredients to final administration to a patient, it is as a result of the Farwell Report that aseptically dispensed preparations are typically given a maximum shelf-life of 7 days, and are not accepted back to pharmacy departments if unwanted. These requirements may mean that wastage of products at ward level increases. There is also a worry that some hospitals may be forced to desist from aseptic dispensing due to the higher resource implications, and it would be regrettable if the consequences of a report designed to increase standards of pharmacy preparation merely shift the workload to nurses and doctors at ward level.

The Drugs and Therapeutics Committee (DTC) and local hospital medication policies

In practice, most of the requirements of the Duthie Report (1988) will be familiar to nurses from their own clinical practice and the policies of the units in which they work. The provisions of the Duthie Report, it will have been observed, are much tighter and more specific than the provisions of the

Medicines and Misuse of Drugs Acts. All nurses responsible for preparing and enforcing procedures should make efforts to obtain a copy of the relevant part(s) of the Duthie Report. Many hospitals publish their own guidelines in an easily retained and accessed format, and all nurses should obtain their own copy. These guidelines are often added to by practice within the hospital. For example, once a CIVAS is established in an NHS Trust, managers may prefer that the CIVAS product is used wherever possible to ensure quality of product and labelling.

In most NHS Trusts, there is a multidisciplinary committee called the Drugs and Therapeutics Committee (DTC). This usually is co-ordinated by the pharmacy department with a senior physician as chair. Nursing, pharmacy, finance, and various clinical input is standard, with co-option of specialist opinion as required. The DTC, wherever its place in the hospital management structure, generally has responsibility for selecting the standard therapies for use in the hospital or other setting, and drawing up the previously mentioned hospital prescribing policies. To avoid difficulties with patient and staff movements in an area, it is increasingly common for several hospitals to share a DTC, and primary-care sector involvement is becoming common.

The UKCC Standards for the Administration of Medicines

In a similar manner to other professional bodies, the United Kingdom Central Council for Nursing, Midwifery and Health Visiting (UKCC) is legally empowered by the Nurses, Midwives and Health Visitors Acts (1979/1992) to register and regulate the conduct of these groups of staff. The *Standards for the Administration of Medicines*, published in 1992 (UKCC, 1992) represent a synthesis of evolving professional practice, the Medicines and Misuse of Drugs Acts and their subsequent regulations, and reports such as the Duthie Report. The *Standards* represent the final major constraint on nurses' professional practice. All nurses should have a copy of the *Standards*, and be familiar with them. The guidelines emphasise that '*(administration of medicines) is not solely a mechanistic task, to be performed in strict compliance with the written prescription of a medical practitioner. It requires thought and the exercise of professional judgement.*' It is not the purpose of this chapter to repeat these standards again, but it is worth drawing the reader's attention to a few points.

- According to the guidelines, nurses must only administer against a clear, complete, unambiguous written prescription, unless a protocol exists to allow telephoned prescriptions in an emergency. Nurses need to know enough about the reason for the prescription and the nature of the medicine to take professional responsibility for their actions, and must *decline any responsibilities or duties unless able to perform them in a safe and skilled manner.*' Therefore, if a nurse is not satisfied that a prescription is appropriate or safe, she or he must refuse to administer it and inform the prescriber.

- If a nurse feels she or he has made a mistake with regard to medicines administration, disclosure should be rapid and honest. If a patient is suspected of having suffered an adverse effect, the prescriber and pharmacist must be informed.

- Nurses may not administer injections prepared previously, unless these have been prepared in their presence or by a pharmacist. (Of course, if a nurse is not sure for how long a product is chemically or microbiologically stable, it should not be given.)

- The guidelines recognise that sometimes a valid prescription may not exist, because nurses have been authorised to administer a medicine without one. In such 'discretionary administration schemes', nurses should still ensure that clear directions exist from a medical practitioner which they can follow in particular cases.

In summary, then, the guidelines stress that nurses are professionally accountable for their actions and must act responsibly in the interests of the patient at all times. For instance, they might ask a doctor to clarify a controlled drug prescription, to revoke the prescription of intravenous antibiotics where these are clearly no longer appropriate, or to explain the use of an unlicensed medicine or a licensed one for an unusual purpose or for use in an unusual way. A close relationship with the relevant pharmacist will be in the interests of both professions as well as the patient.

It should be pointed out that except where the patient is '*sectioned*' under one of the Mental Health Acts, the administration of any medicine must not take place without patient consent. However, in certain medical emergencies, formal consent may be difficult to obtain, and nurses should be guided by the need to ensure appropriate patient care.

In-patient self-administration schemes

The UKCC (1992) guidelines are supportive of patient or parent (in the case of children) administration of medicines, provided safe and secure storage facilities can be provided for the patient. Many nurses have started, or are anxious to start, such schemes, and there is no doubt that patients gain in respect of confidence and empowerment, and problems with medicines use can be identified. Pharmacists are often seen as being lukewarm or even opposed to such initiatives, but they are merely drawing attention to two areas of concern they might have.

- Self-medication schemes invariably impose an extra workload on already stretched hospital pharmacy departments. For example, if only about 20% of the medicines normally needed on the ward are supplied as non-stock items, for patient self administration there will be a fivefold increase in workload. In addition, every time a dose is changed, a fresh supply of medicines with the correct dose will be needed. In the current situation, during an acute medical admission the patient may not be on a stable regimen long enough to make self-medication workloads for nurses and pharmacists worthwhile.

- Hospital legal advisers are well aware of the 'duty of care' that the hospital owes to its vulnerable patients. Self-medication schemes are often proposed for groups such as elderly people or people with chronic mental illness. If the patient selection criteria are not very carefully defined, there is a risk that a patient could be given access to medicines with which they could unintentionally do themselves some harm.

Any attempt to establish a self-medication scheme must therefore involve the pharmacist who may want to refer the matter to the hospital's DTC.

Nurse prescribing schemes in hospital

Many hospitals and community NHS Trusts have discretionary medicines policies which allow nurses to administer remedies without the need for a prior prescription written by a doctor. These policies do not breach the Medicines Act, since the administration of POMs is rarely involved. Neither is any breach of the Duthie recommendations involved, since these schemes are allowed as long as there is an officially approved written policy, and administration is recorded on the prescription card. Some NHS Trusts require the prescription to be countersigned by a doctor within a fixed period, usually 24 hours. Some schemes of this type include the administration of POMs, for example procyclidine in acute reactions in psychiatry, warfarin in anticoagulant clinics, or antibiotics in casualty departments. The law did not really envisage these situations, but nurses acting according to approved protocols are considered to be passing the responsibility back to a medical practitioner. Whether or not a POM is involved, within the NHS Trust situation nurses should ensure that all their actions comply with clearly written local policies. Nurse prescribing according to written protocols is currenly the subject of a Department of Health review. The catalyst for the review was the White Paper *Primary Care: Delivering the Future* (Department of Health, 1996) which announced proposals to review current arrangements for the prescribing, supply and administration of medicines, and to consider whether any changes should be made to existing arrangements. Readers are advised to refer to the forthcoming report from the Department of Health for the most up-to-date information.

Unlicensed medicines

Most hospitals use a small number of medicines which are not licensed under the Medicines Act 1968. Common examples include thalidomide in AIDS, antithymocyte globulins in acute rejection episodes post-renal transplant, and even some specially prepared syrup formulations of commonly available tablets. Sometimes this is simply because a treatment is so new its licence is not yet fully granted, and in other instances it is a lack of commercial demand or good safety data. More commonly, though, a medicine is unlicensed because, while it may be frequently used in a licensed manner, the medical staff wish to use it in an unusual manner. As part of the licence granted to a medicine under the Medicines Act 1968, the indications, normal dosage, contra-indications and other details are approved. If these are breached, the use of that medicine is unlicensed. Nurses can expect that pharmacists will query the prescription of an unlicensed medicine, and pharmacists will generally allow the prescription to proceed unless they feel the patient is being exposed to serious unnecessary risk (UKCC, 1992). In most hospitals, the doctor will be expected to complete documentation to confirm that the prescription is intended and that the medical staff accept full responsibility for the use of the medicine in this manner. Sometimes the hospital will demand informed consent from the patient. In any event, no unlicensed or clinical trial material should be administered to a patient unless the pharmacy department know about it.

The pharmacy profession

It may be appropriate here to mention a little about pharmacists. Their role originated in the preparation and supply of medicines, but this has evolved into a second role in ensuring safe, effective, appropriate and cost-effective therapy. A recent paper outlined their responsibility to provide pharmaceutical care, to *identify drug-related problems* and *potential problems*, and act to *resolve or prevent* them, to achieve *defined outcomes* to improve the patient's quality of life (Hepler & Strand, 1990). All pharmacists today study initially for an honours degree such as a BSc, BPharm or MPharm. This course currently takes 4 years at one of the 15 British Schools of Pharmacy followed by a pre-registration year, generally undertaken in either hospital or community pharmacy. Following this year and satisfactory achievement of the required competencies, there is a further examination organised by the Royal Pharmaceutical Society of Great Britain or its counterpart in Northern Ireland. Registration as a pharmacist then occurs. Most hospital pharmacists then begin further clinical studies which lead to a postgraduate diploma or MSc higher degree, before opting to specialise in an area such as clinical pharmacy, drug information, purchasing, education, technical services or dispensary management. A typical 1000 bed acute hospital might have a staff of up to 80 in its pharmacy department, of whom up to a quarter might be pharmacists, depending on the range of services provided.

Most pharmacists choose to work in a community pharmacy. Increasingly they are employed by one of the large national chains known as *multiples*. Many community pharmacists also study for further qualifications. This artificial split in the profession, which does not exist to the same extent in nursing or medicine, is an area of concern to some pharmacists and may be tackled in the future. Whichever branch of pharmacy a pharmacist works in, however, they are all professionally required to undergo continuing education and a wide variety of course providers and professional organisations exist.

Pharmacists may be removed from their professional register by their registering Society for criminal activity, incompetence, or breach of a very tight code of ethics. Most nurses will have met pharmacists on their wards or in community pharmacies and hopefully will have found them helpful. Pharmacists want to be informed of any concerns nursing staff have about medicines use, and any problems that nurses know that patients are experiencing with their medicines.

Summary

It will have been observed that the actions of nursing staff in relation to medicines administration in the UK do not take place in a procedural vacuum. Rather, nurses are constrained by a comprehensive structure of laws, protocol and professional constraints. There will be times in every health professional's career when this guidance will appear bureaucratic, tedious, unworkable, or typical of advice given by people who do not have direct patient contact in the real world. Another problem is that the regulations are often superseded by advances in medical care and professional roles. The Medicines Act 1968, for example, was brought into force at a time when doctors prescribed, pharmacists supplied, and nurses administered. Whole new areas of nursing responsibility and practice are opening up in advance of controlling legislation.

Nevertheless, it is important to remember that each law, regulation and procedural requirement was introduced for a reason. The experience of history is that professionals' roles are only curtailed following the identification of risk, sadly often tragedy. By working within the limitations of their profession, nurses can remain confident that they are protecting the patient, themselves, and their employers from risks that others have previously failed to manage.

Acknowledgements

The assistance of Mr Christopher Braidwood, Acting Chief Pharmacist of the St. Helens and Knowsley Hospitals Trust, in the preparation of this chapter is gratefully acknowledged.

References

Aitken, J. (1958) *The Report of the Joint Sub-Committee on Control of Dangerous Drugs and Poisons in Hospitals*, HMSO, London.

Applebe, G.E. & Wingfield, J. (1993) *Dale and Appelbe's Pharmacy Law and Ethics*, 5th edn. Pharmaceutical Press, London.

Anon. (1986) CRM update. Cleaning up the nation's medicine chest, *Br. Med. J.* **292**, 333.

Breckenridge, A.M. (1976) *Report of the Working Party on the Addition of Drugs to Intravenous Fluids*. HMSO, London.

Cousins, D.H. & Upton, D.R. (1995) Are aseptic dispensing services risky? *Pharm. Prac.* **5**, 227–8.

Department of Health (1996) *Primary Care: Delivering the Future*. HMSO, London.

Department of Health (1990) *NHS and Community Care Act*. HMSO, London.

Duthie, R.B. (1988) *Guidelines for the safe and secure handling of medicines: A report to the Secretary of State for Social Services by the Joint Sub-committee of the Standing Medical, Nursing and Midwifery, and Pharmaceutical Advisory Committees*. HMSO, London.

Farwell, J. (1995) *Aseptic Dispensing for NHS Patients: A Guidance Document for Pharmacists in the United Kingdom*. HMSO, London.

Gillie, A.C. (1970) *The Report of a Joint Sub-committee of the Standing Medical, Nursing and Pharmaceutical Advisory Committees on Measures for Controlling Drugs on the Wards*. HMSO, London.

Hepler, C.D. & Strand, L.M. (1990). Opportunities and responsibilities in pharmaceutical care. *Am. J. Hosp. Pharm.* **47**, 533–43.

Health and Safety at Work Act (1974) HMSO, London.

Luker, K.A., Wright, K., Ferguson, B., Austin, L., Hogg, C., Jenkins-Clarke, S., Smith, K. & Willock, J. (1997) *Evaluation of Nurse Prescribing Final Report*. University of Liverpool & University of York.

Medicinal Products: Prescription by Nurses etc. Act (1992) HMSO, London.

Medicines Act (1968) HMSO, London.

Mehta, D.K. (1997) *British National Formulary No. 34*. British Medical Association and Royal Pharmaceutical Society of Great Britain, London.

Merrills J. & Fisher J. (1995) *Pharmacy Law and Practice*. Blackwell Science, Oxford.

Misuse of Drugs Act (1971) HMSO, London.

Needle, R. (1995). A survey of hospital centralised intravenous additive services. *Pharm. J.* **255**, 326–7.

Nurses, Midwives and Health Visitors Act (1979/1992) HMSO, London.

Poisons Act (1972) HMSO, London.

Roxburgh, H.L. (1972) *A Report on Control of Medicines in Hospital Wards and Departments*. Scottish Home and Health Department, Scotland.

United Kingdom Central Council for Nursing, Midwifery, and Health Visiting (1992) *Standards for the Administration of Medicines*. UKCC, London.

Chapter 12

The Nurse's Role in Medicines Administration – Operational and Practical Considerations

John A. Sexton and Christopher C. Braidwood

Introduction

When patients present with a medical condition, they are usually expecting a diagnosis (or confirmation of a self-diagnosis), and an intervention to relieve or cure their condition. Traditionally diagnosis is thought to be the domain of the medical profession, and in general nurses and pharmacists simply respond to symptoms. In practice, however, there is an area of overlap, especially in the management of minor conditions. Whilst many interventions are available to treat presenting conditions, e.g. surgery, counselling and radiotherapy, the most common intervention is drug therapy. Before the Second World War most medicinal products were derived from plant materials and were of varying efficacy. After the war a revolution in therapeutics was seen. The medicines on the market today, however, are the extremely potent end-products of decades of research and are capable of doing real harm to patients as well as bringing great relief from suffering and ill-health.

As discussed in Chapter 11, the Duthie Report effectively makes all medicines use in hospitals prescription only, except where discretionary medicines policies exist (Duthie, 1988). All medicines administration must therefore be in accordance with the directions of a medical (or dental) practitioner, either from a clearly written prescription or approved protocol for treatment, in accordance with Section 58 of the Medicines Act 1968 (Applebe & Wingfield, 1993). As a result, the quality administration of a medicine has been commonly described as one in which the *right patient* receives the *right medicine* at the *right time*.

In practice, however, these criteria are too simple because with the increasing complexity of modern prescribing, administration is no longer simply a mechanistic response to a doctor's prescription. Rather, it requires thought and the exercise of professional judgement in a responsible manner (UKCC, 1992).

Nurses should not simply consider the prescription, but the various stages which are involved in the whole therapeutic process, as shown in Fig. 12.1. This will lead to a collaborative, team approach involving the medical staff, pharmacist, nurse and patient which will contribute to assuring quality administration of medicines.

The patient
Indication
Concurrent illness
Size, age, organ function
Preferences and fears

The prescription
Medical staff behaviour
Hospital and ward policy and practice
Therapy choice, dose, route
Monitoring required

The medicine supplied
Pharmacist's opinion and policy
Nature of pharmacy services
Practice in ordering medicines
Practice in unusual supply, e.g. central intravenous additive service (CIVAS),
total parenteral nutrition (TPN), splitting tablets

The nurse
Competence
Experience
Training
Ability to accept responsibility for the administration

Fig. 12.1   The factors behind the prescription which must be considered by the nurse undertaking responsible administration.

Non-Administration Of Medicines

Before any consideration of the errors that can occur during administration, it is noteworthy that the most common problem with medicines administration is that it simply fails to happen. Some common reasons why this occurs include:

- Failure to order the medicine from the pharmacy department, either for stocks which are running low or for non-stock supplies.
- The newly admitted patient has not yet had their medicines supplied from pharmacy, or the ward staff have not quickly unpacked and appropriately stored that which has been sent.
- There are clinical or formulary problems which prevent the pharmacy department from supplying the medicine or have caused nurses to withhold the therapy, or the pharmacy department has simply failed to supply something when requested.
- Patients are transferred between wards without their non-stock medicines.
- The supplied medicines are not recognised by the ward staff (see later).
- Some therapy has been inadvertently omitted on admission, most commonly involving products such as eye-drops and inhalers.
- The patient is nil-by-mouth or away from the ward at the time of medicine administration.
- The patient refuses (as is their right) the administration of the medicine.
- There is no-one available and trained to prepare and/or administer intra-venous medicines at night.

The failure to administer therapy is sometimes the appropriate course of action for the responsible nurse to take. However, if essential therapy is not given then the patient will not derive the expected benefits of treatment. A typical situation is one in which newly admitted patients with unusual prophylactic medicines for angina or epilepsy, for example, are admitted with exacerbations of their condition and paradoxically then fail to receive their usual therapy. The problem seems worse at weekends and all nurses who have accepted professional accountability must be familiar with pharmacy supply systems and support both within and outside working hours. Whenever administration does not take place, for whatever reason, such non-administration must be documented and medical staff advised accordingly.

Responsible administration of medicines

For the nurses involved in the care of a patient, what is considered 'right' will initially be based on what the prescribing doctor has indicated. However, it should not be forgotten that doctors, pharmacy staff and other nurses are not immune from making errors which may not be immediately detected at ward level. Following consideration of their own competence and experience, hospital policy and practice, and an element of common sense, nurses administering medicines should act in concert with medical staff to ensure that patients receive medicines in ways which will produce the most benefit with the lowest risk of harm. The 'right' dose or even medicine may not therefore be that which has been prescribed, and if nurses feel uncertain about a prescription, they should *act in the interests of the patient* and *contact the prescriber without delay* (UKCC, 1992). The subsequent response, which might persuade the nurse involved to administer the medicine or to refuse to participate in such administration, would depend on the nature of the explanation obtained and the nurse's own judgement and that of her or his colleagues. In addition, most nurses would also consider the experience of the prescriber; a reasoned explanation from a consultant physician will naturally be more persuasive than a poor justification from a newly-qualified house officer.

What is clear is that every day, in every hospital, nurses protect patients by querying prescriptions which have raised concern in their minds. It is also clear that wherever drug administration errors have occurred, the failure of nurses to question practice has often been a contributing factor.

The inappropriate administration of medicines may lead to patients not receiving full benefit or receiving harm from their therapy. By considering what can go wrong, it will be observed that there are many things that nurses can do to assure quality of patient care in relation to medicines administration. However, if nurses are to be able to accept responsibility for their actions in relation to the use of medicines, a more suitable definition of a quality administration of a medicine is needed. To modify our initial description, therefore, the criteria used to describe quality administration are listed below.

Medicines administration should ensure that:

- The *correct patient* receives
- The *appropriate medicine*
- In the *appropriate formulation*
- By the *appropriate route*
- At the *appropriate dose*
- At the *appropriate time*
- At the *appropriate rate*
- For the *appropriate duration of therapy*
- With the *appropriate monitoring to ensure safety of therapy*
- With the *appropriate monitoring to ensure efficacy*
- With the *appropriate reporting of adverse drug reactions*

Sources of error: the correct patient

Good administration of medicines involves nurses being certain of the patient's identity (UKCC, 1992). Most nurses will be familiar with situations in which a patient has received, or nearly received, medication intended for another. This could occur when handing out medicines '*to take out/away*' (TTOs/TTAs), or when a clinic prescription has the wrong name and address label attached to it. In the in-patient setting, patients may have similar names, or charts may have been left at the foot of the wrong bed. It should be remembered that some patients are hard of hearing, and many are anxious to please, and when asked questions many tend to nod and agree with what has been said to them. Some independent verification of the patient is therefore required to confirm their identity. In long-stay wards, patient photographs on charts may help ensure that mis-identification is avoided (Williams, 1996).

Sources of error: the appropriate medicine

If nurses feel that the appearance of medicines in a container does not seem quite right, whether that container is the patient's own, ward stock, or newly supplied to the ward by pharmacy, they should consult a pharmacist for guidance. To prevent errors, medicines should *never* be transferred from one container to another in an attempt to make the trolley neater, or separated from their container by 'setting-out' in advance of administration. Neither should labels be altered and defaced except in co-ordination with the ward pharmacist (Williams, 1996). In a similar way, it is against all hospitals' medicines policies for nurses to 'dispense' take-home medicines into envelopes or other containers from ward stock simply because an urgent discharge has been ordered or there has been an oversight. It is much safer to advise the patient or their relatives to call back, or promise to send on the medicines by, for example, a taxi. Nurses should avoid taking actions they know to be professionally unsound and expose themselves and the patient to risk as a result of emotional blackmail from patients, their relatives, or other health professionals. In general, in relation to medicines administration, adherence to hospital protocols, clear thinking and orderly working practices minimise the risk of errors.

There is also the possibility that the patient might be taking their own medicines, including discontinued therapy, without telling medical or nursing staff. If medicines are left in the patient's possession, nursing staff should ensure that local protocols are followed and that medical staff are made aware of any unauthorised self-administration so that appropriate action can be taken.

Generic and proprietary names

Most medicines have at least two names; their proprietary (manufacturer's brand) name and their generic approved name. When a medicine is first marketed, it is under patent and manufacturers will attempt to recoup their development costs by active promotion of their product under its brand name. Eventually, the patent expires and other companies can market their own versions under either the generic name or yet another brand name of their own.

Brand names remain in common use because they are often shorter, catchier, or more descriptive than the generic name, as shown in Table 12.1. The generic name of a medicine may change occasionally to produce internationally approved names. For example, aciclovir has replaced the better known acyclovir. On a more significant level, the internationally used names lidocaine, epinephrine and furosemide may eventually replace the more familiar lignocaine, adrenaline and frusemide (Anon., 1997).

Table 12.1 Some examples of generic, brand and unofficial names

Generic name[a]	Brand name[b] (example)	Unofficial name (to be discouraged)
Aciclovir	Zovirax	
Ranitidine	Zantac	
Ibuprofen	Brufen	
Diamorphine		Heroin
Zidovudine	Retrovir	AZT
Dihydrocodeine	DF118	DFs
Co-proxamol	Distalgesic	DGs
Co-dydramol	Galake	
Some other common compound preparations		
Co-amilofruse	Frumil, Frumil-LS, Frumil Forte, Lasoride	
Co-amilozide	Moduretic, Moduret-25	
Co-amoxiclav	Augmentin	
Co-beneldopa	Madopar	
Co-careldopa	Sinemet	
Co-danthramer	Codalax	
Co-danthrusate	Normax	
Co-fluampicil	Magnapen	
Co-flumactone	Aldactide	
Co-magaldrox	Maalox	
Co-phenotrope	Lomotil	
Co-prenozide	Trasidrex	
Co-tenidone	Tenoretic, Tenoret-50	
Co-triamterzide	Dyazide	
Co-trimoxazole	Septrin, Bactrim	

[a] Different ratios and strengths of many preparations are available.
[b] Some of these brand names are not acceptable on NHS prescriptions.

The Medicines Control Agency ensures through the licensing system that European and British Pharmacopoeial standards are maintained to ensure equivalence of all manufacturers' versions of the product. The generic name of the drug is ideally used to prescribe the drug. In the primary care setting, the community pharmacist can then supply the cheapest brand available of the drug, producing benefits for the NHS. However, patients used to 'own-brands' of provisions in the supermarkets may need reassurance if a prescription is dispensed that their medicine is just as good as an unfamiliar brand. In NHS hospitals, the generic name is the one used on dispensed medicines as a matter of course. The hospital's pharmacists, through purchasing consortia, will be involved in awarding contracts for particular products, usually chosen to ensure the best price once quality factors have been considered. Generally the contracts last for 2 years.

Use of the generic name is important in secondary care because administration errors can arise when medical staff prescribe by brand name in hospitals. Because brand names are much less commonly used in hospitals, when they are specified they may not be recognised. Pharmacists should endorse brand-name prescriptions with the appropriate generic name, but before this happens the medicine may have failed to have been administered because nurses did not know that what they had was the item desired. Alternatively, medical staff may not have known what the item was either, and prescribed the same item twice. The use of unofficial names and abbreviations such as DDI, AZT, and APD is likely to create problems, and has led to disasters in the past due to confusion with other medicines. In a similar way, the use of chemical names and formulae such as acetylsalicylic acid instead of aspirin, or $FeSO_4$ instead of ferrous sulphate should be avoided by prescribing staff.

One exception exists to the generic rule in prescribing. Not all modified release preparations are identical in the manner in which they release their active ingredient into the body. It is therefore more important to dispense and administer the same brand, and hence proprietary names are preferred for prescriptions for modified-release preparations of calcium-channel antagonists such as diltiazem and nifedipine (of which there are many) and theophylline/ aminophylline (Mehta, 1997). Another group of medicines currently causing some debate in this area is the antiepileptic drugs where narrow ranges of acceptable plasma levels are the rule.

Combination products

The generic naming of products began to create problems once manufacturers started to combine different medicines in the same tablet. Common reference sources deprecate the use of combinations because a particular patient may only really need one of the ingredients, for example the frusemide (furosemide) in frusemide/amiloride combinations or the amoxycillin (amoxicillin) in amoxycillin/clavulanic acid combinations. The marketing of combinations thus encouraged the prescription, in effect, of additional and unneeded medicines and the combinations are often much more expensive than the prices of the ingredients as generics. Nevertheless, in many cases combinations of medicines in the same tablet can make administration and compliance much easier, and generic combinations have become available in recent years as co-names have been introduced. However, a large number of names for medicines now all begin co- with the possibility of confusion for nurses and patients, as illustrated in Table 12.1. In general, the stem begins with, or is based on, the first part of the name of the ingredient in lower quantity, followed by the last part of the name of the major ingredient. If more than one combination is available, strengths and other differentiators are needed. For example, the combinations of frusemide (furosemide) and amiloride are known as co-amilofruse 5/40, co-amilofruse 2.5/20, or co-amilofruse 10/80 depending on strength.

Names and errors

The possibility of errors between names is always present during drug prescribing, dispensing and administration, and is especially great if obscure brand names or poor handwriting are employed by the prescriber. Many medicines have long generic names and may be unfamiliar to nursing staff on a particular ward. The rise of the 'sleep-out' or 'outlier' patient, receiving medical treatment on a surgical ward, or a medical ward not generally used for that speciality, makes this ever more likely. Some of the more common examples of similar sounding names with potentially lethal consequences for any errors are listed below. It should be noted that this list can only provide a few examples of common confusions; it is far from exhaustive.

- Quinidine sulphate and quinine sulphate
- Disopyramide and dipyridamole
- De-Nol and Danol or Daonil or danazol
- Dopamine and dobutamine or doxapram
- Chlorpropamide and chlorpromazine
- Slow-K and Slow Sodium
- Co-amilozide and co-amilofruse
- Promazine and promethazine
- Nifedipine and nimodipine or nicardipine
- Ismo and Istin

In practice, however, serious harm can also come from unexpected confusions. Nurses in one hospital administered 600 mg of *Cidomycin* (gentamicin) on two occasions instead of *clindamycin*, though the patient's subsequent death was not attributed to this (Cousins & Upton, 1997). In another case, a community pharmacist dispensed *Daonil* (glibenclamide) instead of *Amoxil*. Damages were subsequently awarded against the pharmacist and general practitioner, who the court felt had contributed to the error with his handwriting (Applebe & Wingfield, 1993). Thus all nurses must consider the appropriateness of the prescription they are about to administer and, if it is in any way illegible, ambiguous, or suspicious, they must seek clarification.

The truly inappropriate item

In addition to nurses administering the wrong item or failing to administer the correct item because of difficulties over names, there remains another source of patients receiving inappropriate medication. This occurs when there is a clear and valid prescription but it is for a clinically inappropriate choice of therapy. Nurses are expected to *'be aware of the patient's current assessment and planned programme of care'* (UKCC, 1992). Thus many nurses would refuse to administer without clarification a prescription for a beta-blocker for an asthmatic patient, or an oral hypoglycaemic agent to a patient with a very low blood glucose. Similarly, they should not continue to give fluids to an obviously fluid-overloaded patient until a medical practitioner has been informed.

Sources of error: the appropriate formulation

Duration of action and strength

Even when the right name has been ascertained, administration errors can still occur when medicines are available in different strengths and formulations. Hopefully, no nurse would administer a prescription calling for 'thioridazine syrup 10 ml' to a patient without checking the strength of preparation that the doctor had in mind when they wrote the prescription. However, just as with names, the prescription of unfamiliar items on hospital wards can cause errors. Many of the ambiguities in prescriptions can only be identified if nurses are familiar with the items in question or have access to information sources.

An example of the possibilities for confusion is the popular antiparkinsonian therapy, co-beneldopa (Madopar). This is a combination of benserazide and levodopa, and is available in three standard strengths, two sustained release strengths, and two soluble strengths. Its close cousin co-careldopa (Sinemet), is available in preparations containing three different ratios of carbidopa and levodopa, as well as sustained release preparations. The previously mentioned three stengths of the frusemide/amiloride combination, co-amilofruse, are available as several brands. The most popular branded product uses slightly different brand names for each strength, but as with a variety of similarly named medicines, one needs to be sure of exactly what is being asked for.

When formulations are considered, the possibilities for confusion are again legion, requiring a thorough understanding of the nature of the therapy under prescription. Many medicines are available in modified or sustained-release preparations designed to simplify therapy or produce a better pharmacokinetic profile. Diltiazem has already been mentioned as an example of a medicine available in a host of non-equivalent once, twice, or three times a day preparations, some of which have the same basic brand name. Morphine sulphate tablets 10 mg are available in two forms, one of which is a sustained-release product designed for twice-daily administration (MST or Oramorph SR) and one is not (Sevredol). Only two letters (SR) in the generic name printed on a hospital-pharmacy label therefore differentiate a medicine which is used for fast relief of breakthrough pain, from one which is intended for use as a baseline maintenance prescription. In addition, there is now a once-daily sustained release preparation (MXL) which must not be confused with the traditional twice-daily preparations. As with all medicines-related problems, the ward or drug-information pharmacists can resolve these types of difficulties very quickly.

Solid and liquid oral dose forms

One of the most common problems seen in administration is that patients often cannot swallow their medicines, and nurses are consequently unable to administer therapy. In these cases, the pharmacy department may be unaware that nurses are having problems, yet can often provide or manufacture a suitable liquid preparation if asked. Sometimes they have to ask nurses to crush tablets or open capsules if a product is unstable in suspension. However, nurses should not attempt to do this without checking with a pharmacist first. It is quite possible that a sustained-release system might be destroyed by crushing or an enteric coating might be damaged, affecting the pharmacodynamics of the dose form considerably. Where no liquid form exists or can be prepared, the pharmacist may be able to suggest an alternative medicine or formulation. This often occurs with elderly patients prescribed isosorbide mononitrate. There is no liquid preparation and the sustained-release preparations cannot be crushed, but a useful approach might be to try a glyceryl trinitrate patch or a buccal tablet. In a similar manner suppositories of domperidone will remove the need for metoclopramide injections in a nauseous patient who is nil-by-mouth.

Where liquid preparations are supplied, nurses should take care to check that high-sugar preparations are not administered to diabetic patients without considering the effect that these will have on blood glucose levels. Many manufacturers of proprietary products are choosing to provide sugar-free formulations of liquids (primarily to protect children's teeth), or alternative preparations such as soluble tablets. However, the choice of cough mixture still needs care, since few low-sugar brands exist and none is commonly stocked on wards.

Sources of error: the appropriate route

It is always important to ensure that the route by which the drug is administered is the appropriate one and not just the one prescribed. Only clear solutions can be injected intravenously and many injections can do serious harm. Phenothiazines such as prochlorperazine and chlorpromazine are too irritant to inject intravenously or even subcutaneously in a syringe driver. Conversely, one popular adult formulation of vitamin K injection (Konakion MM) is not to be given intramuscularly. Another common error is the administration of subcutaneous heparins by injection in the arm, when they are designed to be given in the thighs or abdomen. This can have serious consequences for the patient. As a final example, despite wide awareness of the lethal results of the intrathecal administration of vincristine and vinblastine, and even penicillins, fatalities continue to be reported (Cousins & Upton, 1994, 1995a).

With respect to oral dose formulations, buccal tablets of glyceryl trinitrate or prochlorperazine are designed to be placed under the top-lip, not administered under the tongue, though this is the ideal route for *sublingual* glyceryl trinitrate and buprenorphine. Neither buccal nor sublingual tablets are suitable for swallowing. On a similar note, chlorhexidine mouthwash must be spat out after swilling around the mouth. However, nystatin suspension should be swallowed, though the longer the patient can hold it in their mouth the greater will be the therapeutic effect.

Where liquid formulations are administered through nasogastric or gastrostomy tubes, the tube must be flushed with water or saline solution before and after each medicine has been administered. This prevents blockages and any interaction with feeding fluids being used. For instance, phenytoin solution is well known to interact with nasogastric feeds, resulting in poor absorption and much lower blood levels of phenytoin. As a result, cessation of feeding for short periods before and after administration of phenytoin is generally recommended.

Sources of error: the appropriate dose

Errors by nurses

Frank errors in dosage are uncommon, but undoubtedly do occur during administration by nursing staff. As a general principle, adult doses are typically small numbers of tablets or ampoules, though well known exceptions include mesna and prednisolone. Action was recently brought against nurses who administered a large number of ampoules of intravenous digoxin to a patient who later died; their defence of confirmation of the dose from a senior doctor was not accepted. However, other dose errors are more subtle, though just as potentially dangerous. In the case of the liquid preparations mentioned previously, there is the possibility that errors can occur in dose conversion. For example, if a patient is taking phenytoin capsules 300 mg at night and then converted to syrup, only 270 mg is needed because the capsules contain phenytoin sodium salt rather than phenytoin itself. An attempt to give 300 mg of syrup could produce a toxic blood level. In a similar way, it would be dangerous to administer eight 5 ml spoonfuls of a popular brand of ferrous sulphate syrup, usually quoted as 25 mg ferrous iron/5 ml, in an attempt to give the dose contained in a 200 mg ferrous sulphate tablet, again because like is not being compared with like.

Particular problems with paediatric doses are not covered in detail here, but any administration requiring a calculation or to very young children is prone to error and generally restricted to two-nurse administration techniques. This is because liquid formulations or ampoules might have been designed to administer adult doses, and so fractions of dose forms are needed. The death of a child following the intrathecal administration of the dose of benzylpenicillin normally used for intravenous administration shows that errors can occur even when some effort has been put into calculating the correct dose (Cousins & Upton, 1995a). In another sadly far from unique incident, a child died when doctors administered many times the normal dose of morphine having con-fused the available dose forms (Cousins & Upton, 1996).

In both paediatric and adult prescriptions, dose units must be as clear and unambiguous as the medicine name itself, and abbreviations of terms such as *microgram* and *nanogram* should be avoided.

Failure of nurses to spot inappropriate doses

More commonly, however, errors occur because nurses fail to spot that the dose prescribed is inappropriate for the patient. While this has traditionally been considered a matter for the doctors and pharmacists, nurses have a valuable role to perform here. Where doses are outside the product licence, nurses should, if they feel it appropriate, refuse to administer the prescribed substance (UKCC, 1992). As with many previous examples, familiarity with the pre-scribed drugs makes it more likely that nurses will spot the unusual. For example, methotrexate is usually given weekly, but occasionally gets pre-scribed daily by mistake and deaths have resulted from this. Low molecular weight heparins are designed for once-daily use and hopefully most nurses, especially orthopaedic staff, would query more frequent regimens.

Other examples of inappropriate doses are less obvious: for example, ACE inhibitors, carbamazepine and thyroxine (levothyroxine) must be started at low doses until patient tolerance has been established. Some medicines, such as amiodarone and warfarin, are commenced at high *loading* doses. If these doses are continued beyond the appropriate initiation period, serious harm will probaby result to the patient.

Sources of error: the appropriate time

The problem of hospital medication administration rounds is that they gen-erally take place at fixed times, making it difficult to ensure accurate dose intervals. Studies with antibiotics have shown intervals in a three-times a day regimen varying between 4 and 12 hours. In addition, these rounds often take place between meal servings, which complicates the delivery of 'with-food' regimens, often essential to reduce gastro-intestinal bleeds when using non-steroidal anti-inflammatories.

With regard to the prescription, sedative antidepressants such as ami-triptyline are best given at night (unless in divided doses). The newer anti-depressants such as fluoxetine, however, should be prescribed and administered in the morning because they can cause insomnia. Laxatives such as senna are given at bedtime so that they can work overnight. Most other drugs are given in the morning. Sometimes this is to mimic a natural process, for example with prednisolone, sometimes for patient convenience, as with powerful loop diuretics; but more usually it is simply by convention to establish a routine among patients.

Sources of error: the appropriate rate

With oral therapy, administration tends to take place fairly quickly. However, especially with intravenous therapy, some medicines must be given slowly. Some medicines can be extremely toxic if administered too quickly: a maxi-mum rate of 4 mg/min is recommended for frusemide (furosemide) and 50 mg/min for phenytoin. In a similar manner, ranitidine, if administered too quickly while undiluted, can cause bradycardia. Other medicines, such as aminophylline (after a loading dose), nitrates, dopamine and dobutamine, need slow infusions to maintain a therapeutic level.

Sources of error: the appropriate duration of therapy

Durations of therapy can present problems as well – nurses and pharmacists must press for regular reviews of therapy, especially for antibiotics. As nurses take responsibility off doctors for the administration of intravenous antibiotics, some fear that course lengths and costs will increase because medical staff no longer have the same powerful negative incentive to *step-down* to oral therapy. In a similar way, nurses on ward rounds are in an ideal position to act as the patient's advocate by pressing for the need for review of long-term therapy. Similarly, nurses in GPs' surgeries will often see, as part of health-screening interviews, elderly patients on possibly unneeded continuing therapy.

Sources of error: the appropriate monitoring to ensure safety of therapy

Medicines are often prescribed correctly, but become inappropriate during therapy. All therapies should be monitored for both effect (if they have no effect, there is no justification in continuing therapy in that patient) or toxicity. Medical staff must be informed, for example, if as might be expected, a patient becomes bradycardic during digoxin therapy, or hypotensive after starting ACE inhi-bitors. Most nurses on medical wards are familiar with these medicines and carry out these checks routinely. With other therapies, especially potent cyto-toxic or anti-rheumatic medicines, nurses can make valuable contributions to compliance with protocols, designed to protect patients from harm. These might require periodic blood tests, for example, or patient education about reporting certain possible side effects such as a cough or sore throat.

On general medical wards, one particular group of antibiotics causes special problems. Aminoglycosides such as gentamicin need therapeutic drug moni-toring for peak and trough concentrations, measured pre- and post-dose, on the second day of therapy. If these measurements are not performed then the continued administration of gentamicin may cause serious harm. Nurses should not continue to administer aminoglycosides unless therapeutic drug levels are being checked *and acted on*. In a similar way, the continued administration of newly prescribed warfarin is unwise unless clotting times are being checked. As a final example, hopefully it would be hard to find nursing staff administering isosorbide dinitrate infusions without keeping a close eye on blood pressure.

Sources of error: the appropriate monitoring to ensure efficacy

Most nurses will routinely be involved in reporting back to prescribers if therapy is ineffective or only partially effective. In addition, just as infusions of nitrates, theophyllines and insulin are monitored to prevent harm to the patient, nurses will be familiar with the increasing of flow rates of these medicines either within protocols or by contacting the doctor, if the patient needs more of the therapy to obtain the desired outcome.

Sources of error: the appropriate reporting of adverse drug reactions

As a minimum level of professional practice, the relevant medical staff *must* be informed if a patient is observed to have suffered (or possibly suffered, or reports suffering) an adverse effect to a medicine. This report should ideally be recorded in writing to further protect the patient and nurse. As discussed in Chapter 13, there may be a hospital adverse drug reaction (ADR) reporting scheme as well, and this should be used where appropriate to do so. In the case of frank allergy, nurses should ensure that the report has been clearly docu-mented in the medical notes to prevent re-exposure to the medicine.

Sources of error: summary

At its simplest level, administration of medicines involves checking the name, strength, formulation, expiry date and route of administration against the prescription. However, administration needs more thought to avoid the risk of errors. A current copy of the *British National Formulary* must be available on every ward if nurses are to be able to discharge their professional responsibilities in drug administration. Very occasionally situations arise where it is clear that the medical staff involved did not actually know the nature of the prescriptions they had written. But how much more often do nurses administer therapy they have not used before without the knowledge, experience or support needed to assure quality administration? Nurses must ensure they are competent to perform the tasks involved if the quality administration of medicines is to be responsibly performed (UKCC, 1992).

Parenteral therapy problems

The administration of parenteral therapy presents particular problems for the nurse. The drugs which are given by injection or infusion are often more potent, and errors and harm can result from inappropriate routes, concentrations, carrier and diluent fluids, and rates of administration. In particular, though, problems of compatibility and microbiological and chemical stability may present additional risks that nurses must consider.

Fluid replacement regimens

At the simplest level, patients commonly receive fluid replacement regimens through peripheral intravenous or subcutaneous cannulae. The two most common fluids available on hospital wards are the isotonic preparations of glucose (dextrose) 5% and sodium chloride (saline) 0.9%. Each of these is commonly available in a range of sizes from 50 ml to 1000 ml. Since these bags all cost roughly the same price, pharmacy departments tend to prefer wards to use the largest size available, which also makes administration easier for nurses, since fewer bag changes are needed.

Potassium administration

Potassium is best added to bags at the manufacturing stage. If added at ward level extreme care needs to be taken to avoid '*layering*', in which dense potassium chloride does not mix with the diluting fluid. On commencement of the infusion, therefore, the patient initially receives a concentrated potassium solution and this can be as dangerous to the heart as giving the undiluted injection as a bolus injection. Because the very presence of potassium ampoules on wards and in theatres is a potential source of harm (ampoules have been mistaken for sodium chloride 0.9% or water and used to reconstitute, for example, antibiotics, with tragic consequences), many hospitals have made parenteral potassium preparations subject to the same restrictions as controlled drugs. If stronger solutions than those supplied by pharmacy are needed, an additional 40 mmol of potassium may be added to a 1000 ml bag so long as the bag is then mixed well. Stronger solutions need pumps and cardiac monitoring, and are best left to specialist units.

Intravenous administration of medicines

Nurses are commonly expected to administer medicines intravenously. As a general principle, the NHS has long advised that additions of medicines to fluids should preferably be carried out in an aseptic environment in a pharmacy department. This ensures low levels of microbial contamination and the choice of appropriate fluids and volumes for dilution. Some medicines are unstable in certain fluids due to the pH (acidity/alkalinity) of the fluid. For example, the traditional formulation of colloidal amphotericin is unstable in sodium chloride 0.9% and must be infused in glucose solution with a pH greater than 4.2.

Resource and practical considerations, however, often mean that the addition has to be carried out on the ward by medical and nursing staff. Many hospitals restrict these functions to those staff who have been additionally certified, or to a defined range of products. As well as checking the expiry date, strength and identity of the medicine to be added to the fluid, the following points must be observed:

- The initial diluent used to reconstitute the vial of medicine must be the appropriate one. In addition, if the contents of the reconstituted injection are to be added to a bag of fluid for infusion, the fluid chosen must be known to be compatible with the medicine to be added. This information can be found in the package insert, Appendix 6 in the *BNF*, or from pharmacy.

- Two medicines must never be mixed in the same syringe, bag, or line unless they are known to be compatible. Some combinations, for example gentamicin with penicillins or cephalosporins, will render the product useless.

- The volume of the fluid used must be appropriate for the medicine. Many antibiotics can be administered as bolus injections, but the use of a small volume bag will dilute the product and make it less irritating to the veins. Some preparations, notably erythromycin, vancomycin and sodium fusidate, must be diluted in quite large volumes of fluid and given slowly, to avoid serious harm to the patient. These large volumes may then necessitate a reduction in the other fluids prescribed for the patient, especially in fluid restricted patients.

- Good aseptic technique must be used, assembled products labelled with the contents and time of addition, and any hospital policies, such as who is allowed to give the first dose, followed. Most hospitals prohibit the addition of medicines to fluids such as blood, parenteral nutrition, mannitol or sodium bicarbonate.

- The container used may itself be a cause of problems. Nitrates are adsorbed onto soft PVC infusion bags and must be given in either a syringe or rigid infusion container such as a *Polyfusor*.

- For paediatric doses, nurses will generally be familiar with the principle of *displacement value*. The addition of 10 ml of fluid does not mean that 10% of the dose will then be present in a 1 ml fraction of the vial. Fortunately, the increasing provision of central intravenous additive services (CIVAS) means that these corrections are increasingly done elsewhere by other staff.

- Apart from bags made in pharmacy, administration must begin immediately after the addition of the fluid. This is because as soon as the product has been reconstituted chemical and microbiological deterioration will begin. No nurse should administer a product that they did not see assembled (unless it came from pharmacy) (UKCC, 1992).

If in any doubt about the safety or appropriateness of any step during intravenous administration, advice should be sought from more experienced colleagues. It should never be assumed that 'it will be all right'.

Cytotoxic medication administration

Many cytotoxic therapies are administered intravenously. The medicines involved are often extremely toxic, both immediately to the patient and nurse if not handled and administered correctly, and subsequently in what they do to the patient. In addition, few have doses that can be easily confirmed using the *BNF*. Most of these medicines are administered as part of clinical trials, in complex combinations, and often have doses which are based on surface area and clinical condition. If nurses are fortunate to work in a unit with excellent interdisciplinary relationships, few problems will result. Where pharmacy services provide the infusions in appropriate volumes and fluids, and check all preparation and prescription, including rates and days of administration against protocols, unexpected risk to staff and patients is very unlikely.

If staff are asked to reconstitute cytotoxic therapy before administration, then all reasonable steps should be taken to protect both the staff and the product. No nurse should reconstitute cytotoxics unless the fluid choice and volume have been defined in writing, along with administration directions. In one well known case, pharmacists continued to prepare, and nurses to administer, an unclear prescription for a cytotoxic each day that was only intended for weekly administration.

Other injections

Nurses are familiar with intramuscular and subcutaneous injections. Though more painful than intravenous therapy, they are more suited to some products, especially for short periods. Each hospital has a policy about who can give, and into which sites, intramuscular and subcutaneous injections. In general, subcutaneous low molecular weight heparins should not be given into the arm, but rather in the abdomen or thigh to avoid bruising.

Insulins are generally given subcutaneously, and sites should be rotated to avoid lipotrophy with resulting erratic absorption. Some particular problems commonly occur with insulin administration.

- Insulins often have similar names which disguise different preparations, for example *Human Mixtard* which is available in five different ratios of short/long acting insulins. In addition, this particular product is also available as *Pork Mixtard*, and, if the origin is not specified, the prescriber needs to clarify the prescription.

- If insulins are to be mixed in the same syringe, the short acting (clear) insulin should be drawn up first to avoid contamination of the vial.

- In hospitals where insulins are supplied as stock, and not labelled for individual patients, it is important that vials are dated when first used so that they can be discarded after an appropriate period. Even though the vials are preserved, most manufacturers recommend disposal after 4 weeks of use.

- Insulin must be stored securely under lock and key.

Syringe drivers

These are most commonly used for the subcutaneous infusion of medicines in palliative care, or the administration of heparins and nitrates. Whatever the reason for their use, deaths and injury result when the nature of the pump has not been fully understood. Some are volumetric, and measure the *volume* of fluid infused, though nurses should check against what period the volume is set on the pump (Cousins & Upton, 1995b). Most terminal-care drivers deliver fluid based on the *distance* that a plunger moves in a time period, however. With these drivers, it is essential to check whether the distance set is *per hour* or *per 24 hours.* It is also important to check that any protocols laid down by the hospital are followed. Sometimes these assume that the same syringe brand and size is always used, and so can define volumes of reconstituting fluid to be used, which will produce a known length for the syringe driver plunger to travel. Again, care must be taken that confusion does not arise over what is being asked for.

Parenteral nutrition

In most hospitals, total parenteral nutrition (TPN) bags are now supplied ready-made from pharmacy, thus making obsolete former bottle-based systems which were more likely to lead to errors, infections, and nutritional waste if amino acids were not administered simultaneously with carbohydrate. That is not to say that TPN administration has become easy; sepsis is the greatest risk and can be greatly reduced by nursing practice. The lowest sepsis rates are found where staff are familiar with TPN, follow infection-control protocols when changing and caring for the line, and are supported in their role by specialist infection-control and nutrition nurses.

Nurses should ensure that the line, once changed, is protected and not broken again until the next 24-hour bag and line change, to prevent infection.

Any break in feeding, including line blockage, will mean that the blood-glucose level will become unstable, which is why feeding should always be discontinued gradually. Nothing should *ever* be added to the bag once it has been supplied from pharmacy. Quite apart from the infection risk, the bag may become unstable; once the lipid emulsion has '*cracked*' and the fat component separated, the TPN fluid may not be administered.

The most important contribution that nurses can make to successful TPN administration is in their holistic clinical care of the patient. Frequent checks of temperature, pulse, respiration, and blood glucose are needed in the early stages of TPN. Any signs of infection such as redness at the infusion site, fever, or restlessness must be reported and acted upon. If the patient is becoming fluid overloaded, the medical staff and pharmacists involved in formulating the bag must be informed so that adjustments can be made in subsequent bags. The best nurses go further than this. Often nurses point out to the TPN for-mulators (who may not include the medical staff directly caring for the patient), that some blood or albumin, for example, are due to be administered in the near future.

Topical and inhaled medication

The administration of topical and inhaled medicines is usually straightforward, but a few problems do present from time to time. Creams containing steroids should always be applied sparingly and the patient similarly encouraged to use the least amount possible. Antifungal creams such as clotrimazole are often prescribed in the '*prn*' section of the prescription chart. However, to be effec-tive, like antibiotics, they need to be used regularly, two or three times a day.

Patients with inhalers may need assistance with technique. Patients will not derive any benefit if the dose is merely being deposited on the back of their throats, and in the case of steroid inhalers this may lead to oral candidiasis. It should never be assumed that patients are able to use their inhalers properly. Different staff such as doctors, physiotherapists and pharmacists are often involved in this observation, as are specialist chest nurses, but there is no substitute for the primary nurse reinforcing good technique on every occasion. Pharmacists and other staff can suggest spacer devices or automatic inhalers, for those patients who have difficulty with standard metered-dose aerosols, and there is a wide variety of different inhalers to suit different patients' needs, though possibly at a price. It is important that nurses are familiar with the device that a patient is using, if they are going to be able to offer constructive advice.

Other useful interventions that nurses can make include advice on candidiasis prevention. Once correct technique has been established, the additional practices of using a spacer device and rinsing the mouth after use often prevent the infection from troubling patients. In relation to nebuliser therapy, nurses should take care that vapours from anticholinergic therapy such as ipratropium do not get into the eyes of patients with glaucoma. In addition, nebulised therapy for patients with long-term chronic bronchitis should generally be delivered in air, not oxygen. This is because chronically hypoxic patients rely on their hypoxia to provide their respiratory stimulus, and high strength oxygen can suppress respiration.

Summary

This chapter does not cover all the things that can go wrong during medicines administration. Quality medicines administration is maintained by care and thought by medical staff and pharmacists as well as nurses. Where errors have occurred, they must be reported as quickly as possible and remedial action taken. It is good practice not to develop a culture of blame, as this discourages honesty. Consideration of what went wrong and training are more likely to prevent recurrence of mistakes.

The *Standards for the Administration of Medicines* (UKCC, 1992) provide the best guidance on the responsibilities in therapy delivery which should be accepted by nurses, and those which should not. All nurses should have a copy, and use it to guide their practice. Few administration errors result from a single mistake; in the errors mentioned in this chapter and reported elsewhere, actions and omissions by doctors and pharmacists have often been contributory or even causal factors to the error. However, this does not remove the ultimate responsibility of the nurse who actually administers a medicine to be accountable for her or his actions (UKCC, 1992).

References

Anon. (1997) Five year transition period for name changes for high-risk drugs, *Pharm J.* **259**, 668–9.

Applebe, G.E. & Wingfield, J. (1993) *Dale and Appelbe's Pharmacy Law and Ethics*, 5th edn. Pharmaceutical Press, London.

Cousins, D.H. & Upton, D.R. (1994) Chemotherapy errors can kill. *Pharm. Pract.* **4**, 311–12.

Cousins, D.H. & Upton, D.R. (1995a) Penicillin injections can kill. *Pharm. Pract.* **5**, 29.

Cousins, D.H. & Upton, D.R. (1995b) Make infusion pumps safer to use. *Pharm. Pract.* **5**, 401–6.

Cousins, D.H. & Upton, D.R. (1996) Prevent drug overdose tragedies. *Pharm. Pract.* **6**, 135.

Cousins, D.H. & Upton, D.R. (1997) How to prevent IV drug errors. *Pharm. Pract.* **7**, 310–12.

Duthie, R.B. (1988) *Guidelines for the safe and secure handling of medicines: A report to the Secretary of State for Social Services by the Joint Sub-committee of the Standing Medical, Nursing and Midwifery, and Pharmaceutical Advisory Committees.* HMSO, London.

Mehta, D.K. (1997) *British National Formulary No. 34.* British Medical Association and Royal Pharmaceutical Society of Great Britain, London.

United Kingdom Central Council for Nursing, Midwifery and Health Visiting (1992) *Standards for the Administration of Medicines.* UKCC, London.

Williams, A. (1996). How to avoid mistakes in medicines administration. *Nursing Standard* **92**, 40–1.

Chapter 13
Adverse Drug Reactions

Chris Green

Introduction

Risk–benefit ratio

No drug is completely without side effects, although some are perceived as being 'safer' than others. In general, a drug should be prescribed on the basis of its risk–benefit ratio, that is, the risk of adverse effects associated with the drug's use are outweighed by the therapeutic benefits the patient will potentially receive. The risks presented by a drug are often unrelated to the indication for which it is required, a complicating element in evaluating any risk–benefit ratio. The aim of this chapter is to discuss the origins of drug safety, pharmacovigilance, the detection and management of adverse drug reactions (ADRs) and risk factors associated with their occurrence.

Why adverse drug reactions are a problem

Adverse drug reactions have been defined by the World Health Organization (WHO, 1975) as a response to a drug which is noxious and unintended and which occurs at doses normally used in man for the prophylaxis, diagnosis or therapy of disease or for the modification of a physiological function.

ADRs are a problem because they may complicate existing disease, cause hospital admissions, affect quality of life and may delay cure of the disease which the drugs were intended to treat. ADRs may mimic numerous other disease states and result in inappropriate treatment of unrecognised, drug-induced problems. Furthermore, it is estimated that ADRs cost the NHS in excess of one billion pounds a year. ADRs can also impair a patient's willingness to take prescribed medicines, which in turn may lead to poor compliance and consequently treatment failure. It is not surprising, therefore, that ADRs can result in a loss of confidence by patients in their health care professionals.

Pharmacovigilance

Development of pharmacovigilance in the UK

Thalidomide was first marketed in 1956 in Germany as Distival and promoted as a treatment for insomnia and nausea in pregnancy. Reports of fetal abnormalities thought to have been caused by thalidomide were first published in the medical literature in 1961, and it is now estimated that over 8000 babies were born with thalidomide-related deformities. Almost 40 years after this tragedy, thalidomide remains a household name synonymous with adverse and undesirable effects of drugs.

As a result of the thalidomide tragedy and other less publicised but not dissimilar incidents, many countries decided that drug safety should become a priority. Until this point, drugs could be marketed with little regard to their safety and efficacy. The UK was no exception and with the co-operation of the Association of the British Pharmaceutical Industry (ABPI) and the Proprietary Association of Great Britain, the Committee on Safety of Drugs (CSD) was established in 1963, becoming operational on 1 January 1964. Under the chairmanship of Sir Derek Dunlop, the Committee's function was to monitor drug safety throughout the UK, to monitor and approve the introduction of new drugs and to collect and act upon reports of ADRs.

In 1968, the Medicines Act brought into effect several new laws relating to the marketing of therapeutic and diagnostic agents. In September 1971, under Section 4 of the Medicines Act 1968, the Committee on Safety of Drugs was replaced by the Committee on Safety of Medicines (CSM). Although the membership of the committee did not greatly alter, the new committee now had statutory backing and authority.

Aims of post marketing surveillance

The aims of post marketing surveillance are to detect the occurrence of previously unrecognised ADRs, to identify risk factors for ADRs in individual patients, to collate data concerning recognised ADRs and ultimately to determine the safety of drugs. It may be used to encourage the safe and effective use of drugs which have been licensed.

Adverse drug reactions: the size of the problem

Due to various problems associated with ADRs, which will be discussed within this chapter, it is extremely difficult to accurately define the extent to which they affect the population. Suggested incidences of ADRs vary for a number of reasons. The population in question will affect the incidence of reported ADRs, for example, young patients requiring minor surgery and taking few medicines are less likely to suffer an ADR than an elderly patient experiencing several clinical conditions and polypharmacy. Other factors which affect the reported incidence of ADRs include variation in the precise definition of an ADR: many ADRs are unreported or unidentified, sample sizes in surveys vary greatly and specific specialities, for example an excess of surgical or renal patients, may greatly influence the results of such estimates.

A review of studies examining ADR-related admissions to hospitals found that reported rates varied from 0.2% to 21.7% with an average rate of 5.5% (Einarson, 1993). Studies examining the incidence of ADRs in the hospitalised population have proposed incidences of between 1% and 28%, although most studies suggest between 10% and 20% (Lawson, 1991).

Clinical trials

Clinical trials have numerous purposes and, especially, aim to demonstrate a drug's effectiveness and safety. However, they have a number of limitations. In order to fully investigate the agent in question, large numbers of patients are required. The quantity of patients involved in clinical trials is often limited due to the complexity of the investigations, monitoring of patients, co-ordination of trials and ultimately, cost. Patients are selected for clinical trials using certain criteria and it is likely that many different concurrent pathologies and drug therapies will not be encountered. The detection of certain drug–disease and drug–drug interactions is also unlikely to occur until after the drug has been marketed. Furthermore. as the length of these trials is limited, long term side effects of drug therapy may not become apparent for a number of years after marketing. Trials may also fail to obtain substantial data about the use of the agent concerned in very young or very old patients. Due to the limits placed on the numbers of patients involved, clinical trials are also ineffective at detecting very rare ADRs, and it is thought that those with an incidence of less than 1 in 250 are unlikely to be detected. As few as 1000 patients may have been exposed to a new therapeutic agent or device prior to its marketing (Rawlins & Jefferys, 1993). In order to verify that drugs are as safe as clinical trials have suggested, it is therefore vital that post marketing surveillance is carried out to monitor the safety of these agents.

The yellow card scheme

In 1964 the Committee on Safety of Drugs provided doctors and dentists with pre-paid yellow postcards with which to report adverse reactions to drugs, thus creating the yellow card scheme. Nurses were not officially allowed to report as part of the scheme, although many became indirectly involved in ADR reporting. Pharmacists were also excluded from official participation in the scheme until 1997. Yellow cards may be found in NHS prescription pads, the *British National Formulary* (BNF), the *Compendium of Data Sheets and Summaries of Product Characteristics* (formerly the *ABPI Data Sheet Compendium*), *Monthly Index of Medical Specialities* (MIMS) or may be obtained from the CSM.

Over 300 000 yellow card ADR reports have now been made to the CSM and stored in their database. These reports are made to the CSM in confidence and personal details of reporters and patients are neither published nor used for purposes of litigation. Data collected by the yellow card scheme are not only used for national drug safety surveillance but also for international surveillance. Along with several other countries, the UK submits reports of ADRs to the WHO's Adverse Drug Reaction Collaborating Centre where data are collated for international use.

Action taken by the CSM

Once a specific problem has been identified with regard to a certain product, the CSM may take action in a number of ways. The CSM may choose to advise individual doctors as to the adverse effects of certain drugs. They may also publish their findings and advice to prescribers in *Current Problems in Pharmacovigilance*, a communication used to disseminate information about ADRs to doctors and pharmacists. Analysis of ADR reports received by the CSM may also result in the withdrawal of drugs from the market. For example, remoxipride was withdrawn by its manufacturer on a worldwide basis following a number of yellow card reports of aplastic anaemia. Terfenadine (Triludan/ Seldane), an antihistamine used in the treatment of hay fever, has been withdrawn in the USA and its use has recently been reviewed in the UK. This is due to the findings that terfenadine may have arrhythmogenic effects when taken by patients with cardiac disorders, hepatic impairment and those taking certain antibiotics and antifungal agents.

The CSM may also choose to amend product licences in response to reported ADRs. For example, azapropazone (Rheumox) has recently had its product licence amended. It is now recommended for use only when other drugs in its class (non steroidal anti inflammatory drugs or NSAIDs) have been tried and failed, in reduced dosage for elderly people and in specific medical conditions such as ankylosing spondylitis. The CSM may also publish warnings in the *BNF* to highlight particular aspects of drug safety. Examples of this include warnings about the use of beta-blockers in asthmatics, the risks of developing agranulocytosis with carbimazole and the need to monitor hepatic function with cyproterone acetate.

Under-reporting of ADRs

Under-reporting of ADRs is considered to be a long-standing problem with several reasons thought to contribute to its persistence. It is estimated that the incidence of under-reporting of serious ADRs is in the order of 10% and for non-serious ADRs it is estimated at 2–4% (Rawlins, 1994). The data obtained from the yellow card scheme are therefore incomplete, and indeed many serious and fatal reactions are never brought to the attention of the regulatory authorities. Factors considered to dissuade potential reporters from completing an ADR report are listed here (Inman, 1980).

- Reaction not severe enough
- Reaction well known
- Familiarity with the suspect drug concerned
- Concern over potential legal implications
- Reaction may be predictable or expected
- Ignorance of how to report an ADR
- Lack of time, lethargy or complacency
- Lack of feedback following previous reports
- Lack of awareness of the existence of an ADR
- Guilt because of patient suffering
- Lack of confidence in making a report.

The data collected in the yellow card scheme are also open to significant bias. Reports of reactions appearing in the medical or lay press may result in numerous similar reports being submitted to the CSM, which in turn may result in a 'false positive' or 'true positive' sign that a problem exists. An example of a false positive is the association of suicidal ideation with fluoxetine (Prozac), a myth perpetuated by the media and refuted by the authorities in pharmacovigilance (Rawlins, 1994). An example of a true positive is the association of paroxetine (Seroxat), an antidepressant, with acute withdrawal symptoms in patients stopping therapy. This was found on further analysis to be substantiated (Rawlins, 1994).

The lessons of the practolol-induced oculomucocutaneous syndrome are worth noting. Following publication of a report on this syndrome in the medical press, over 200 reports of a similar nature were subsequently submitted to the CSM. Before the publication of the first report, only one report had been made to the CSM in 4 years (Inman, 1980). This case has been described as a failure of the yellow card scheme.

Successes of the yellow card scheme

The CSM has been responsible for the identification of a multitude of important ADRs. Examples of successes of the scheme are outlined in Table 13.1 (Rawlins, 1994). The yellow card scheme has provided important information concerning factors which may predispose patients to ADRs; for example, age, concurrent disease and concurrent medication. The yellow card scheme has also allowed comparison between drugs in the same class; for example, the comparison between different NSAIDs to identify those with the greater risk of different adverse effects (CSM, 1994). However, as discussed earlier, under-reporting and biased reporting can distort true comparisons between different drugs. As stated earlier, nurses are not usually involved in completing the yellow card, but they have a part to play in identifying and documenting the

Table 13.1 Successes of the yellow card scheme since 1993.

Drug (Trade name)	ADR reporting	Action taken
Clozapine (Clozaril)	Myocarditis	Additional warnings in summary of product characteristics
Remoxipride (Roxiam)	Aplastic anaemia	Worldwide withdrawal by manufacturers
Rifabutin (Myobutin)	Uveitis/drug interactions	Additional warnings and dose reduction
Tiaprofenic acid (Surgam)	Severe cystitis	Additional warnings augmented and contraindications altered
Cyproterone acetate (Cyprostat, Androcur)	Hepatotoxicity	Indications restricted and requirements for hepatic monitoring introduced
Alendronate (Fosamax)	Severe oesophageal reactions	Additional warnings and altered dosing instructions
Tacrolimus (Prograf)	Hypertrophic cardiomyopathy	Additional warnings, dose reduction and monitoring required
Tramadol (Zydol)	Psychiatric reactions	Additional warnings

side effects of drug therapy. In many cases the nurse may be the first to hear of the patient's new symptoms and is instrumental in seeking a medical opinion.

Intensive monitoring of newly marketed agents

Once a new medicine or device has been awarded a product licence and marketed, it is placed under intensive surveillance by the CSM. This also applies to new formulations of established agents. For example, pilocarpine eye *gel* has been recently introduced and is under intensive monitoring despite the fact that eye *drop* formulations have been in use for many years. As discussed, limitations of clinical trials mean that it is important to monitor drugs once marketed to detect any potential problems with their safety. For this reason, new drugs are flagged with an inverted black triangle in the *BNF, MIMS* and the *Compendium of Data Sheets and Summaries of Product Characteristics*, and on all promotional materials. Agents normally remain under intensive surveillance for approximately 2–3 years.

The CSM requests that all suspected reactions to black triangle drugs be reported via yellow cards to the CSM. They should be reported even if the relationship between the suspect drug and the reaction is uncertain, and regardless of the severity of the suspected reaction.

Monitoring of established drugs

Once drugs are no longer under intensive surveillance, the black triangle is removed and the emphasis on ADR surveillance alters. Instead of seeking reports on all reactions, the CSM requests that only serious or unusual reactions be reported. Relatively minor or well documented reactions become less significant. Any reaction which is fatal, is life threatening, disabling, incapacitating, or which results in, or prolongs, hospitalisation should be reported, even if well recognised. These data are especially of value when comparing drugs in the same class and identifying risk factors for individual ADRs. Examples of 'serious' reports which are of particular interest to the CSM are listed below.

- Anaphylaxis
- Blood disorders
- Endocrine disturbances
- Effects on fertility
- Haemorrhage from any site
- Hepatic abnormalities
- Jaundice
- Ophthalmic disorders
- Renal abnormalities
- Severe CNS effects
- Severe skin reactions.

Other methods of pharmacovigilance

Other methods employed in pharmacovigilance include case control studies, cohort studies, case register studies and prescription event monitoring. These methods, rather than relying on spontaneous reports, are focused on individual drugs with the aim of identifying ADRs. Alternatively, these studies may be focused on selected clinical conditions to identify potential relationships with individual drugs.

Local ADR reporting schemes

Several in-house or local ADR reporting schemes have been implemented in hospitals throughout the UK. These schemes are not designed to replace the yellow card scheme, but to supplement it by increasing awareness and encouraging reporting of ADRs within hospitals. Some of the factors listed earlier, in the section on under-reporting of ADRs, which deter potential reporters from making an ADR report, are negated by these schemes, for example, reports are simpler to make, reducing pressures on time. Descriptions of examples of local reporting schemes have been published in the literature and although methods of reporting may vary between institutions, most operate on similar principles (Green *et al.*, 1997). In most cases, reporting may be made by different health care professions and some schemes allow reporting by any member of hospital staff. In general, a central location, usually the pharmacy department, is informed of the ADR, either by a reporting card or verbally. The co-ordinators of the scheme then investigate the ADR and collect all the necessary details to evaluate the ADR report and decide whether a report to the CSM is appropriate.

Problems with CSM data

Although the data received by the CSM are of great value with regard to pharmacovigilance, there are problems associated with them. For example, reporting rates for drugs tend to be at their highest following their introduction onto the market, particularly as they are marked with black triangles. In order for a meaningful comparison of two drugs to be made, comparable periods of time post marketing need to be used. It is not uncommon for unusual or unexpected reactions to be reported at the expense of well recognised, albeit more serious, reactions. Furthermore, due to under-reporting and because the sample size in which a drug is used in unknown, it is impossible to calculate the incidence of specific ADRs. It is only possible to hypothesise about identified problems.

Monitoring and management of ADRs

Documentation and communication of ADRs

Given their importance, it is surprising that many serious ADRs are incompletely documented in patients' notes and never communicated to the patients' GPs. It is an important part of ADR monitoring and management that information concerning ADRs is appropriately disseminated to health care providers. Without such information, patients may be inadvertently exposed to drugs to which they have had a previous ADR, and again suffer similar and potentially life threatening reactions. In instances where a patient has suffered a minor ADR or one of doubtful causality, it may be possible to safely represcribe the suspect drug for the patient, provided appropriate precautions are taken. Therefore, unless information is made available to those health professionals caring for the patient, patients could be denied important medicines which, although they may have suffered a previous ADR, could still be safely prescribed.

It is therefore important to ensure that ADR information is carefully documented in the patient's medical records, communicated to the patient's GP and pharmacist, and recorded in the nursing records.

Difficulties in detecting ADRs

There are few clinical or laboratory methods of testing for ADRs. Laboratory data may assist in the identification of clinical abnormalities, but often provide few clues as to their cause. In instances of suspected drug toxicity, high blood drug concentrations of agents with narrow therapeutic indices may explain the reason for some patients' symptoms (see Chapter 3). ADRs may masquerade as other diseases; for example, water retention secondary to the use of NSAIDs may be clinically similar to the symptoms of cardiac failure. In other instances a patient's clinical condition may not be associated with the ADR profile of current medication, especially if the adverse effects of newer or lesser known drugs are not well known. Consequently, patients' carers may not have considered the possibility that the patient may be suffering an ADR, resulting in potentially inappropriate treatment.

Identification of ADRs

A number of factors may assist in the identification of ADRs; for example, drug history, timing, professional experience, published literature, alternative aetiologies such as the patient's concurrent disease state, placebo effect or excipients. Certain drugs may be used to treat the adverse effects of other agents. For example, in instances of heparin overdose, protamine may be used to reverse the effects of heparin should a patient become overly anticoagulated. Similarly vitamin K may be used to treat the effects of warfarin toxicity. Dermatological reactions may be treated with corticosteroid creams or with oral antihistamines. Further examples of these 'antidote' drugs are listed in Table 13.2.

Table 13.2 Presented drugs that may suggest the patient has suffered an ADR.

Antidote drug	Adverse effect
Antacids	Indigestion
Benzodiazepines	Insomnia
Chlorpheniramine (chlorphenamine)/hydroxyzine	Skin rashes
Corticosteroids	Inflammatory/allergic reactions
Hydrocortisone injection/cream	Inflammatory/allergic reactions
Metoclopramide	Nausea
Procyclidine	Drug induced extra-pyramidal effects
Protamine	Heparin overdose
Vitamin K	Warfarin overdose

ADRs may occur at various times during or after drug therapy. For example, anaphylaxis may occur during an infusion of penicillin, blood dyscrasias may occur during the first few months of treatment with carbimazole, cholestatic jaundice secondary to co-amoxiclav may occur up to 6 weeks after the cessation of therapy, while osteoporosis secondary to the use of corticosteroids may not become clinically apparent for several years.

Obtaining an accurate drug history from the patient is therefore of great importance. As discussed above, the drugs to which a patient has been exposed in the near or even distant past are equally as important as the drugs that the patient is currently taking. Drug histories should not be limited to prescribed medicines, but should also include over the counter (OTC) remedies bought in pharmacies, herbal products and illicit drug use.

A strong indicator that an ADR has occurred is the improvement of the condition on 'dechallenge' or withdrawal of the suspect drug. If the patient were to recover from the condition, it is suggestive that an ADR has occurred and the possibility of 'rechallenging' the patient exists. Should the reaction recur on rechallenge then it is highly likely that the drug caused the reaction. Should there be no recurrence of the patient's symptoms, then an ADR is less likely. However, rechallenge is rarely ethical if other alternatives exist.

Patients' disease states also need to be considered. While it is true that ADRs are great mimics of disease, there is some truth in the reverse, with diseases mimicking ADRs. It is important to exclude the patient's condition as a cause of a suspected ADR. For example, water retention and cardiac failure may be induced by NSAID use.

Many patients will also suffer ADRs which arise as a result of a placebo effect. Studies investigating this occurrence have found that patients not taking medicines may report similar symptoms to those taking medication (Reidenberg and Lowenthal, 1968). Consequently it may be the case that many drugs are unfairly blamed for adverse effects suffered by the patients in whom they have been used.

Further assistance in the identification of ADRs may be found in Appendix 2 and in the medical literature. A number of sources of general information about drugs is available and *Martindale: The Extra Pharmacopoeia* and the *Compendium of Data Sheets and Summaries of Product Characteristics* are widely available and are useful sources of information. Information sources and texts of particular relevance to ADR reporting are listed below.

- British National Formulary
- Compendium of Data Sheets and Summaries of Product Characteristics
- Davies' Textbook of Adverse Drug Reactions
- Drug information centres
- Industry/pharmaceutical manufacturers
- Martindale: The Extra Pharmacopoeia
- Medline
- Meyler's Side Effects of Drugs (Dukes, 1996)

- Royal Pharmaceutical Society of Great Britain
- Specialist centres, for example, children's hospitals
- The Internet.

A number of algorithms have been published, which may assist in the evaluation of an adverse drug reaction (Naranjo *et al.*, 1981; Kramer *et al.*, 1979; Karch & Lasagna, 1977). These algorithms are a number of questions, for example, concerning the drugs the patient has been taking, effects of dechallenge, concurrent disease states and other relevant information.

Options in management of an ADR

Depending on the reaction concerned, different options are open to the health care professional. Examples of options are given in Table 13.3. Drugs may be stopped, doses reduced, appropriate monitoring may be introduced, treatment may be introduced to counteract the adverse effect, the timing of the dose may be altered or the drug may be continued to see if the adverse effect is transient.

Table 13.3 Examples of options available in the treatment of ADRs.

Option	Example
Add an additional agent to counteract the adverse effects of another agent	Addition of amiloride to loop diuretics to reduce the risk of hypokalaemia
Alter the timing of a dose	Amitriptyline may cause drowsiness, therefore give at night
Continue drug treatment to see if adverse effect is transient	Anti-parkinson agent induced nausea may wear off after a few days
Introduce monitoring	Raised liver enzymes with anti-tuberculous agents
Reduce dose	Bendrofluazide (bendroflumethiazide) induced diabetes
Withdraw drug	Carbimazole-induced agranulocytosis

Classification of ADRs

Traditionally, ADRs have been classified into two distinct categories (Table 13.4). Type A reactions tend to be extensions of a drug's pharmacological effects. Examples include hypoglycaemia in response to an antidiabetic agent and bradycardia secondary to the use of beta-blockers. Conversely, Type B reactions tend to be more bizarre in nature as they are idiosyncratic, unpredictable and unrelated to the pharmacological action of a drug. Currently, this classification is under review, primarily because the two groups are somewhat

Table 13.4 Classification of adverse drug reactions (adapted from Bateman and Chaplin, 1988).

Reaction type	Nature of reaction	Example of reaction type
Type A	These reactions may be predicted from the pharmacological actions of the drug and are usually dose dependent. These reactions tend to be mild, have low mortality and may be alleviated by a reduction in dose	Dry mouth with anti-cholinergics, hypoglycaemia with anti-diabetics
Type B	These reactions are unpredictable from the pharmacology of the drug and are not dose-dependent. These reactions have a higher mortality rate than Type A reactions	Anaphylactic reactions of penicillin, hepatotoxicity with sulphasalazine (sulfasalazine)

restrictive. Further subtypes of ADR under consideration are those caused by long term use of a drug, those caused by drug–drug interactions, ADRs resulting in carcinogenicity or teratogenicity, and ADRs occurring as a result of an overdose.

Predisposing and risk factors for ADRs

Drug related factors in ADRs

The indication for which a drug is used may determine whether its effects are adverse or otherwise. Many ADRs are dose related; for example, at doses of 900 mg or above, demeclocycline induces a predictable and reversible diabetes insipidus. The route of administration of a drug also affects the manifestation of ADRs. Inhaled steroids, often used in the treatment of asthma, may be used regularly with minimal adverse systemic effects in comparison to oral steroids taken by patients for the same condition.

ADRs may arise as a result of drug–drug interactions (often referred to as adverse drug interactions or ADIs). Warfarin toxicity may result from an erythromycin–warfarin interaction. ADRs may also be caused by the method of drug administration. 'Red man' syndrome may result if vancomycin is administered at a rapid rate (although the reaction may still occur at normal administration rates). Drugs may also decompose into toxic by-products and is the reason that some drugs have limited shelf lives. Pharmaceutical variation also has an important role to play in drug toxicity as many dosage forms have differing bioavailability (see Chapter 3).

ADRs may sometimes be attributable to the formulation of the dosage form rather than to the therapeutic agent it is designed to deliver. Osmosin, a modified release preparation of indomethacin, was withdrawn from use after reports of gastro-intestinal haemorrhage. These were found to be due the formulation of the product which resulted in local damage to the mucosa of the stomach. As well as the therapeutic agent itself, many dosage forms contain excipients or agents designed to assist the delivery of the agent into the area in which it is required. Many dosage forms contain preservatives, buffering agents, controlled release matrices, flavourings and stabilisers, all of which may result in adverse events in certain individuals. Dosage forms may also result in local irritation. For example, transdermal patches may cause skin irritation, injections may result in thrombophlebitis and eye drops may result in ocular irritation.

Age

Neonates and infants may have immature metabolic systems and as such may have difficulty metabolising and excreting drugs, and are thus at risk of toxic effects. Inefficient renal filtration, immature enzyme function, differing organ sensitivity and inadequate detoxifying systems all expose the neonate to an increased risk of ADRs. Examples of drugs required to be used with caution in young children and neonates are barbiturates, chloramphenicol, morphine and its derivatives, sulphonamides, vitamin K and analogues.

Elderly people have decreased functional and homeostatic reserve. For example, the ability to regulate blood glucose levels and blood pressure may be impaired. Drugs affecting parameters such as blood pressure may have a more pronounced effect, because the natural response mechanisms are slow to react to such changes. Elderly patients are also susceptible to alterations in pharmacodynamic properties, that is, an alteration in their sensitivity to some agents. In particular, the elderly are more sensitive to the effects of benzodiazepines, and an increase in susceptibility to warfarin, heparin and narcotic analgesics has been noted. Reduction in dose may be appropriate for many drugs, and avoidance of polypharmacy may help to reduce the incidence of ADRs in the elderly.

A further risk factor, which often relates to elderly people, may be the existence of concurrent disease states. An increasing number of clinical conditions often results in the patient taking a correspondingly increasing number of drugs. Therefore, it is logical to assume that the risk of drug–drug and drug–disease interactions will increase accordingly. Elderly patients are also at risk of ADRs as drugs may be prescribed inappropriately. The estimated rate of ADR-related hospital admissions in elderly people is thought to be as high as 10% (Williamson & Chopin, 1980).

A large proportion of ADRs are dose related. Therefore, age-related reductions in pharmacokinetic capacity may result in a greater risk of ADRs in elderly people. Renal and hepatic function tend to deteriorate with age, and reduced drug metabolism and excretion increase the risk of adverse effects. It is thought that moderate decreases in hepatic function have little impact on drug metabolism. However, even modest reductions in renal function may have significant implications for drug excretion. Elderly people are more susceptible to the adverse effects of nephrotoxic drugs. Examples of drugs that are frequently associated with ADRs in elderly people are antihypertensives, benzodiazepines, digoxin, diuretics, NSAIDs and psychotropics.

Concurrent disease states

Patients with certain disease states may be at an increased risk of ADRs. Hepatic, renal, cardiac and thyroid dysfunction may have a significant impact on the metabolism and excretion of many drugs. In such individuals, it may be appropriate to avoid certain drugs completely, to reduce the dose of other drugs, and to be especially cautious of drug interactions. Drugs to be used with caution in renal impairment include digoxin and the aminoglycoside antibiotics. Phenothiazines should be used with great caution in hepatic impairment.

Immunological risk factors

Individuals suffering from infectious mononucleosis (glandular fever), when given ampicillin, develop a skin rash. This is thought to be due to an immunological abnormality induced by the disease. Similarly, HIV positive patients appear to be at greater risk of developing rashes secondary to co-trimoxazole and are also more susceptible to anaphylactic reactions. Patients, having had a previous ADR, are more likely to suffer a further ADR. A history of allergic conditions, such as eczema or hay fever, may also predispose the patient to an increased risk of an ADR.

Gender

Women are thought to be at greater risk of ADRs than men. Studies have shown that the frequency of ADRs in women is significantly higher than that of ADRs in men. In addition, the nature of ADRs experienced by males and females appears to be different. In one study, women experienced more gastrointestinal and cutaneous reactions than men, whereas men suffered more electrolyte disturbances, despite the fact that drugs causing the ADRs in both groups were similar. In this study, age and the numbers of drugs administered did not account for the differences (Kando *et al.*, 1995). A further factor is that drugs are not usually prescribed on a body-weight basis. Women may therefore be exposed to higher blood concentrations of drugs than men, and so be at greater risk of Type A reactions.

Racial and genetic factors

Increasing knowledge in genetics in recent years has had an impact on several areas of interest related to ADRs. Examples of inherited characteristics of interest are the subtyping of cytochrome P450 (an enzyme involved in the metabolism of many drugs), glutathione reductase deficiency, and susceptibility to malignant hyperthermia.

Acetylation is a process important in the metabolism of isoniazid, procainamide and other agents. Individuals may be classified into two main groups, fast acetylators and slow acetylators. Rapid acetylator status tends to predominate in the Inuit and the Japanese, while slow acetylator status predominates among Mediterranean Jews. Thus slow acetylators, while they may benefit therapeutically from high blood concentrations of drug, are more likely to develop peripheral neuropathy with isoniazid than fast acetylators. Fast acetylators metabolise, and subsequently excrete, isoniazid at a faster rate than slow acetylators, reducing the risk of dose related side effects.

Glucose-6-phosphate dehydrogenase (G6PD) is an enzyme involved in another important metabolic pathway. Individuals with G6PD deficiency may be found in several races including Africans and some Mediterranean groups. It is relatively uncommon in other races. G6PD is important for the viability of erythrocyte membranes and its absence predisposes erythrocytes to haemolysis by certain drugs including nitrofurantoin, quinolone antibiotics and methylene blue.

Multiple drug therapy (polypharmacy)

It has been shown that as the number of drugs a patient takes increases, the likelihood that an ADR will occur increases. An investigation into this area in the general population suggests that the risk of an ADR in patients taking between one and five drugs is approximately 4%, while in those taking 11–15 medicines the risk increases to 24% (Lucas & Colley, 1991). In comparison, a further study found that the incidence of ADRs in elderly patients taking one drug was of the order of 11% and this rose to 27% in those taking six drugs (Williamson & Chopin, 1980). An increasing number of drugs also contributes to increasing problems with poor compliance and its consequences, especially in populations such as the elderly, who may be easily confused.

Drug–drug interactions

As a patient is prescribed an increasing number of drugs, the possibility that a drug–drug interaction will occur increases accordingly. Some drug interactions are of little clinical significance, while others are potentially fatal. Drug interactions may be pharmacokinetic or pharmacodynamic in nature. Alternatively, drug combinations may have an additive toxic effect to a target organ; for example, use of phenytoin and carbamazepine may lead to an increase in the risk of hepatotoxicity. Further information on this topic is given in Chapter 14.

Drug–disease interactions

Various disease states may predispose the patient to ADRs. Drug–disease interactions may affect the metabolism and excretion of various drugs, augmenting their toxic potential. For example, metformin is contra-indicated in cardiac failure following reports of life threatening acidosis. Phenothiazines should be used with caution in hepatic disease as they may cause the patient to become comatose. Other drug–disease interactions arise as a result of pharmacological interactions. For example, patients with obstructive airways disease receiving beta blockers may experience bronchospasm.

Therapeutic drug monitoring

The concept of the therapeutic window is demonstrated in Chapter 3, Fig. 3.5. The effects of numerous drugs are dependent upon whether they reach a certain concentration in the blood or tissues. Many drugs have very large therapeutic windows; for example, ibuprofen and propranolol. However, other drugs have a very narrow therapeutic window, and it is critical that these drugs are carefully monitored when given to patients. Examples of drugs with narrow therapeutic windows or indices are digoxin, gentamicin, theophylline, aminophylline, vancomycin and phenytoin.

When ADRs are not necessarily 'adverse'

Medical history is littered with 'accidental' discoveries which have had a significant impact on treatment of numerous diseases; for example, the discovery of penicillin. The identification of a number of ADRs has led to the use of certain drugs, not for the purpose for which they were designed but for their 'adverse' effects. The importance of such uses may range from the treatment of diarrhoea with codeine to the treatment of the potentially life threatening syndrome of inappropriate anti-diuretic hormone secretion (SIADH) with demeclocycline. Minoxidil, a potent vasodilator, is indicated for use in severe hypertension and is noted for its potential to cause excessive hair growth. This drug has subsequently been successfully marketed as a remedy for male pattern baldness and is available for sale in community pharmacies. Dothiepin (dosulepin) is a commonly used antidepressant which, as a side effect, may cause drowsiness. However, as a common symptom of depression is insomnia, dothiepin taken at night may be used to treat depression, but may also alleviate the patient's insomnia. Examples of 'beneficial' uses of ADRs are shown in Table 13.5.

Table 13.5 Beneficial use of the adverse drug reactions.

Drug	Intended use	Adverse effect	Use of adverse effect
Codeine	Analgesia	Constipation	Diarrhoea
Demeclocycline	Infection	Diabetes insipidus	Syndrome of inappropriate anti-diuretic hormone secretion (SIADH)
Dothiepin (dosulepin)	Depression	Drowsiness	Insomnia
Minoxidil	Hypertension	Hair growth	Male pattern baldness
Phenytoin	Epilepsy	Skin hypertrophy	Wound healing

The role of the nurse

Nurses have an important role to play in ADR monitoring. In the clinical setting nurses are in a good position to become involved in pharmacovigilance. As nurses tend to spend much time in contact with patients, they are in a useful position to monitor patients for ADRs. This may be achieved by monitoring patients at risk of ADRs (see earlier), monitoring drugs with known toxic effects, and monitoring newly marketed agents. Any potential ADRs should be brought to the attention of, and discussed with, pharmacists and doctors. Nurses should also participate in local ADR reporting schemes wherever possible.

Nurses also have an important role to play in counselling patients and in informing them of potential adverse effects they may experience from their medication. Advice needs to be clear, concise and in a format that the patient may understand. It is also important that the patient understands what is required of them in a given scenario. For example, on developing signs of infection while taking carbimazole, which may cause a decrease in the patient's white blood cell count, patients should be aware that they need to seek medical assistance immediately.

Summary

Adverse drug reactions have a significant impact on patient care, morbidity, mortality and NHS resources. Efforts to monitor, manage and report ADRs must therefore be a priority in patient care. The benefits from the use of any therapeutic agent may be outweighed by the unwanted and adverse effects it may produce in the patient. An evaluation of the risk–benefit ratio should therefore be performed before the initiation of drug therapy.

Several risk factors may predispose patients to the occurrence of an ADR. In particular, patients with concurrent disease states and multiple drug therapy are at a greater risk of ADRs and should be closely monitored. In practical terms, documentation and communication of ADRs are important processes which may ultimately protect both the patient and their carers from inadvertent re-exposure to medicines which have previously caused an ADR. In clinical settings, nurses have an important role to play in ADR monitoring. Any potential ADRs should be brought to the attention of, and discussed with, pharmacists and doctors.

The development of pharmacovigilance since the thalidomide tragedy has led to improved drug safety in the UK and worldwide. The role performed by the Committee on Safety of Medicines (CSM) in the operation of the yellow card scheme is of great importance, particularly when considering the limitations associated with clinical trials. Intensive monitoring of newly marketed agents and monitoring of established drugs are important roles for nurses and other health care professionals. The yellow card scheme has had numerous successes. Undeniably, problems with CSM data exist and are largely due to under-reporting of ADRs. It is therefore vital that post-marketing surveillance receives the support of health care professionals in a position to identify ADRs.

References

Bateman, D.N. & Chaplin, S. (1988) Adverse Reactions I. *Br. Med. J.* **296**, 761–4.

Committee on Safety of Medicines (1994) Comparison of non-aspirin NSAIDs. *Curr. Prob. Pharmacovigilance* **20**, 9–11.

Dukes, M.N.G. (ed.) (1996) *Meyler's Side Effects of Drugs*, 13th edn. Elsevier, Amsterdam.

Einarson, T.R. (1993) Drug related hospital admissions, *Ann. Pharmacother.* **27**, 832–9.

Green, C.F., Mottram, D.R., Brown, A.M. & Rowe, P. (1997) Setting up a hospital pharmacy based local adverse drug reaction monitoring scheme, *Hosp. Pharm.* **4**, 75–8.

Inman, W.H.W. (1980) In: *Monitoring for Drug Safety*, (ed. W.H.W. Inman), MTP Press, Lancaster.

Kando, J.C., Yonkers, K.A. & Cole, J.O. (1995) Gender as a risk factor for adverse events to medications. *Drugs* **50**(1), 1–6.

Karch, F.E. & Lasagna, L. (1977) Toward the operational identification of adverse drug reactions, *Clin. Pharmacol. Ther.* **21**(3), 247–54.

Kramer, M.S., Leventhal, J.M., Hutchinson, T.A. & Feinstein, A.R. (1979) An algorithm for the operational assessment of adverse drug reactions: 1. Background, description, and instructions for use. *J. Am. Med. Assoc.* **242**, 623–32.

Lawson, D.H. (1991) Epidemiology. In: *Textbook of Adverse Drug Reactions*, 4th edn. (ed. D.M. Davies) Oxford University Press, Oxford.

Lucas, L.M. & Colley, C.A. (1991) Recognizing and reporting adverse drug reactions. *West. J. Med.* **156**, 172–5.

Naranjo, C.A., Busto, U., Sellars, E.M., Sandor, P., Ruiz, I., Roberts, E.A., Janecek, E., Domecqu, C. & Greenblatt, D.J. (1981) A method for estimating the probability of adverse drug reactions. *Clin. Pharmacol. Ther.* **30**, 239–45.

Rawlins, M.D. & Jefferys, D.B. (1993) United Kingdom Product Licence applications involving new active substances, 1987–1989: their fate after appeals. *Br. J. Clin. Pharmacol.* **35**, 599–602.

Rawlins, M.D. (1994) Pharmacovigilance: paradise lost, regained or postponed. *J. R. Coll. Physicians London* **29**(1), 41–9.

Reidenberg, M.M. & Lowenthal, D.T. (1968) Adverse non drug reactions. *N. Engl. J. Med.* **279**(13), 678–9.

Williamson, J. & Chopin, J.M. (1980) Adverse reactions to prescribed drugs in the elderly: a multicentre investigation, *Age Ageing,* **9**(2), 73–80.

World Health Organization (1975) Requirements for adverse drug reaction reporting, WHO, Geneva.

Further reading

Davies, DM, (1991) (ed.) (1991) *Textbook of Adverse Drug Reactions,* 4th edn. Oxford University Press, Oxford.

Chapter 14
Drug Interactions

Neil A. Caldwell

Introduction

A common problem for both nurses and pharmacists is that many drugs or medicines interact with each other. One of the most difficult tasks for a pharmacist is to gauge the clinical significance of any purported interaction between combined therapies. The significance of the interactions traverses a broad line between potentially fatal to relatively trivial. The challenge for the nurse, who is often the professional in closest contact with the patient, is to detect and report drug interactions.

A drug interaction occurs when the effects of one drug are changed by the presence of another drug, chemical, environmental agent or foodstuff. Interactions may be harmful and produce iatrogenic illness. If alcohol is consumed with benzodiazepines, marked central nervous system depression may result, possibly impairing the individual's ability to drive or operate machinery. Such combinations may also increase hospitalisation through an association with hip fracture in older people, or may necessitate the recipient to make lifestyle adjustment and take account of the exaggerated sedative effect.

Some interactions may be inconsequential and produce very little change in clinical outcome. The proton pump inhibitor omeprazole, which decreases gastric acid release, may inhibit the metabolism of benzodiazepines such as diazepam. Increased sedation, which could have serious consequences, may result, but because the duration of effect of diazepam is so long, it will probably have little effect on clinical response. Indeed the patient may be unaware of the interaction taking place.

Other drug interactions may be positively beneficial. As a result a number of drug combinations are used specifically for their additive effect. Paracetamol is a very good analgesic but shows limited usefulness in the treatment of migraine. Gastric stasis, which may accompany the attack, slows gastro-intestinal absorption and thus prevents the analgesic from reaching the pharmacological site of action within the brain. Metoclopramide, an antiemetic, speeds up gastric transit and can propel paracetamol to the small intestine where it may be quickly absorbed and thus resolve the migrainous attack. The clinical usefulness of the paracetamol/metoclopramide combination is supported by the fact that a combined preparation is commercially available as a prescription only medicine.

The probability of a drug interaction occurring increases with the number of drugs taken by each particular individual. It is thus a sobering thought that administration of more than one medicine is the norm within the hospital setting rather than the exception.

When we consider drug interactions in our daily practice we must remember that interactions are not inherently harmful; indeed some may be positively beneficial in terms of therapeutic outcome.

Object or precipitant

- The drug whose effect, or action, is altered by the introduction of another agent is known as the object drug
- The drug which alters or precipitates a change in the effect of the other drug is known as the precipitant

Certain drugs are strong contenders for Champion Interactor of the Year, in that when they are used in combination with other medicines, it is certain that an interaction will occur. One example is that of cimetidine, an H_2-receptor antagonist used in peptic ulcer disease, and the bronchodilator theophylline.

Cimetidine can inhibit the liver enzymes responsible for the metabolism and clearance of theophylline, such that its effects are prolonged and increased. A rise in theophylline concentration of about 30% has been reported, which in certain individuals may give rise to clinical signs of toxicity. This is no reason to ban the combination altogether because whether the clinical signs of toxicity are evident or not will be influenced by the time frame in which each respective treatment is introduced. Two possible scenarios are illustrated.

A 72 year old asthmatic patient (Ms Bee) has been stabilised on inhaled corticosteroid as a preventer, inhaled salbutamol as required for relief of acute breathlessness, and theophylline tablets for nocturnal dyspnoea. Her theophylline serum concentration was usually around 18 to 20 mg/l (target range 10–20 mg/l). Following diagnosis of a gastric ulcer her GP commenced an 8 week course of cimetidine tablets 400 mg twice daily. Within 10 days of starting the new treatment Ms Bee was admitted to hospital with nausea, vomiting, tremor, anxiety and tachycardia. Her theophylline concentration on admission was 28 mg/l. Her symptoms were all ascribed to theophylline toxicity.

Mr Jay was a 67 year old patient with chronic bronchitis and a history of peptic ulcer disease. His usual drug treatment comprised cimetidine 400 mg *nocte* long term for prophylaxis, salbutamol breath activated inhaler 4 hourly, ipratropium bromide breath activated inhaler three times daily and intermittent courses of antibiotic. Due to increasing shortness of breath his doctor decided to introduce theophylline. He commenced Uniphyllin 200 mg twice daily and was asked to return to see the GP in 7 days time. A week later the dose was increased to 300 mg twice daily because his symptoms had not improved. Two weeks later Mr Jay felt much improved and had no side effects of which to complain.

If the precipitant therapy is introduced to someone successfully stabilised on a dose of object drug, a significant drug interaction may occur. However, if the patient is taking the precipitant medicine long term, the object drug is usually introduced and its dose will be fine tuned according to the individual patient response. In such circumstances a significant drug interaction is less likely to present. In commenting on the significance of any drug interaction, recognition must therefore be paid to which drug came first.

Which drugs are involved?

On reviewing the cause and effect of drug interactions, one is constantly astonished at the sheer number of drugs which have been reported as precipitant and object. With new medicines marketed every year it is becoming increasingly difficult to remember which drugs interact with which. Useful summaries of the potential for drug interaction are listed in Appendix 1 of the *British National Formulary (BNF)*.

When we consider drug interactions it would be useful to draw a distinction between clinically significant events, and those which are merely of academic or theoretical interest. Unfortunately, creating such a divide is hampered by the very fact that what appears inconsequential in one individual may produce major symptomology in someone else. Every drug interaction, or potential interaction, must be judged on individual merit. Generalisations must be viewed in the light of this truism.

Drugs most likely to show a change in clinical or therapeutic response, in consequence of the introduction of a precipitant therapy, are those with a low toxic: therapeutic ratio. Any drug with a very narrow therapeutic window, such that a slight increase in drug concentration will produce side effects and a small decrease will cause therapeutic failure, is susceptible to influence by drug interactions. Examples of these object drugs are numerous and some of the more common ones are listed below.

- Cyclosporin (ciclosporin) (immunosuppressant)
- Digoxin (antiarrhythmic)
- Lithium (antimanic)
- Monoamine oxidase inhibitors (antidepressants)
- Oral contraceptives (birth control)
- Phenytoin and carbamazepine (anticonvulsants)
- Theophylline (bronchodilator)
- Warfarin (anticoagulant)

Which patients are most susceptible?

Certain patient groups are more susceptible to drug interactions. These would include:

- Patients on multiple drug therapy or polypharmacy (as mentioned previously drug interactions are more likely as the number of drugs consumed increases)
- Elderly people who have less physiological reserve to counter any adverse effects which may result from an interaction
- Critically ill patients who often have major organ dysfunction and are prescribed many parenteral therapies
- Patients who have chronic illness, such as diabetes, epilepsy, asthma or chronic obstructive airways disease. Such patients tend to be on drug therapy long term and any change in treatment may produce side effects or a recurrence of symptoms

Drug interactions may be explained in terms of:

- Pharmacokinetic interaction
- Pharmacodynamic interaction
- Pharmaceutical incompatibility

In this chapter we shall explore each of these processes and illustrate some of the important examples.

It must be emphasized that drug interactions do not occur in all individuals who receive combination therapy. Certain drug combinations are very likely to produce a change in clinical effect, but in any one individual this in itself may or may not necessitate a change in therapy. All drug interactions must be examined in the light of the individual patient response and clinical findings. Knowledge of the various mechanisms of drug interaction, and commonly implicated drugs, will allow one to predict the significance of each combination and inform the patient accordingly.

Pharmacokinetic interactions

The pharmacokinetic process describes the time course of drug moving from formulated medicine into the body, and its subsequent metabolism and elimination. When two drugs interact they can do so at any point in this transition. Hence interactions can be explained in terms of changes in absorption, distribution, metabolism or elimination. Changes in any, or all, of these four parameters may alter the concentration of drug within the body, and consequently influence the individual's physiological response.

Absorption

Most absorption interactions occur as a result of decreased absorption within the gastro-intestinal tract. An important distinction must be drawn between *rate* and *extent* of absorption. When patients are on chronic therapies, such as the cardiovascular agents warfarin or digoxin, the rate at which drug reaches the bloodstream is usually unimportant, provided the total amount remains unchanged. An alteration in the extent of drug absorbed, however, may produce a different or sometimes inadequate pharmacological response. Consider the case of medicines which are used on an as required basis, such as analgesics and hypnotics. If the rate of absorption is slowed for medicines used predominantly as rescue treatment, that is for an immediate effect, there may be therapeutic failure. Which analgesic would you personally prefer? One that relieved symptoms in 10 minutes or one that worked, hopefully, within about 2 hours of ingestion?

Absorption of drugs can be reduced by chemical reactions which produce a less soluble substance. Both tetracycline antibiotics (e.g. oxytetracycline) and quinolone antibiotics (e.g. ofloxacin) chelate with metal ions from antacids and iron supplements. This results in the formation of an insoluble salt and as a result less of the antibiotic will be absorbed. With less drug in the bloodstream, a smaller proportion of the medicine will reach the focus of infection, and efficacy may be compromised. Such interactions are easily avoided by leaving a suitable time period between administration of the antibiotic and the antacid: 60 minutes is probably a sufficient time gap.

Certain medicines can bind other drugs in the gut and reduce their bio-availability. For most agents this is not a problem, but for drugs with a narrow therapeutic range, such as digoxin, warfarin or the hormone thyroxine (levo-thyroxine), a small reduction in amount absorbed can dramatically reduce therapeutic response. Cholestyramine, an anion-exhange resin used in the management of hyperlipidaemia, also binds the aforementioned drugs and so reduces their clinical effect. To avoid such interactions it is recommended that drugs be given to such patients at least 1 hour before or at least 4–6 hours after ingestion of the resin. As the resin stays in the intestinal tract for a number of hours after ingestion, the time frame in which one can reliably take another medicine is considerably longer after taking the resin, than it is if the other medicine is taken before the resin's consumption.

Any agent which alters the rate of stomach emptying will influence the time it takes medicines to reach their site of absorption, which is commonly within the small intestine. Many medicines, including opiate analgesics and tricyclic antidepressants, slow gastric transit and consequently may reduce the speed with which other medicines are absorbed. If such patients require rapid symptom relief, it may be advisable to try other routes of drug administration, such as the sublingual route, which do not rely on passage through the stomach.

Changes in the acidity of the stomach can affect whether some medicines dissolve and can thus be absorbed from the lower gut. The influence of the many agents which we administer to reduce stomach pH, including antacids, H_2-receptor antagonists like nizatidine, and proton pump inhibitors such as omeprazole, have not been shown to have a major influence on drug absorption. One medicine, however, the antifungal ketoconazole, requires an acid environment to aid absorption. Patients are always advised to take the medicine with food. This is because when we consume food the body's natural response is to release lots of acid into the stomach to facilitate digestion. If ketoconazole is taken concurrently with an antacid, or soon after a meal, its absorption may be reduced significantly. This is another example of the importance of adhering to the supplementary information given with medicines by all pharmacists.

Some drugs undergo a recycling process whereby the drug is conjugated in the liver and excreted via the bile into the gut. Bacteria in the large intestine break down the drug–conjugate complex, thus freeing the previously excreted drug and allowing it to be reabsorbed. Certain medicines demonstrate a longer clinical effect by being recycled into the bloodstream. Broad spectrum antibiotics, or any other therapy which interferes with the balance of commensal bacteria within the gut, can alter the recycling process. Oestrogens undergo enterohepatic recycling. Failure of the oral contraceptive pill has frequently been blamed on antibiotic therapies which may wipe out gut bacteria and remove the potential for oestrogen recycling. Such failures could possibly be avoided if patients were advised of the necessity to follow alternative methods of contraception during the course of antibiotic therapy and for a suitable time period after completion.

Distribution

Within the body a drug exists in two main forms. A proportion is bound to plasma proteins or is distributed out of the bloodstream and is essentially pharmacologically inactive. The rest is unbound and is known as free drug. This free proportion exerts the pharmacological, or therapeutic, effect by binding to the appropriate receptors. An equilibrium exists within the body between these two states of free and active with bound and inactive.

Drug interactions were previously thought to occur if one drug could displace another drug from the binding sites on plasma proteins and thus increase the free proportion of drug which was available to interact with the receptors. However, free drug is also more readily metabolised and eliminated. Displacement is no longer considered to be a significant mechanism of drug interaction.

Metabolism

Metabolic processes within the body aim to convert foreign materials, including drugs, into more water soluble substances which can then be excreted, primarily, though not exclusively, in the urine. Most metabolism within the human body occurs within the liver. The liver contains many different enzyme systems which metabolise and break down foreign waste. Various drugs and environmental agents can induce or increase the liver's capacity to metabolise drugs. Other medicines may do the reverse and inhibit or decrease the body's capacity to remove exogenous substances.

Enzyme induction

A diverse array of chemicals is commonly implicated in enzyme induction reactions. Examples are barbiturates (e.g. phenobarbitone), carbamazepine, chronic ethanol, phenytoin, primidone, rifampicin and tobacco smoke. The only relation between the wide-ranging group is that they are commonly lipid (or fat) soluble in nature. A simple overview suggests that if the enzymes responsible for the metabolic breakdown of a drug are induced, or stimulated, the concentration of the object drug will decrease.

A solution to induction interactions may thus appear obvious. If the metabolic clearance of a medicine is increased why don't we simply give more of the same product? Unfortunately life is not so simple.

Enzyme induction interactions do not tend to occur immediately. They tend to have a slow onset before clinical signs of a reduction in drug concentration become apparent. Induction is often explained by the body making more enzyme to cope with the presence of the inducing chemical. Manufacture of biological proteins is obviously not an instantaneous response and may take a number of days, or perhaps longer to evidence.

When combination therapy is discontinued, it may similarly take some time for enzyme induction to disappear, or for the clinical signs of the interaction to dissipate. Clearly the induced enzymes will not return to their non-induced state overnight.

A serious concern arises in the event of patients who have had therapy increased because of the prescription of a concurrent enzyme inducer. If the inducing agent is subsequently withdrawn, and no recognition is taken of the fact that maintenance therapy with the affected drug had been increased, when metabolism returns to normal the unfortunate patient may suffer drug overdose. This may best be illustrated by a clinical example.

A 63 year old retired academic with a prosthetic heart valve was normally well maintained on 6 mg of warfarin. His international normalised ratio (INR), an indicator of the extent of anticoagulation, consistently ranged between 3 and 3.5. Following the introduction of rifampicin and flucloxacillin for an unusual staphylococcal chest infection his INR plummeted to 1.2. Subsequently his warfarin dose was escalated to 11 mg to achieve a stable INR of around 3. Mr Lee completed a 16 day course of antibiotics and he thought nothing more of it. However on his next anticoagulant clinic review, around 10 days after finishing the rifampicin, his INR was reported as 7.3. Warfarin was omitted for 2 days and he recommenced therapy on his usual dose of 6 mg daily which again appeared to give satisfactory INRs.

The case readily illustrates the caution that is required both when enzyme inducers are introduced and also when they are subsequently discontinued.

Now consider what might have happened had Mr Lee been maintained on the enzyme inducer long term and warfarin commenced. The dose of warfarin would have been individualised, according to INRs, to take account of his induced liver enzymes. This is another example which illustrates the importance of defining which drug came first, object or precipitant.

The clinical significance of one inducing agent is commonly overlooked. Tobacco smoke can induce liver enzymes to such an extent that drug treatment with agents such as theophylline, the bronchodilator, will require a different dose in smokers compared with non-smokers. Tobacco smoke increases the rate of theophylline clearance by up to 2.5 times. Smokers may thus require larger doses of theophylline to account for their significantly increased clearance.

Enzyme inhibition

Inhibition of the enzymes responsible for breakdown of another drug is probably the most common type of drug interaction reported. The clinical outcome of enzyme inhibition is a reduced metabolism or rate of drug clearance, with subsequent increase in concentration of the object drug. As the concentration rises, the risk or probability of adverse symptoms or dose related side effects also increases. Medicines frequently associated with the inhibition of drug metabolising enzymes are listed below.

- Acute ethanol
- Allopurinol
- Amiodarone
- Chloramphenicol
- Cimetidine
- Ciprofloxacin
- Dextropropoxyphene
- Diltiazem
- Erythromycin
- Isoniazid
- Itraconazole
- Metronidazole
- Omeprazole
- Oral contraceptives
- Sodium valproate
- Sulphonamides
- Verapamil

The time course of enzyme inhibition is slightly different from induction. Inhibition tends to be faster in onset as the body does not have to manufacture new enzymes. At the end of inhibition, again this change will occur quite quickly. Inhibition interactions can be managed by reducing the dose of the affected drug.

Consider the case of a 56 year old man (Mr Mee) with a 15 year history of chronic obstructive airways disease (COAD). His usual medical management comprises nebulised salbutamol 2.5 mg four times daily and *pro re nata,* beclomethasone (beclometasone) 250 µg inhaler three puffs twice daily via a spacer device and theophylline (Uniphyllin) tablets 400 mg twice daily. Frequent exacerbations of his COAD are usually managed by a 14 day course of antibiotics, either erythromycin or co-amoxiclav. Previous experience has taught Mr Mee that within 4 or 5 days of commencing erythromycin he will tend to feel quite sick, with his heart almost jumping out of his chest and a noticeable tremor. These symptoms usually last until 2 or 3 days after stopping the erythromycin. They do not happen when he takes a course of co-amoxiclav, so Mr Mee simply blames his symptoms on the side effects of erythromycin. He is almost, but not quite, correct.

Erythromycin will commonly cause symptoms of nausea and vomiting, but is rarely associated with tachycardia and tremor. Elevated concentrations of theophylline, however, are strongly associated with all three symptoms. An upset stomach because of erythromycin usually occurs within the first few days of therapy. What has probably happened in this case is that the erythromycin, a common enzyme inhibitor, has reduced the metabolic clearance of theophylline such that his concentrations have risen to produce toxic symptoms, or side effects.

Two methods of avoiding the unpleasant symptoms experienced in the above case would be in future to use another antibiotic which does not act as an enzyme inhibitor, or advise Mr Mee to reduce his dose of Uniphyllin, perhaps to 300 mg twice daily, whenever he commences a course of erythromycin. He must remember, however, to increase the dose back to 400 mg twice daily on completion of the course.

Once again we must recognise that enzyme inhibition interactions are not always bad news. Sometimes we positively welcome them. For many years management of Parkinson's disease has relied on combination therapies. The pathological abnormality in Parkinson's disease is a deficiency of the neuro-transmitter dopamine. Levodopa, the amino acid precursor of dopamine, is converted to dopamine both within the brain and in the nervous tissue of the periphery. Outside the brain dopamine gives rise to side effects including nausea, vomiting, postural hypotension and cardiac arrhythmias, with little clinical benefit. Co-careldopa, also known as Sinemet, and co-beneldopa, brand name Madopar, contain levodopa plus carbidopa and benserazide, respectively. Carbidopa and benserazide are both peripheral dopa-decarboxylase inhibitors, which limit the conversion of levodopa to dopamine in the peripheral tissues. By using such combination therapy the incidence of side effects is greatly reduced, and clinical benefit increased.

Following the introduction of enzyme inhibitors, concentrations of the affected drug may rise. Conversely when enzyme inhibitors are discontinued, concentrations of the affected drug may fall. As is the case with enzyme inducing agents, therefore, great caution is recommended whenever drugs known to inhibit drug metabolising enzymes are introduced or discontinued. Patients should be monitored very closely around these times and for a suitable time period afterwards.

Elimination

Most drugs are excreted or eliminated either via biliary excretion or in the urine. Other drugs can alter the rate of excretion via both of these routes.

The influence of broad-spectrum antibiotics on enterohepatic recycling of the oral contraceptive pill is described earlier in this chapter. Unwanted pregnancy could be reduced if all such at-risk patients were given specific instruction to follow alternative methods of contraception while on interacting drugs.

Certain chemicals within the body, notably prostaglandins, dilate the veins which supply blood to the kidneys. Non-steroidal anti-inflammatory drugs (NSAIDs) inhibit the production of prostaglandins, and in certain predisposed individuals can induce renal impairment. Lithium salts, used in the management of mania and manic-depressive illness, are cleared from the body predominantly by the kidney. Indomethacin, a potent NSAID, can reduce lithium excretion and raise lithium concentrations, it is assumed by altering renal vasodilatation. If recognition is not taken of this potential drug interaction, toxicities, including seizures, coma and cardiovascular collapse, may result from the lithium.

Aspirin can inhibit the tubular secretion of the cytotoxic agent methotrexate, which finds diverse use in the management of malignancy, rheumatoid arthritis and psoriasis. It does so by competing with the methotrexate for elimination. Toxicity has been reported following combination therapy. This clearly emphasizes the fact that drug interactions are not restricted solely to prescription only medicines (POMs). Certain over the counter (OTC) or General Sale List (GSL) medicines can have a dramatic effect on other concomitantly used therapies. It should be stressed to patients at every opportunity to seek the advice of a pharmacist when purchasing medicines. Further details can be found in Appendix 1 to the *BNF* (Mehta, 1997).

Pharmacodynamic interactions

Pharmacodynamic interactions occur when the effect of the object drug is altered at its site of action by the presence of the precipitant. This can occur through competition at the receptor site, or may happen if both drugs act on the same physiological system. Interactions may result from antagonism, where the effect of the object drug is inhibited. They can be additive where the effect of combined therapy may be expressed as the sum of its component parts. Or it may be synergism, where the result is much greater than the simple sum of each part.

Drug interactions which can be explained from a pharmacodynamic perspective tend to be of a more predictable nature than pharmacokinetic interactions. They are usually explained through an understanding of each medicine's pharmacological method of action, or from an appreciation of what side effects they normally produce in the clinical setting. It is very easy to remember what a drug is meant to do within the body and ignore the predictable side effects which may readily give rise to a pharmacodynamic interaction when combined with a drug with a similar side effect profile. If not anticipated beforehand, these interactions tend to appear blindingly obvious in retrospect.

If an interaction occurs with one member of a therapeutic class of drug, it is likely to recur and give rise to the same symptoms if therapy is changed to a closely related medicine from the same therapeutic group.

The most obvious illustration of a pharmacodynamic drug interaction is that of antagonism. Consider the use of a beta-blocker such as atenolol in any individual who maintains airways patency with an inhaled bronchodilator, for example salbutamol. The Committee on Safety of Medicines has warned both prescribers and pharmacists that, 'beta-blockers, even those with apparent cardioselectivity should not be used in patients with asthma or a history of obstructive airways disease, unless no alternative treatment is available'. In such cases the risk of inducing bronchospasm should be appreciated and appropriate precautions taken. (Mehta, 1997).

It would appear obvious that the pharmacological effect of atenolol which blocks the beta-receptor (the antagonist) and salbutamol which stimulates beta-receptors (the agonist) would be opposite in nature. Hopefully this interaction will always be noticed before the event, rather than when the patient experiences irreversible bronchospasm.

An example of an additive pharmacodynamic drug interaction is that of an elderly patient prescribed both amitriptyline, a tricyclic antidepressant, and the antihistamine chlorpheniramine (chlorphenamine). Both medicines are sedatives. Both medicines have antimuscarinic activity and produce dry mouth, urinary retention and blurred vision. Whether the symptoms experienced by any patient on such a combination are due simply to the sum of effects or due to synergy is difficult to answer. Overall, however, this would not be a wise combination for an elderly patient who will be more susceptible to side effects and adverse events.

Pharmacodynamic interactions occur commonly in clinical medicine. If they are anticipated and expected from a review of the relevant pharmacology they present no major problem.

Again not all pharmacodynamic interactions are bad news. Sometimes we actively pursue the clinical benefit of additive effect because monotherapy is insufficient to control the patient's symptoms. It is not uncommon to treat resistent hypertension with a combination of two or three antihypertensive therapies. This is implemented in a bid to maximise the drop in blood pressure while minimising the occurrence of side effects.

Drug–food interactions

The clinical response to drugs can be influenced by ingestion of certain foodstuffs. The most noticeable food–drug interactions occur with products that contain vitamin K and their effect on warfarin anticoagulation, and the dramatic influence of tyramine-containing foodstuffs on patients treated with monoamine oxidase inhibitors.

Vitamin K is required for the liver to synthesize blood clotting factors II, VII, IX and X. Warfarin inhibits the production of these vitamin K dependent clotting factors, and consequently is used as an anticoagulant. The clinical effects of warfarin can be reversed with phytomenadione, a vitamin K analogue, a practice sometimes undertaken if a patient has a bleeding episode or a markedly elevated INR. A range of foodstuffs has been reported to inhibit the anticoagulant effect of warfarin, perhaps by providing an alternative source of vitamin K. Green vegetables such as spinach, Brussels sprouts and broccoli, liver and certain liquid dietary supplements are rich in vitamin K (Stockley, 1996). Patients prescribed warfarin should be counselled to avoid dramatic changes to their diet which may influence anticoagulation.

If patients who are prescribed warfarin do change their dietary intake significantly, for example if they commence a nasogastric feed, close monitoring of the INR is necessary until a new maintenance dose is found.

The enzyme monoamine oxidase (MAO) is involved in the metabolic breakdown of a number of the body's chemical transmitters including adrenaline (epinephrine), noradrenaline (norepinephrine), dopamine and 5-hydroxytryptamine. MAO inhibitors, such as phenelzine, are still occasionally used in the treatment of depressive illness. The most important interaction with MAO inhibitors is that with amines, particulary tyramine from food which may produce an acute hypertensive crisis that is potentially fatal. Patients must be informed about such interactions. They should be given a warning card listing examples of what foods to avoid, such as cheese, Bovril or other meat or yeast extract, and certain medicines, and should be given full supportive counselling.

Drug–alcohol interactions

One of the most frequently asked questions from patients to their pharmacist is, 'Is it all right to drink with this medicine?' Now we all appreciate the great difficulty presented by trying to swallow a tablet with no liquid to wash it down, but what the patient is actually enquiring on is the safety, or otherwise, of combining their medication with one or two or ten alcoholic drinks. What does the pharmacist then say in reply when there is no obviously correct response? For the majority of medicines small quantities, that is one or two small measures of alcohol, will do little harm. However, certain drug–alcohol combinations are worth mentioning in more detail.

Ingestion of alcohol by patients who take disulfiram, a medicine used as adjunctive treatment in the management of alcoholism, will produce classic symptoms of flushing and fullness of the face and neck, tachycardia, dyspnoea, hypotension, nausea and vomiting. This is known as the disulfiram reaction. Alcohol is normally metabolised in the liver to acetaldehyde which is broken down into carbon dioxide and water. Disulfiram inhibits the breakdown and there is build up of acetaldehyde which gives rise to symptoms. Metronidazole, an antibiotic used for anaerobic infection, and alcohol can produce a similar disulfiram-like reaction. Patients are thus always advised to avoid alcoholic drink during the course of antibiotic treatment.

Patients treated with warfarin for coagulopathies often ask most questions about 'having a drink'. This may be because alcohol is mentioned specifically in the warfarin booklet. Mild intake of alcohol will have no effect on anti-coagulation, but heavy intake or binge drinking will affect the INR such that good control of results is very difficult to achieve. This is because large and irregular ingestion of alcohol will inhibit liver enzymes in a very unpredictable fashion. Sometimes it is possible to reach a compromise with such patients if anticoagulation is to continue for a fixed time period, for example 3 months. If the patient sees light at the end of the darkened tunnel of abstinence, they may moderate their behaviour in the short term.

The gut wall does more than simply separate intestinal content from the bloodstream. It contains a number of enzyme systems which can metabolise drugs. One enzyme, alcohol dehydrogenase, breaks down a proportion of ethanol before it can reach the systemic circulation and exert its pharma-cological effect. Aspirin has been shown to increase the amount of alcohol entering the bloodstream after ingestion of standardised drinks, perhaps by inhibiting the activity of alcohol dehydrogenase (Roine *et al.*, 1990).

When enquiring on a patient's drug history, it is very important to ask questions regarding OTC preparations and not just focus on POMs. In addition, one must recognise the influence of both food and alcohol on the clinical consequences of drug therapy.

Pharmaceutical incompatibilities

Pharmaceutical incompatibilities occur as a consequence of chemical or phy-sical interactions between drugs or fluids. Incompatibility may result in immediate precipitation of either drug product or may occur over a prolonged time period such that the therapeutic effect may decline despite administration of the 'same dose of medicine'. Incompatibility may result in loss of potency, increased toxicity, or other adverse effects. Certain medicines, however, are commonly used as mixtures, but it is nevertheless important to seek further information before adopting such practice as routine.

Nebulised bronchodilators are often used in the treatment of severe short-ness of breath. If patients fail to respond to salbutamol or terbutaline, both beta-agonist bronchodilators, ipratropium bromide, an anticholinergic bronchodi-lator, may be added to the prescription. Some individuals encourage the administration of these two agents as separate solutions because of the lack of information on their chemical compatibility. Separate administration may take 30 minutes to complete. Others suggest mixing the two nebuliser solutions immediately before administration such that the process may be completed within 10–15 minutes and thus greatly improve patient compliance. Obtaining detail on the compatibility of different drugs and solutions often requires an extensive search of the literature before one can reach an informed opinion. No simple answer will cover all eventualities. Drug information departments of local hospitals are suitable sources of unbiased commentary.

When patients are treated with multiple intravenous therapies a common question raised is that of compatibility. Whether two intravenous infusions are compatible and safe to administer at the same time cannot be judged purely on visual appearance. Just because there is no obvious precipitation or cloudiness when solutions are mixed does not guarantee that the chemical integrity of the drug has not been altered. It is possible that a drug may be inactivated by mixing without an obvious visual change in solution. Infusions must however be checked regularly for signs of precipitation, crystallisation, colour change or any other change in physical nature, as this is a clear indicator of possible incompatibility which necessitates discontinuation of a potentially hazardous infusion.

Incompatibility, or the potential for inactivation of a drug, may be influenced by a number of factors including exposure time and the number of drugs mixed.

Exposure time

The longer time period that interacting drugs are in contact with each other the greater the likelihood of an interaction taking place. If drugs are mixed in the same infusion bag they will remain in high concentration together until administered into the patient and diluted by the individual's blood volume. Whenever drugs are added to an infusion container the product should be labelled with the time and date of the addition. The chance of the interaction happening may be significantly decreased if the mixture is made immediately before administration.

If two separate infusions are run concurrently through a Y-connector, drugs will mix along the entire length of tubing from the point of entry into the blood stream to the Y-site where the solutions mix. If the administration line is short the contact time will be decreased relative to that which would occur with a longer line. If the solutions are infused slowly, likewise, this will increase the contact time and may increase the chance of incompatibility. As an interaction can occur at any point in the infusion fluid pathway, if infusions are to be mixed, then the point at which they do so should be as close to the administration site as is physically possible.

Number of drugs mixed

Incompatibility will be greater as the number of drugs and fluids infused into the same administration line increases, or as the number of drugs added to the same infusion fluid rises. Also more than one drug should not be added to the same infusion fluid because it then becomes impossible to individualise the dose of each drug.

Certain parenteral drugs are commonly associated with problems of incompatibility. Most medicines which are given by injection tend to be water soluble. Some medicines are poorly soluble in water and have to be formulated in emulsions, that is mixtures of fat and water, or with other chemicals which act as solvents and help retain the drug in solution. Examples of drugs which are poorly soluble and hence more liable to compatibility problems include diazepam (available as an emulsion), phenytoin (formulated in propylene glycol and alcohol), and vitamin K (recently reformulated as a colloidal solution). Whenever any of these medicines are administered with other parenteral therapies great attention must be paid to possible interactions.

Incompatibility is not simply a problem that relates to parenteral therapies; it applies equally to all routes of administration. Certain drugs are broken down in an acid environment. To protect them from hydrochloric acid in the stomach, they may be formulated with an enteric coating which dissolves in less acid surroundings such as the small intestine. Examples of pH-sensitive medicines include omeprazole, the proton pump inhibitor used in peptic ulcer disease, and pancreatic enzyme supplements prescribed in exocrine deficiency states. If the capsules of either preparation are opened and the contents sprinkled on alkaline foods or milk the enteric coating may dissolve and provide no protection from gastric acid. The end result may be inactivation or breakdown before the drug reaches the site in the lower intestine from which it is usually absorbed.

For further information on compatibility, useful sources include Appendix 6 of the *BNF*, or local drug information centres.

Summary

Drug interactions commonly occur, and their frequency increases as the number of medicines consumed rises. Many interactions cause no perceptible change in the individual patient but a number can result in therapeutic failure or clinical toxicity. The chapter highlights the significance of a wide range of drug interactions illustrated by clinical example.

The difference between object and precipitant drug, and the expected time course of purported interaction is reviewed. Drugs most commonly involved and patients who are at most risk are highlighted.

Drug interactions arise by three major mechanisms. Firstly, interactions may be explained by changes in the pharmacokinetic handling of medicines. Altered drug absorption, distribution, metabolic enzyme induction or inhibition, or elimination may change the pharmacological response. Secondly, interactions may be explained by pharmacodynamic changes. Finally, pharmaceutical incompatibilities may result from chemical or physical interaction between drugs or fluids.

The clinical response to certain medicines may be influenced by the ingestion of foods and alcohol: the chapter illustrates some of the important examples.

The pivotal role of clinical nurses in making informed choices about how to minimise potential toxicity and optimise outcomes in those patients requiring polypharmacy is discussed.

References

Mehta, D.K. (1997) *British National Formulary No. 34.* British Medical Association and Royal Pharmaceutical Society of Great Britain, London.

Roine, R., Gentry, T., Hernandez-Munoz, R., Baraona, E. & Lieber, C.S. (1990) Aspirin increases blood alcohol concentrations in humans after ingestion of alcohol, *J. Am. Med. Assoc.* **264**, 2406–8.

Stockley, I.H. (1996) *Drug Interactions: A Source Book of Adverse Interactions, Their Mechanisms, Clinical Importance and Management,* 4th edn. Pharmaceutical Press, London.

Further reading

Anon. (1997) A knowledge of potential drug–food interactions is important. *Drug Ther. Perspect.* **9**, 12–15.

Grahame-Smith, D.G. & Aronson, J.K. (1992) *Oxford Textbook of Clinical Pharmacology and Drug Therapy,* 2nd edn. Oxford University Press, Oxford.

Hansten, P.D. & Horn, J.R. (1993) *Drug Interactions and Updates.* Applied Therapeutics Inc., Vancouver.

Lee, A. & Stockley, I.H. (1994) Drug interactions. In: *Clinical Pharmacy and Therapeutics* (eds R. Walker & C. Edwards). Churchill Livingstone, Edinburgh.

Mason, P. (1995) Diet and drug interactions, *Pharm. J.* **255**, 94–7.

Appendix 1

Nurse Prescriber's Formulary

Nurse Prescriber's Formulary Appendix

(Appendix NPF). List of preparations approved by the Secretary of State which may be prescribed on forms FPIO(CN) and FPIO(PN) (forms GPIO(CN) and GPIO(PN) in Scotland) by Nurses for National Health Service patients.

Preparations on this list which are not included in the BP or BPC are described on p. 691 of the British National Formulary.

Medicinal preparations

Almond Oil Ear Drops, NPF
Aqueous Cream, BP
Arachis Oil Enema, NPF[1]
Aspirin Tablets, Dispersible, 300 mg, BP
Bisacodyl Suppositories, BP (includes 5-mg and 10-mg strengths)
Bisacodyl Tablets, BP
Cadexomer-Iodine Ointment, NPF
Cadexomer-Iodine Paste, NPF
Cadexomer-Iodine Powder, NPF
Calamine Cream, Aqueous, BP
Calamine Lotion, BP
Calamine Lotion, Oily, BP 1980
Carbaryl Lotion, BP, alcoholic containing at least 0.5%
Carbaryl Lotion, BP, aqueous containing at least 0.5%
Carbaryl shampoos containing at least 0.5%[2]

Catheter Maintenance Solution, Chlorhexidine, NPF
Catheter Maintenance Solution, Mandelic Acid, NPF
Catheter Maintenance Solution, Sodium Chloride, NPF
Catheter Maintenance Solution, 'Solution G', NPF
Catheter Maintenance Solution, 'Solution R', NPF
Clotrimazole Cream 1%, BP
Co-danthramer Capsules, NPF
Co-danthramer Capsules, Strong, NPF
Co-danthramer Oral Suspension, NPF
Co-dandiramer Oral Suspension, Strong, NPF
Co-danthrusate Capsules, BP
Co-danthrusate Oral Suspension, NPF
Dextranomer Beads, NPF

Dextranomer Paste, NPF

Dimethicone barrier creams containing at
  least 10%

Docusate Capsules, NPF

Docusate Enema, NPF

Docusate Enema, Compound, NPF

Docusate Oral Solution, NPF[3]

Docusate Oral Solution, Paediatric, NPF[3]

Emulsifying Ointment, BP

Glycerol Suppositories, BP

Hydrous Ointment, BP

Ispaghula Husk Granules, NPF

Ispaghula Husk Granules, Effervescent,
  NPF

Ispaghula Husk Powder, NPF

Ispaghula Husk Powder, Effervescent,
  NPFI

Lactitol Powder, NPF

Lactulose Powder, NPF

Lactulose Solution, BP

Lignocaine Gel, BP

Lignocaine Ointment, NPF

Lignocaine and Chlorhexidine Gel, BP

Magnesium Hydroxide Mixture, BP

Magnesium Sulphate Paste, BP

Malathion alcoholic lotions containing at
  least 0.5%

Malathion aqueous lotions containing at
  least 0.5%

Malathion shampoos containing at least
  1%[2]

Mebendazole Tablets, NPF

Mebendazole Oral Suspension, NPF

Miconazole Oral Gel, NPF

Nystatin Oral Suspension, BP

Nystatin Pastilles, NPF

Olive Oil Ear Drops, NPF

Paracetamol Oral Suspension, BP
  (includes 120 mg/5 mL and 250 mg/5
  mL strengths – both of which are
  available as sugar-free formulations)

Paracetamol Tablets, BP

Paracetamol Tablets, Soluble, BP

Permethrin Cream, NPF

Permethrin Cream Rinse, NPF

Phenothrin Alcoholic Lotion, NPF

Phosphates Enema, BP

Piperazine Citrate Elixir, BP

Piperazine and Senna Powder, NPF

Povidone-Iodine Aqueous Solution, NPF[4]

Senna Granules, Standardised, BP

Senna Oral Solution, NPF

Senna Tablets, BP

Senna and Ispaghula Granules, NPF

Sodium Chloride Solution, Sterile, BP

Sodium Citrate Compound Enema, NPF

Sterculia Granules, NPF

Sterculia and Frangula Granules, NPF

Streptokinase and Streptodornase Topical
  Powder, NPF

Thymol Glycerin, Compound, BP 1988

Titanium Ointment, NPF

Zinc and Castor Oil Ointment, BP

Zinc Oxide and Dimethicone Spray, NPF

Notes:
1 This preparation has now been introduced into the BP
2 No longer prescribable under NHS
3 May no longer be available
4 This preparation has now been introduced into the BP as Providone-Iodine Solution

This list is currently **only** for the purposes of the **Nurse Prescribing demonstration
scheme** which involves nurses with a District Nurse (DN) or Health Visitor (HV)
qualification.

Appliances and Reagents (including Wound Management Products)

Chemical Reagents

The following as listed in Part IXR of the Drug Tariff (Part 9 of the Scottish Drug Tariff):

Detection Tablets for Glycosuria
Detection Tablets for Ketonuria
Detection Strips for Glycosuria
Detection Strips for Ketonuria
Detection Strips for Proteinuria
Detection Strips for Blood Glucose

Fertility (Ovulation) Thermometer as
listed under Contraceptive Devices in Part IXA of the Drug Tariff (Part 3 of the Scottish Drug Tariff)

Film Gloves, Disposable, EMA as listed
under Protectives in Part IXA of the Drug Tariff (Part 2 of the Scottish Drug Tariff)

Elastic Hosiery including accessories as
listed in Part IXA of the Drug Tariff (Part 4 of the Scottish Drug Tariff)

Hypodermic Equipment

The following as listed in Part IXA of the Drug Tariff (Part 3 of the Scottish Drug Tariff):

Hypodermic Syringes – U100 Insulin
Hypodermic Syringe Carrying Case[1]
Screw cap to convert Hypodermic Syringe Carrying Case for use with Pre-set U100 Insulin Syringe[1]
Hypodermic Syringe – Single Use or Single-patient Use, U100 Insulin with Needle
Hypodermic Needles – Sterile, Single-use
Lancets – Sterile, Single-use
Needle Clipping Device

Incontinence Appliances as listed in Part
IXB of the Drug Tariff (Part 5 of the Scottish Drug Tariff)

Pessaries, Ring as listed in Part IXA of the
Drug Tariff (Part 3 of the Scottish Drug Tariff)

Stoma Appliances and Associated
Products as listed in Part IXC of the Drug Tariff (Part 6 of the Scottish Drug Tariff)

Urethral Catheters as listed under
Catheters in Part IXA of the Drug Tariff (Part 3 of the Scottish Drug Tariff)

Urine Sugar Analysis Equipment as
listed in Part IXA of the Drug Tariff (Parts 3 and 9 of the Scottish Drug Tariff)

Wound Management and Related
Products (including bandages, dressings, gauzes, lint, stockinette, etc)

The following as listed in Part IXA of the Drug Tariff (Part 2 of the Scottish Drug Tariff):

Absorbent Cottons
Absorbent Cotton Gauzes
Absorbent Cotton and Viscose Ribbon Gauze, BP 1988
Absorbent Lint, BPC
Arm Slings
Cellulose Wadding, BP 1988
Cotton Conforming Bandage, BP 1988
Cotton Crêpe Bandage, BP 1988
Cotton, Polyamide and Elastane Bandage
Crêpe Bandage, BP 1988
Elastic Adhesive Bandage, BP
Elastic Web Bandages
Elastomer and Viscose Bandage, Knitted
Gauze and Cellulose Wadding Tissue, BP 1988[1]
Gauze and Cotton Tissues
Heavy Cotton and Rubber Elastic Bandage, BP
High Compression Bandages (Extensible)
Knitted Polyamide and Cellulose Contour Bandage, BP 1988
Knitted Viscose Primary Dressing, BP, Type 1
Multiple Pack Dressing No. 1

Multiple Pack Dressing No. 2
Open-wove Bandage, BP 1988, Type 1
Paraffin Gauze Dressing, BP
Perforated Film Absorbent Dressing[2]
Polyamide and Cellulose Contour
   Bandage, BP 1988
Povidone–Iodine Fabric Dressing,
   Sterile
Skin Closure Strips, Sterile
Sterile Dressing Packs
Stockinettes
Surgical Adhesive Tapes
Suspensory Bandages, Cotton
Swabs
Titanium Dioxide Elastic Adhesive
   Bandage, BP[1]
Triangular Calico Bandage, BP 1980
Vapour-permeable Adhesive Film
   Dressing, BP
Vapour-permeable Waterproof Plastic
   Wound Dressing, BP, Sterile
Wound Management Dressings
   (including gel, colloid and foam)
Zinc Paste Bandages (including both
   plain and with additional
   ingredients)

Notes: 1   May no longer be available
          2   Now named Absorbent, Perforated Plastic Film Faced Dressing

In the Drug Tariff Appliances and Reagents which may **not** be prescribed by Nurses are annotated Ⓧ
In the Scottish Drug Tariff Appliances and Reagents which may **not** be prescribed by Nurses are annotated **Nx**

This list is currently **only** for the purposes of the **Nurse Prescribing demonstration scheme** which involves nurses with a District Nurse (DN) or Health Visitor (HV) qualification.

Details of NPF preparations

Preparations on the Nurse Prescribers' Formulary which are not included in the BP or BPC are described as follows in the pilot edition of the Nurse Prescribers' Formulary which has been produced for the Nurse Prescribing demonstration scheme.

Although brand names have sometimes been included for identification purposes preparations on the list should be prescribed by non-proprietary name.

Almond Oil Ear Drops, almond oil 10 mL supplied in a multidose container fitted with an appropriate applicator
Arachis Oil Enema (proprietary product: *Fletchers' Arachis Oil Retention Enema*), arachis oil
Cadexomer–Iodine Ointment (proprietary product: *Iodosorb Ointment*), cadexomer–iodine containing iodine 0.9% in an ointment basis

PoM **Cadexomer–Iodine Paste** (proprietary product: *Iodoflex*), cadexomer–iodine containing iodine 0.9% in a paste basis
PoM **Cadexomer–Iodine Powder** (proprietary product: *Iodosorb Powder*), cadexomer–iodine containing iodine 0.9%
NHS **Carbaryl shampoos** (proprietary product: *Carylderm Shampoo*), carbaryl 1% in a shampoo basis

Catheter Maintenance Solution, Chlorhexidine (proprietary products: *Uro-Tainer Chlorhexidine; Uriflex C*), chlorhexidine 0.02%

Catheter Maintenance Solution, Mandelic Acid (proprietary product: *Uro-Tainer Mandelic Acid*), mandelic acid 1%

Catheter Maintenance Solution, Sodium Chloride (proprietary products: *Uro-Tainer Sodium Chloride; Uriflex-S*), sodium chloride 0.9%

Catheter Maintenance Solution, 'Solution G' (proprietary products: *Uro-Tainer Suby G, Uriflex G*), citric acid 3.23%, magnesium oxide 0.38%, sodium bicarbonate 0.7%, disodium edetate 0.01%

Catheter Maintenance Solution, 'Solution R' (proprietary products: *Uro-Tainer Solution R, Uriflex R*), citric acid 6%, gluconolactone 0.6%, magnesium carbonate 2.8%, disodium edetate 0.01%

PoM **Co-danthramer Capsules**, co-danthramer 25/200 (danthron 25 mg, poloxamer '188' 200 mg)

PoM **Co-danthramer Capsules, Strong**, co-danthramer 37.5/500 (danthron 37.5 mg, poloxamer '188' 500 mg)

PoM **Co-danthramer Oral Suspension** (proprietary product: *Codalax*), co-danthramer 25/200 in 5 mL (danthron 25 mg, poloxamer '188' 200 mg/5 mL)

PoM **Co-danthramer Oral Suspension, Strong** (proprietary product: *Codalax Forte*), co-danthramer 75/1000 in 5 mL (danthron 75 mg, poloxamer '188' 1 g/ 5 mL

PoM **Co-danthrusate Oral Suspension** (proprietary product: *Normax*), co-danthrusate 50/60 (danthron 50 mg, docusate sodium 60 mg/5 mL

Dextranomer Beads (proprietary product: *Debrisan Beads*), dextranomer

Dextranomer Paste (proprietary product: *Debrisan Paste*), dextranomer in a soft paste basis

Dimethicone barrier creams (proprietary products: *Conotrane Cream*, dimethicone '350' 22%; *Siopel Barrier Cream*, dimethicone '1000' 10% *Vasogen Barrier Cream*, dimethicone 20%), dimethicone 10–22%

Docusate Capsules (proprietary product: *Diocyl Capsules*), docusate sodium 100 mg

Docusate Enema (proprietary product: *Norgalax Micro-enema*), docusate sodium 120 mg in 10 g

Docusate Enema, Compound (proprietary product: *Fletchers' Enemette*), docusate sodium 90 mg, glycerol 3.78 g/5 mL with macragol and sorbic acid

Docusate Oral Solution, docusate sodium 50 mg/5 mL [*Note*. May no longer be available]

Docusate Oral Solution, Paediatric, docusate sodium 12.5 mg/5 mL [*Note*. May no longer be available]

Ispaghula Husk Granules (proprietary products: *Isogel*), ispaghula husk 90%

Ispaghula Husk Granules, Effervescent (proprietary product: *Fybogel Granules*), ispaghula husk 3.5 g/sachet

Ispaghula Husk Powder (proprietary product: *Konsyl*), ispaghula husk 3.4 g or 6 g per sachet

Ispaghula Husk Powder, Effervescent (proprietary product: *Regulan Powder*), ispaghula husk 3.6 g/6.4 g sachet [*Note*. May no longer be available]

Lactitol Powder, lactitol 10 g/sachet

Lactulose Powder (proprietary products: *Lactulose Dry, Duphalac Dry*), lactulose 10 g/sachet

Lignocaine Ointment (proprietary product: *Xylocaine Ointment*), lignocaine 5%

Malathion alcoholic lotions (proprietary products: *Prioderm Lotion; Suleo-M Lotion*), malathion 0.5% in an alcoholic basis

Malathion aqueous lotions (proprietary products: *Derbac-M Liquid; Quellada M Liquid*), malathion 0.5% in an aqueous basis

NHS **Malathion shampoos** (proprietary products: *Prioderm Cream Shampoo; Quellada M Cream Shampoo*), malathion 1% in a shampoo basis

PoM[1] **Mebendazole Tablets** (proprietary products: *Ovex, Vermox*), mebendazole 100 mg

1. for exemption, see p. 294

PoM **Mebendazole Oral Suspension** (proprietary product: *Vermox*), mebendazole 100 mg/5 mL

PoM[2] **Miconazole Oral Gel** (proprietary product: *Daktarin Oral Gel*), miconazole 24 mg/mL

2. For exemption, see p. 274

PoM **Nystatin Pastilles** (proprietary product: *Nystan Pastilles*), nystatin 100 000 units

Olive Oil Ear Drops, olive oil 10 mL supplied in a multi-dose container fitted with an appropriate applicator

Permethrin Cream (proprietary product: *Lyclear Dermal Cream*), permethrin 5%

Permethrin Cream Rinse (proprietary product: *Lyclear Cream Rinse*), permethrin 1%

Phenothrin Alcoholic Lotion (proprietary product: *Full Marks Lotion*), phenothrin 0.2% in a basis containing isopropyl alcohol

Piperazine and Senna Powder (proprietary product: *Pripsen Oral Powder*), piperazine phosphate 4 g, sennosides 15.3 mg/sachet

Povidone–Iodine Aqueous Solution (proprietary product: *Betadine Antiseptic Solution*), povidone–iodine 10%

Senna Oral Solution (proprietary product: *Senokot Syrup*), sennosides 7.5 mg/5 mL

Senna and Ispaghula Granules (proprietary product: *Manevac Granules*), senna fruit 12.4%, ispaghula 54.2%

Sodium Citrate Compound Enema (proprietary products: Fleet Micro-enema; *Micolette Micro-enema; Micralax Micro-enema; Relaxit Micro-enema*), sodium citrate 450 mg with glycerol, sorbitol and an anionic surfactant

Sterculia Granules (proprietary product: *Normacol Granules*), sterculia 62%

Sterculia and Frangula Granules (proprietary product: *Normacol Plus Granules*), sterculia 62%, frangula (standardised) 8%

PoM **Streptokinase and Streptodornase Topical Powder** (proprietary product: *Varidase Topical*), streptokinase 100 000 units, streptodornase 25 000 units

Titanium Ointment (proprietary product: *Metanium Ointment*), titanium dioxide 20%, titanium peroxide 5%, titanium salicylate 3%, titanium tannate 0.1%

Zinc Oxide and Dimethicone Spray (proprietary product: *Sprilon*), dimethicone 1.04%, zinc oxide 12.5% in a pressurised aerosol unit

---

Note: Page numbers given refer to those in the British National Formulary.

Appendix 2
Adverse Reactions to Drugs

Christine Proudlove

The following table lists some of the reactions reported in association with drug therapy. It illustrates the fact that drugs can cause a wide range of adverse reactions, affecting every organ system of the body. It also demonstrates that reactions can vary between relatively trivial symptoms through to life-threatening or even fatal disease.

The table has been compiled principally from the *British National Formulary No. 32* (September 1996) with some additional reference to the manufacturers' Data Sheets or Summary of Product Characteristics. It is not comprehensive. It contains only a selection of adverse reactions, and not all available drugs are included. By its very nature, the table is now out of date since new drugs, with their own particular adverse reaction profiles, are being marketed, and new reactions to established drugs are occasionally recognised. It is important, therefore, that this table is not used as a sole reference source on adverse drug reactions.

Inclusion of a reaction in the table gives no indication of the frequency with which the reaction occurs; the table includes both common and rarely reported effects. However, entries for nausea, vomiting and headache have been omitted because they are reported with such a wide range of drugs that compilation would not be helpful.

The table lists adverse reactions to individual drugs and, where appropriate, to therapeutic groups. Therapeutic groups are in *italics*. Where a therapeutic group is listed, individual drugs within that class are not listed separately.

Adverse reaction	Drug	
Cardiovascular disorders		
Angina or myocardial ischaemia	*ACE inhibitors* Bicalutamide Carvedilol Dopexamine Ergotamine	Methysergide Sumatriptan Thyroxine Vasopressin
Arrhythmias	*ACE inhibitors* Adrenaline Aminophylline Amphotericin *Anthracycline cytotoxics* *Antihistamines* Atropine Azathioprine Bicalutamide *Butyrophenones* *Calcium salts* Carbamazepine Cisapride Digoxin Dopexamine Enoximone Ephedrine Flecainide Ganciclovir Gemfibrozil Hydralazine Interferon-alfa	Levodopa *Macrolide antibiotics* *MAOI antidepressants* Methylphenidate Mexiletine Milrinone Moracizine Ondansetron Oxybutynin Paclitaxel Pentamidine *Phenothiazines* Probucol Propafenone Quinidine Sotalol Sumatriptan Theophylline Thyroxine Tocainide *Tricyclic antidepressants*
Bradycardia	Adenosine Amiodarone Atropine *Beta-blockers* *Calcium salts* Clonidine Diltiazem Epoprostenol *H_2-receptor antagonists* Lignocaine	Lofexidine Mefloquine Ondansetron *Opioids* Paclitaxel Peppermint oil Propafenone Protamine Sumatriptan Tropisetron
Cardiac failure	Amsacrine *Beta-blockers* Bicalutamide Carbenoxolone	Moracizine Procainamide Quinidine

Adverse reaction	Drug	

Cardiovascular disorders (contd.)

Adverse reaction	Drug	
Cardiomyopathy	Anthracycline cytotoxics Dexamphetamine	Tacrolimus
Conduction disorders	Amiodarone *Beta-blockers* Bicalutamide Carbamazepine Digoxin Diltiazem Disopyramide	*H_2-receptor antagonists* Mefloquine Metoclopramide Mexiletine Paclitaxel Propafenone
Hypertension	Allopurinol Carbenoxolone Cyclosporin Dexamphetamine Dobutamide Dopamine Epoetin Ganciclovir Interferon-alfa	Levodopa Mefloquine Methylphenidate Mycophenolate Pamidronate Phentermine Sodium bicarbonate Tramadol Venlafaxine
Hypotension	*ACE inhibitors* *Adrenergic neurone* *blockers* *Alpha-blockers* Aminoglutethimide *Antihistamines* Apomorphine Azathioprine Baclofen *Benzodiazepines* Bromocriptine *Butyrophenones* Carvedilol Co-dergocrine Dexfenfluramine Diltiazem Dipyridamole Disopyramide *Diuretics* Docetaxel Dopamine Enoximone Epoprostenol Fenfluramine Ganciclovir	Interferon-alfa Labetalol Levodopa Lignocaine Lofexidine Losartan Lysuride *MAOI antidepressants* Mefloquine Mesna Methysergide Mexiletine Milrinone Mycophenolate Nabilone Nefazodone Nicardipine Nicorandil *Nicotinic acid derivatives* Nimodipine *Nitrates* Ondansetron *Opioids* Paclitaxel Pamidronate

Adverse reaction	Drug	
Cardiovascular disorders (contd.)		
Hypotension *(contd.)*	Pentamidine	*SSRI antidepressants*
	Pergolide	Sumatriptan
	Phenothiazines	Tetrabenazine
	Propafenone	*Tricyclic antidepressants*
	Protamine	Vancomycin
	Selegiline	Venlafaxine
Oedema	*Adrenergic neurone blockers*	Lansoprazole
	Amantadine	Lithium
	Anabolic steroids	*MAOI antidepressants*
	Aspirin	Mesterolone
	Bicalutamide	Methyldopa
	Calcium channel blockers	Methysergide
	Carbamazepine	Mycophenolate
	Chorionic gonadotrophin	*NSAIDs*
	Clonidine	*Oestrogens*
	Cyclosporin	Omeprazole
	Danazol	*Progestogens*
	Desmopressin	Quinagolide
	Docetaxel	Rifampicin
	Doxazosin	Sodium bicarbonate
	Fludarabine	Sodium valproate
	Flutamide	Somatotropin
	Formestane	Tamoxifen
	Ganciclovir	Terazosin
	Gestrinone	Testosterone
	Hydralazine	Tibolone
	Itraconazole	Toremifene
		Vigabatrin
Palpitations	*ACE inhibitors*	Methylphenidate
	Alpha-blockers	Mexiletine
	Aminophylline	Moracizine
	Antihistamines	Nicorandil
	Atropine	Nicotine
	Beta-2 agonists	*Opioids*
	Buspirone	Phentermine
	Cabergoline	Sodium nitroprusside
	Calcium channel blockers	*SSRI antidepressants*
	Dexamphetamine	Theophylline
	Gonadorelin analogues	Thyroxine
	Indapamide	Venlafaxine
Pulmonary hypertension	Dexfenfluramine	Fenfluramine

Adverse reaction	Drug	
Cardiovascular disorders (contd.)		
Sudden death	*Antipsychotics*	*Tricyclic antidepressants*
Tachycardia	Adrenaline	Methysergide
	Alpha-blockers	Mycophenolate
	Aminophylline	Nabilone
	Antimuscarinics	Nefopam
	Beta-2 agonists	*Nitrates*
	Buspirone	Ofloxacin
	Butyrophenones	*Opioids*
	Ciprofloxacin	Oxpentifylline
	Dexamphetamine	Pergolide
	Dobutamine	*Phenothiazines*
	Dopamine	Phentermine
	Dopexamine	Riluzole
	Ephedrine	Sumatriptan
	Levodopa	Tacrolimus
	Mefloquine	Theophylline
	Mesna	Thyroxine
	Methylphenidate	*Tricyclic antidepressants*

Disorders of the ear

Hearing loss	*Aminoglycosides*	*Loop diuretics*
	Amphotericin	*Macrolide antibiotics*
	Aspirin	Tacrolimus
	Capreomycin	Teicoplanin
	Cisplatin	Vancomycin
	Ganciclovir	
Tinnitus	*Aminoglycosides*	Nicardipine
	Aspirin	Norfloxacin
	Capreomycin	*NSAIDs*
	Carboplatin	Quinine
	Cisplatin	Tacrolimus
	Loop diuretics	Teicoplanin
	Mefloquine	Vancomycin

Endocrine, metabolic or nutritional disorders

Appetite decreased/anorexia	Amantadine	Dexamphetamine
	Aminoglutethimide	Digoxin
	Amphotericin	*Fibrate antilipaemics*
	Anastrozole	Ganciclovir
	Bicalutamide	Indapamide
	Carbamazepine	Interferon-alfa
	Dantrolene	Levodopa
	Dapsone	Lithium

Adverse reaction	Drug	

Endocrine, metabolic or nutritional disorders (contd.)

Adverse reaction	Drug	
Appetite decreased/anorexia *(contd.)*	Mefloquine Metformin Methylphenidate Nabilone Naltrexone Nitrofurantoin Pamidronate Penicillamine Pyrazinamide Quinagolide	*Quinolone antibiotics* Rifampicin *SSRI antidepressants* Terbinafine Topiramate Toremifene Venlafaxine Vitamin D Zalcitabine Zidovudine
Appetite increased	*Corticosteroids* Flutamide	Pizotifen Sodium valproate
Hypercalcaemia	Mesterolone Testosterone	*Thiazide diuretics*
Hyperglycaemia	Bicalutamide Clozapine Indapamide Isoniazid *Loop diuretics* Mycophenolate	*Nicotinic acid derivatives* Pentamidine *SSRI antidepressants* Tacrolimus *Thiazide diuretics* *Tricyclic antidepressants*
Hyperkalaemia	*ACE inhibitors* Amiloride Aminoglutethimide Cyclosporin Epoetin Losartan	Pentamidine Potassium citrate Spironolactone Tacrolimus Triamterene
Hyperlipidaemia	Anastrozole Crisantaspase Cyclosporin	*Loop diuretics* Mycophenolate *Thiazide diuretics*
Hypernatraemia	Carbenoxolone *MAOI antidepressants*	Pamidronate
Hyperprolactinaemia	Metoclopramide Domperidone	*Phenothiazines* *Tricyclic antidepressants*
Hyperthyroidism	Amiodarone	Interferon-alfa
Hyperuricaemia	Cyclosporin *Loop diuretics*	Pancreatin *Thiazide diuretics*
Hypocalcaemia	Clodronate Etidronate Foscarnet	Pamidronate Pentamidine Phenytoin

Adverse reaction	Drug	
Endocrine, metabolic or nutritional disorders (contd.)		
Hypoglycaemia	Aminoglutethimide	Pentamidine
	Disopyramide	Quinine
	Foscarnet	*SSRI antidepressants*
	Ganciclovir	*Sulphonylureas*
	Insulins	*Tricyclic antidepressants*
	Mycophenolate	
Hypokalaemia	Amphotericin	*Loop diuretics*
	Beta-2 agonists	Milrinone
	Carbenicillin	Pamidronate
	Carbenoxolone	*Stimulant laxatives*
	Glucagon	Tacrolimus
	Indapamide	*Thiazide diuretics*
	Itraconazole	
Hyponatraemia	*ACE inhibitors*	*Diuretics*
	Aminoglutethimide	*MAOI antidepressants*
	Atovaquone	Moclobemide
	Carbamazepine	*SSRI antidepressants*
	Chlorpropamide	*Tricyclic antidepressants*
	Desmopressin	Vincristine
Hypothyroidism	Aminoglutethimide	Interferon-alfa
	Amiodarone	Somatotropin
Lactic acidosis	Metformin	Zidovudine
Osteomalacia	Phenytoin	Spironolactone
Weight gain	*Antipsychotic agents*	Lithium
	Astemazole	*MAOI antidepressants*
	Clomiphene	Methysergide
	Corticosteroids	Mycophenolate
	Cyclosporin	*Oestrogens*
	Cyproheptadine	Piracetam
	Cyproterone	Pizotifen
	Danazol	*Progesterones*
	Gabapentin	Sodium valproate
	Gestrinone	Tibolone
	Gonadorelin analogues	Toremifene
	Indoramin	*Tricyclic antidepressants*
	Isradipine	Venlafaxine
	Ketotifen	Vigabatrin
Weight loss	Ethosuximide	Topiramate
	Gonadorelin analogues	Vitamin D
	SSRI antidepressants	Zalcitabine
	Thyroxine	

Adverse reaction	Drug	

Eye/vision disorders

Cataract	*Corticosteroids* Tacrolimus	Tamoxifen
Conjunctivitis	Chlormethiazole	Pamidronate
Corneal disorders	Amiodarone Chloroquine *Corticosteroids* Flecainide	*Phenothiazines* Tamoxifen Toremifene
Eye pain	Ganciclovir Interferon-alfa	Nifedipine
Increased intraocular pressure	*Antimuscarinics* *Corticosteroids*	*Tricyclic antidepressants*
Nystagmus	Baclofen Gabapentin *MAOI antidepressants* Mexiletine	Phenytoin Topiramate Vigabatrin
Optic neuritis	Amiodarone Chloramphenicol	Ethambutol Isoniazid
Retinal disorders	Chloroquine Ganciclovir Interferon-alfa	*Phenothiazines* Tamoxifen Vigabatrin
Uveitis	Pamidronate	Rifabutin
Visual disturbance	Amantadine Amphotericin *Antihistamines* *Antimuscarinics* *Benzodiazepines* *Butyrophenones* Carbamazepine Chloroquine Clomiphene Colistin Dantrolene Dexamphetamine Dexfenfluramine Digoxin Disopyramide Fenfluramine Flecainide Flutamide	Gabapentin Ganciclovir Gemfibrozil *Gonadorelin analogues* Indapamide Lamotrigine Lansoprazole Lithium *MAOI antidepressants* Mefloquine Nabilone Nefazodone Nefopam Omeprazole Ondansetron Oxitropium Oxybutynin Pergolide

Adverse reaction	Drug	

Visual disturbance *(contd.)*

Phenothiazines	Tamoxifen
Phenytoin	*Tetracyclines*
Pirenzepine	Tibolone
Primidone	Topiramate
Propafenone	*Tricyclic antidepressants*
Quinine	Venlafaxine
Quinolone antibiotics	Vigabatrin
Somatotropin	Zolpidem

Gastrointestinal disorders

Abdominal pain

Acamprosate	Mefloquine
Acarbose	Meropenem
ACE inhibitors	Mesalazine
Alendronate	Methylphenidate
Amphotericin	Misoprostol
Auranofin	Mycophenolate
Aztreonam	Nabilone
Bicalutamide	Naftidrofuryl
Cabergoline	Naltrexone
Cephalosporins	Nedocromil
Cisapride	Olsalazine
Clindamycin	Omeprazole
Clomiphene	Oxybutynin
Colchicine	Pamidronate
Digoxin	Pancreatin
Ergotamine	Pergolide
Etidronate	Probucol
Fibrate antilipaemics	Quinagolide
Fluconazole	Quinine
Flutamide	*Quinolone antibiotics*
Ganciclovir	Risperidine
Gonadorelin analogues	Sodium nitroprusside
Iron preparations	*SSRI antidepressants*
Itraconazole	*Stimulant laxatives*
Labetalol	Sulphasalazine
Lactitol	Terbinafine
Lactulose	Tiludronate
Lansoprazole	Tropisetron
Loperamide	Vasopressin
Lysuride	Venlafaxine
Macrogols	Vitamin E
Macrolide antibiotics	Zalcitabine
Magnesium salts	Zidovudine
Mebendazole	*Zinc salts*

Adverse reaction	Drug	

Gastro-intestinal disorders (contd.)

Colitis	*Antibiotics*	Mesalazine
	Cyclosporin	*NSAIDs*
	Gold preparations	Sulphasalazine

| Colonic stricture | Pancreatin | |

Constipation	Alendronate	Mexiletine
	Aluminium salts	Mycophenolate
	Aminoglutethimide	Naltrexone
	Antimuscarinics	Nefazodone
	Antipsychotic agents	Omeprazole
	Bicalutamide	Ondansetron
	Bismuth salts	*Opioids*
	Bromocriptine	Oxitropium
	Carbamazepine	Oxybutynin
	Cholestyramine	Pamidronate
	Clonidine	Pergolide
	Colestipol	Phentermine
	Dantrolene	Pizotifen
	Etidronate	Propafenone
	Formestane	*SSRI antidepressants*
	Gonadorelin analogues	Statins
	Granisetron	Sucralfate
	Indapamide	Toremifene
	Ipratropium	*Tricyclic antidepressants*
	Iron preparations	Tropisetron
	Itraconazole	Venlafaxine
	Lansoprazole	Verapamil
	Lysuride	*Vinca alkaloids*
	MAOI antidepressants	Zalcitabine

Diarrhoea	Acamprosate	Cisapride
	Acarbose	Clindamycin
	ACE inhibitors	Co-trimoxazole
	Alendronate	Colchicine
	Aminoglutethimide	Colestipol
	Amphotericin	Dantrolene
	Anastrazole	Dexfenfluramine
	Atovaquone	Didanosine
	Auranofin	Digoxin
	Aztreonam	Dipyridamole
	Carbamazepine	Enoximone
	Cephalosporins	Ergotamine
	Chenodeoxycholic acid	Etidronate
	Chloramphenicol	Fenfluramine
	Cholestyramine	Fluconazole

Adverse reaction	Drug	
Gastro-intestinal disorders (contd.)		
Diarrhoea *(contd.)*	Flucytosine	Phenindione
	Flutamide	Piperazine
	Fosfomycin	Piracetam
	Ganciclovir	Probucol
	Glucagon	Procainamide
	Guanethidine	Proguanil
	Imipenem	Propafenone
	Indapamide	*Proton pump inhibitors*
	Lithium	Quinagolide
	Macrolide antibiotics	Quinidine
	Magnesium salts	*Quinolone antiobiotics*
	Mebendazole	Rifampicin
	Mefloquine	*SSRI antidepressants*
	Meropenem	*Statins*
	Mesalazine	Sucralfate
	Mesna	Teicoplanin
	Metformin	Terbinafine
	Methyldopa	*Tetracyclines*
	Misoprostol	Thymoxamine
	Mycophenolate	Thyroxine
	Naltrexone	Tiludronate
	Nicoumalone	Tranexamic acid
	Nitrofurantoin	Tropisetron
	NSAIDs	Ursodeoxycholic acid
	Nystatin	Vitamin D
	Olsalazine	Vitamin E
	Oxybutynin	Warfarin
	Pamidronate	Zalcitabine
	Penicillins	Zolpidem
	Pergolide	
Dry mouth	*Alpha-blockers*	Fenfluramine
	Amiloride	Ganciclovir
	Antihistamines	Indoramin
	Antimuscarinics	Ipratropium
	Antipsychotic agents	Ketotifen
	Baclofen	Lansoprazole
	Bicalutamide	Lofexidine
	Bromocriptine	*MAOI antidepressants*
	Buspirone	Methyldopa
	Clonidine	Methylphenidate
	Dexamphetamine	Moxonidine
	Dexfenfluramine	Nabilone
	Disopyramide	Nefazodone
	Ephedrine	Nefopam

Adverse reaction	Drug	
Gastro-intestinal disorders (contd.)		
Dry mouth *(contd.)*	Opioids Oxitropium Oxybutynin Phentermine Pirenzepine Pizotifen Propafenone	*SSRI antidepressants* Sucralfate Triamterene *Tricyclic antidepressants* Venlafaxine Zopiclone
Dyspepsia/heartburn	*ACE inhibitors* Amantadine Aspirin Bicalutamide Cholestyramine Ciprofloxacin Colestipol *Corticosteroids* Disopyramide Fosfomycin Gabapentin Ganciclovir Indapamide Itraconazole Lansoprazole Methysergide Misoprostol	Nedocromil Nicotine *NSAIDs* Olsalazine Pamidronate Peppermint oil Pergolide Proguanil Risperidone Sodium valproate *SSRI antidepressants* Stanozolol Sucralfate Venlafaxine Vigabatrin Zidovudine *Zinc salts*
Dysphagia	Alendronate Ciprofloxacin Dantrolene	Ganciclovir Zalcitabine
Flatulence	Acarbose Alendronate Bicalutamide *Bulk-forming laxatives* Chloral hydrate Cholestyramine Ciprofloxacin Colestipol	Fluconazole Guar gum Lactitol Lactulose Misoprostol Probucol *Proton pump inhibitors*
Gingival hyperplasia	*Calcium channel blockers* *(except diltiazem)* Cyclosporin	Ethosuximide Phenytoin
GI ulceration/haemorrhage	Aspirin Colchicine *Corticosteroids* Ganciclovir	Levodopa *NSAIDs* Sulphinpyrazone Warfarin

Adverse reaction	Drug	
Gastro-intestinal disorders (contd.)		
Glossitis	Chloramphenicol Clarithromycin	Co-trimoxazole
Mouth ulcers/stomatitis	*ACE inhibitors* Amsacrine Aztreonam Chloramphenicol Clarithromycin Ganciclovir	Mycophenolate Omeprazole Proguanil Sodium aurothiomalate Zalcitabine
Mucositis	Amsacrine *Anthracycline cytotoxics* Bleomycin	Fluorouracil Methotrexate
Oesophagitis	Alendronate *Corticosteroids* Potassium chloride	Tetracyclines Zalcitabine
Pancreatitis	*ACE inhibitors* Azathioprine Cimetidine Co-trimoxazole *Corticosteroids* Cyclosporin Didanosine Gemfibrozil *Loop diuretics* Mesalazine Nitrofurantoin	*NSAIDs* Olsalazine Paracetamol Pentamidine Sodium valproate *Statins* Sulphasalazine *Tetracyclines* *Thiazide diuretics* Warfarin Zalcitabine
Peritoneal fibrosis	Bromocriptine Ergotamine	Methysergide
Salivation	Clozapine	Nicardipine
Taste disturbance	*ACE inhibitors* Allopurinol Amiodarone Auranofin Aztreonam Calcitonin Cefpirome Clarithromycin Ganciclovir Imipenem Losartan	Metronidazole Omeprazole Penicillamine Pentamidine Propafenone *Quinolone antibiotics* Salcatonin Terbinafine Tinidazole Topiramate Zopiclone

Adverse reaction	Drug	
Haematological disorders		
Agranulocytosis	*ACE inhibitors*	Nitrofurantoin
	Aminoglutethimide	*NSAIDs*
	Antipsychotic agents	Ofloxacin
	Carbamazepine	Penicillamine
	Carbimazole	Phenindione
	Cephalosporins	Phenytoin
	Cimetidine	Pirenzepine
	Chloroquine	Procainamide
	Clindamycin	Propylthiouracil
	Co-trimoxazole	Quinidine
	Dapsone	Sulphasalazine
	Ethosuximide	*Sulphonylureas*
	Etidronate	Tocainide
	Gold preparations	*Tricyclic antidepressants*
	Griseofulvin	Vancomycin
	Isoniazid	
Aplastic anaemia	Captopril	Mesalazine
	Carbamazepine	Nitrofurantoin
	Cephalosporins	*NSAIDs*
	Chloramphenicol	Penicillamine
	Chloroquine	Phenytoin
	Cimetidine	Probenecid
	Ethosuximide	Sulphasalazine
	Flucytosine	*Sulphonylureas*
	Gold preparations	Tocainide
Bone marrow depression	Azathioprine	Ganciclovir
	Chloroquine	*Loop diuretics*
	Cytotoxic agents	Trimethoprim
	Enalapril	Zidovudine
Clotting disorders	Amiodarone	Colestipol
	Aspirin	*Quinolone antibiotics*
	Carbenicillin	Sodium valproate
	Cholestyramine	
Eosinophilia	Apomorphine	*Quinolone antibiotics*
	Cephalosporins	Rifabutin
	Clindamycin	Rifampicin
	Co-trimoxazole	Teicoplanin
	Dapsone	*Tricyclic antidepressants*
	Ganciclovir	Tryptophan
	Meropenem	Vancomycin

Adverse reaction	Drug	

Haematological disorders (contd.)

Haemolytic anaemia	Flutamide	Penicillamine
	Hydralazine	*Phenothiazines*
	Methyldopa	Quinidine
	NSAIDs	Rifampicin
Leucopenia	Azithromycin	Metronidazole
	Aztreonam	Mycophenolate
	Capreomycin	Omeprazole
	Captopril	Pamidronate
	Carbamazepine	Pemoline
	Carbimazole	Penicillamine
	Carvedilol	*Penicillins*
	Cephalosporins	Pentamidine
	Chloral hydrate	Phenindione
	Clindamycin	Phenytoin
	Co-trimoxazole	Propylthiouracil
	Danazol	*Quinolone antibiotics*
	Enalapril	Rifabutin
	Etidronate	Rifampicin
	Flucytosine	Sodium valproate
	Ganciclovir	Sulphasalazine
	Griseofulvin	Tamoxifen
	Interferon-alfa	Teicoplanin
	Lamotrigine	*Thiazide diuretics*
	Lansoprazole	Tinidazole
	MAOI antidepressants	*Tricyclic antidepressants*
	Mefloquine	Vancomycin
	Meropenem	Zalcitabine
	Mesalazine	Zidovudine
	Methylphenidate	
Thrombocytopenia	*ACE inhibitors*	Cyclosporin
	Aminoglutethimide	Danaparoid
	Amiodarone	Danazol
	Aspirin	Flucytosine
	Aztreonam	Ganciclovir
	Bicalutamide	*Gold preparations*
	Capreomycin	Heparin
	Carbamazepine	Indapamide
	Carvedilol	Lamotrigine
	Cephalosporins	Lansoprazole
	Chloroquine	Mefloquine
	Cimetidine	Meropenem
	Clindamycin	Mesalazine
	Co-trimoxazole	Methylphenidate

Adverse reaction	Drug	

Haematological disorders (contd.)

Thrombocytopenia *(contd.)*	Moracizine	Quinidine
	Mycophenolate	Quinine
	Naltrexone	Rifabutin
	Nicardipine	Sodium valproate
	Nimodipine	Sulphasalazine
	Nitrofurantoin	*Sulphonylureas*
	NSAIDs	Tamoxifen
	Omeprazole	Teicoplanin
	Pamidronate	*Thiazide diuretics*
	Penicillamine	Tocainide
	Penicillins	*Tricyclic antidepressants*
	Pentamidine	Vancomycin
	Phenytoin	Zalcitabine
	Pirenzepine	Zidovudine
	Quinolone antibiotics	

Hepatic disorders

Abnormal liver function tests	Aciclovir	Lamotrigine
	Amphotericin	Lansoprazole
	Anabolic steroids	Levodopa
	Antipsychotic agents	Losartan
	Atovaquone	*MAOI antidepressants*
	Azathioprine	Mefloquine
	Bicalutamide	Meropenem
	Capreomycin	Methyldopa
	Carvedilol	Moclobemide
	Cephalosporins	Moracizine
	Chenodeoxycholic acid	Mycophenolate
	Chlormethiazole	Naltrexone
	Cisapride	*Nicotinic acid derivatives*
	Clindamycin	*Oestrogens*
	Crisantaspase	Omeprazole
	Cycloserine	Ondansetron
	Cyclosporin	Pamidronate
	Danaparoid	Pemoline
	Diltiazem	Pentamidine
	Ethosuximide	*Quinolone antibiotics*
	Flecainide	Rifabutin
	Fluconazole	Rifampicin
	Ganciclovir	Riluzole
	Granisetron	*SSRI antidepressants*
	H_2-receptor antagonists	Sulphinpyrazone
	Imipenem	Sumatriptan
	Indapamide	Tamoxifen

Adverse reaction	Drug	

Adverse reaction	Drug	
Abnormal liver function tests (contd.)	Teicoplanin Tibolone Tocainide *Tricyclic antidepressants*	Venlafaxine Verapamil Zalcitabine Zidovudine
Gall bladder disorders	Ceftriaxone	Clofibrate
Hepatitis	Allopurinol Amiodarone Aztreonam Carbamazepine *Cephalosporins* Ciprofloxacin Clarithromycin Co-amoxiclav Cyproterone Dapsone Diltiazem Flucloxacillin Flucytosine Isoniazid Itraconazole Lansoprazole Mesalazine Methyldopa Mexiletine	Mycophenolate Naftidrofuryl Nitrofurantoin *NSAIDs* Omeprazole Phenindione Phenytoin Pyrazinamide Quinidine Stanozolol *Statins* Sulphasalazine Sulphinpyrazone Tamoxifen Terbinafine *Tetracyclines* Thymoxamine Tocainide
Hepatocellular damage	Bicalutamide Co-trimoxazole Cyproterone Disulfiram Flucytosine Flutamide Labetalol *MAOI antidepressants*	Naftidrofuryl *Nicotinic acid derivatives* Probenecid Pyrazinamide Sodium valproate *Tetracyclines* Zalcitabine
Jaundice	*ACE inhibitors* Aminoglutethimide Amsacrine *Antipsychotic agents* Azathioprine Aztreonam *Benzodiazepines* Bicalutamide Carbamazepine Carbimazole	*Cephalosporins* Ciprofloxacin Clarithromycin Clindamycin Co-amoxiclav Co-trimoxazole Cyproterone Danazol Disopyramide Flecainide

Adverse reaction	Drug

Hepatic disorders (contd.)

Jaundice *(contd.)*

Flucloxacillin
Flutamide
Gemfibrozil
Itraconazole
Lansoprazole
Macrolide antibiotics
MAOI antidepressants
Methyldopa
Mexiletine
Moracizine
Nicoumalone
Nitrofurantoin
NSAIDs
Oestrogens
Omeprazole
Phenindione
Progestogens

Propylthiouracil
Pyrazinamide
Rifabutin
Rifampicin
Sodium aurothiomalate
Sodium fusidate
Stanozolol
Sulphinpyrazone
Sulphonylureas
Terbinafine
Thymoxamine
Tocainide
Toremifene
Tricyclic antidepressants
Warfarin
Zalcitabine

Immunological disorders

Allergic or hypersensitivity reactions

ACE inhibitors
Allopurinol
Aminoglutethimide
Anistreplase
Antihistamines
Antimuscarinics
Aspirin
Azathioprine
Barbiturates
Beta-2 agonists
Bleomycin
Capreomycin
Cephalosporins
Cimetidine
Corticosteroids
Danaparoid
Dapsone
Docetaxel
Finasteride
Glucagon
Gonadorelin
Interferon-alfa
Interferon-beta
Isoniazid
Ispaghula
Itraconazole
Levodopa

Lignocaine
Mebendazole
Mesna
Nicoumalone
NSAIDs
Ondansetron
Paclitaxel
Pancreatin
Penicillins
Peppermint oil
Phenindione
Piperazine
Probenecid
Procarbazine
Propafenone
Quinine
Rifabutin
SSRI antidepressants
Statins
Streptokinase
Sulphonylureas
Thiazide diuretics
Tropisetron
Vasopressin
Warfarin
Zopiclone

Adverse reaction	Drug	

Immunological disorders (contd.)

Anaphylaxis

Aminoglutethimide	Imipenem
Amiodarone	Interferon-beta
Anistreplase	Metronidazole
Antihistamines	*Penicillins*
Cephalosporins	*Quinolone antibiotics*
Chlormethiazole	Streptokinase
Corticosteroids	Sumatriptan
Crisantaspase	Teicoplanin
Epoetin	Tramadol
Fluconazole	Vancomycin
Heparin	

Musculoskeletal disorders

Arthropathy

Alendronate	Naltrexone
Amphotericin	Nitrofurantoin
Azathioprine	Olsalazine
Carbamazepine	Omeprazole
Carbimazole	Pamidronate
Cephalosporins	*Penicillins*
Cimetidine	Propylthiouracil
Fluoxetine	Pyrazinamide
Formestane	*Quinolone antibiotics*
Lansoprazole	Sodium cromoglycate
Mefloquine	Somatotropin
Mesna	Sucralfate
Methylphenidate	Terbinafine
Mianserin	Zalcitabine

Gout

Cyclosporin	Thiazide diuretics
Loop diuretics	

Myalgia or myopathy

ACE inhibitors	*Fibrate antilipaemics*
Alendronate	Fluoxetine
Amiodarone	Ganciclovir
Amphotericin	Gemfibrozil
Antihistamines	*Gonadorelin analogues*
Azathioprine	Indapamide
Baclofen	Lansoprazole
Beta-2 agonists	Lithium
Bumetanide	Mefloquine
Cimetidine	Methysergide
Colchicine	Naltrexone
Corticosteroids	Nicotine
Cyclosporin	Omeprazole
Ergotamine	Paclitaxel

Adverse reaction	Drug	
Musculoskeletal disorders (contd.)		
Myalgia or myopathy *(contd.)*	Pamidronate	Terbinafine
	Quinolone antibiotics	Thyroxine
	Rifampicin	Tryptophan
	Somatotropin	Zalcitabine
	Stanozolol	Zidovudine
	Statins	
Osteoporosis	*Corticosteroids*	Danaparoid
	Cyproterone	Heparin
SLE-like syndrome	*Antipsychotic agents*	Nitrofurantoin
	Ethosuximide	Penicillamine
	Flutamide	Phenytoin
	Griseofulvin	Procainamide
	Hydralazine	Propafenone
	Isoniazid	Propylthiouracil
	Mesalazine	Quinidine
	Methyldopa	Sulphasalazine
	Minocycline	Tocainide
Tendonitis or tendon rupture	*Corticosteroids*	*Quinolone antibiotics*

Nervous system disorders

Convulsions	Aciclovir	Isoniazid
	Amantadine	Lignocaine
	Aminophylline	*MAOI antidepressants*
	Amphotericin	Mefloquine
	Antihistamines	Meropenem
	Antipsychotic agents	Metronidazole
	Baclofen	Mexiletine
	Chloroquine	Nalidixic acid
	Cisapride	Ondansetron
	Clomiphene	Pamidronate
	Cycloserine	Propafenone
	Cyclosporin	*SSRI antidepressants*
	Dantrolene	Sumatriptan
	Dexamphetamine	Theophylline
	Didanosine	Tinidazole
	Epoetin	Tocainide
	Flucytosine	Tramadol
	Foscarnet	*Tricyclic antidepressants*
	Gabapentin	Venlafaxine
	Imipenem	Vigabatrin
	Interferon-alfa	Zidovudine
	Interferon-beta	

Adverse reaction	Drug	

Nervous system disorders (contd.)

Adverse reaction	Drug	
Co-ordination disorders	Aminoglutethimide	Lithium
	Amiodarone	Metronidazole
	Anticonvulsants	Mexiletine
	Baclofen	Nabilone
	Barbiturates	Nefazodone
	Benzodiazepines	Ofloxacin
	Carbamazepine	Peppermint oil
	Chloral hydrate	Piperazine
	Flecainide	Tinidazole
	Ganciclovir	Zolpidem
	Griseofulvin	Zopiclone
Dizziness	*ACE inhibitors*	Ganciclovir
	Aciclovir	*Gonadorelin analogues*
	Alpha blockers	Griseofulvin
	Alprostadil	*H_2-receptor antagonists*
	Alverine citrate	Indapamide
	Amantadine	Itraconazole
	Aminoglutethimide	Ketotifen
	Azathioprine	Lamotrigine
	Baclofen	Levodopa
	Barbiturates	Lignocaine
	Bicalutamide	Losartan
	Bromocriptine	Lysuride
	Buspirone	*MAOI antidepressants*
	Calcium channel blockers	Mefloquine
	Carbamazepine	Methylphenidate
	Carvedilol	Methysergide
	Celiprolol	Metronidazole
	Cephalosporins	Minocycline
	Clozapine	Misoprostol
	Clomiphene	Moclobemide
	Clonidine	Moracizine
	Co-dergocrine	Moxonidine
	Cycloserine	Mycophenolate
	Danazol	Naltrexone
	Dexamphetamine	Nefazodone
	Dexfenfluramine	Nicorandil
	Ethosuximide	Nicotine
	Fenfluramine	*Nicotinic acid derivatives*
	Fibrate antilipaemics	*Nitrates*
	Flecainide	Ondansetron
	Flutamide	Oxpentifylline
	Formestane	Oxybutynin
	Gabapentin	Pamidronate

Adverse reaction	Drug	

Nervous system disorders (contd.)

Dizziness *(contd.)*	Pentamidine	Sumatriptan
	Phentermine	Tacrolimus
	Phenytoin	Teicoplanin
	Piperazine	Thymoxamine
	Pizotifen	Tibolone
	Probenecid	Tiludronate
	Propafenone	Tinidazole
	Proton pump inhibitors	Topiramate
	Quinolone antibiotics	Tocainide
	Riluzole	Toremifene
	Risperidone	Tropisetron
	Sodium nitroprusside	Venlafaxine
	Spectinomycin	Zalcitabine
	SSRI antidepressants	Zolpidem
	Sucralfate	Zopiclone
Drowsiness	*Adrenergic neurone blockers*	Lofexidine
	Allopurinol	Lysuride
	Alpha blockers	*MAOI antidepressants*
	Aminoglutethimide	Methyldopa
	Antihistamines	Methylphenidate
	Apomorphine	Methysergide
	Baclofen	Metoclopramide
	Barbiturates	Metronidazole
	Benzodiazepines	Mexiletine
	Bromocriptine	Nabilone
	Buspirone	Nefopam
	Carbamazepine	Nicardipine
	Clonidine	*Opioids*
	Cycloserine	Oxybutynin
	Dexfenfluramine	*Phenothiazines*
	Digoxin	Piperazine
	Disulfiram	Pizotifen
	Ethosuximide	Primidone
	Fenfluramine	*SSRI antidepressants*
	Flucytosine	Sucralfate
	Formestane	Sumatriptan
	Ganciclovir	Tetrabenazine
	Gonadorelin analogues	*Tricyclic antidepressants*
	Ketotifen	Tryptophan
	Lamotrigine	Vigabatrin
	Levodopa	Zolpidem
	Lignocaine	Zopiclone

Adverse reaction	Drug	

Nervous system disorders (contd.)

Adverse reaction	Drug	
Extrapyramidal symptoms	*Antihistamines*	Methylphenidate
	Antipsychotic agents	Metoclopramide
	Apomorphine	Ondansetron
	Bromocriptine	Pergolide
	Cisapride	Phenytoin
	Dexamphetamine	Piracetam
	Domperidone	*SSRI antidepressants*
	Ethosuximide	Tetrabenazine
	Indoramin	*Tricyclic antidepressants*
	Levodopa	
Hiccups	*Corticosteroids*	Ondansetron
	Ethosuximide	
Intracranial hypertension	Amiodarone	*Quinolone antibiotics*
	Corticosteroids	Somatotropin
	Danazol	*Tetracyclines*
	Nitrofurantoin	
Light headedness	Adenosine	Cisapride
	Apomorphine	Nefazodone
	Baclofen	Nefopam
	Benzodiazepines	Tamoxifen
	Buspirone	Tryptophan
	Chloral hydrate	Zopiclone
Memory impairment	*Benzodiazepines*	Vigabatrin
	Gabapentin	Zolpidem
	Topiramate	Zopiclone
Migraine	Ganciclovir	Tacrolimus
	Gonadorelin analogues	Tibolone
Myasthenic syndrome	*Aminoglycosides*	Ganciclovir
	Fibrate antilipaemics	Penicillamine
Neuroleptic malignant syndrome	*Antipsychotic agents*	*SSRI antidepressants*
	Metoclopramide	*Tricyclic antidepressants*
	Pergolide	
Paraesthesia	*ACE inhibitors*	Cyclosporin
	Allopurinol	Etidronate
	Antihistamines	Ganciclovir
	Baclofen	*Gonadorelin analogues*
	Calcitonin	Indapamide
	Carbamazepine	Lansoprazole
	Carvedilol	Lignocaine
	Colistin	*MAOI antidepressants*

Adverse reaction	Drug	

Nervous system disorders (contd.)

Adverse reaction	Drug	
Paraesthesia *(contd.)*	Mefloquine	Salcatonin
	Meropenem	Sumatriptan
	Methysergide	Topiramate
	Mexiletine	Tocainide
	Nalidixic acid	Venlafaxine
	Nefazodone	Vigabatrin
	Ofloxacin	*Vinca alkaloids*
	Omeprazole	Zidovudine
	Riluzole	
Peripheral neuropathy or neuritis	Allopurinol	Griseofulvin
	Amiodarone	Isoniazid
	Amphotericin	Itraconazole
	Carboplatin	Levodopa
	Chloramphenicol	*MAOI antidepressants*
	Cisplatin	Mefloquine
	Colchicine	Metronidazole
	Cyclosporin	Nitrofurantoin
	Dapsone	Ofloxacin
	Didanosine	Paclitaxel
	Disulfiram	Phenytoin
	Docetaxel	Stavudine
	Ethambutol	Tinidazole
	Etidronate	*Vinca alkaloids*
	Flecainide	Zalcitabine
	Fludarabine	
Tardive dyskinesia	*Antipsychotic agents*	Metoclopramide
Tremor	Aciclovir	*MAOI antidepressants*
	Adrenaline	Mexiletine
	Amiodarone	Milrinone
	Antihistamines	Mycophenolate
	Antipsychotic agents	Nabilone
	Apomorphine	Ofloxacin
	Baclofen	Peppermint oil
	Beta-2 agonists	Phenytoin
	Ciprofloxacin	Sodium valproate
	Cycloserine	*SSRI antidepressants*
	Cyclosporin	Thyroxine
	Dexamphetamine	Tocainide
	Dopexamine	Toremifene
	Ephedrine	*Tricyclic antidepressants*
	Gabapentin	Venlafaxine
	Ganciclovir	Vigabatrin
	Lamotrigine	Zolpidem
	Lithium	

Adverse reaction	Drug	

Vertigo	Amiodarone	Minocycline
	Aspirin	Nabilone
	Benzodiazepines	*NSAIDs*
	Capreomycin	Omeprazole
	Chloral hydrate	*Opioids*
	Colistin	Riluzole
	Cycloserine	Sucralfate
	Doxazosin	Toremifene
	Ergotamine	Vitamin D
	Fibrate antilipaemics	Zolpidem
	Flucytosine	

Psychiatric disorders

Aggression	*Benzodiazepines*	Sodium valproate
	Carbamazepine	Vigabatrin
	Ethosuximide	Zopiclone
	Lamotrigine	
Agitation	Aciclovir	Pamidronate
	Antipsychotic agents	Phentermine
	Carbamazepine	Selegiline
	Lamotrigine	Tacrolimus
	Levodopa	Topiramate
	MAOI antidepressants	Venlafaxine
	Moclobemide	Vigabatrin
	Omeprazole	
Anxiety	Adrenaline	Norfloxacin
	Ephedrine	Ofloxacin
	Interferon-beta	Risperidone
	Mefloquine	*SSRI antidepressants*
	Naltrexone	Tacrolimus
	Nicotine	Venlafaxine
Confusion	Aciclovir	*Cephalosporins*
	Amiloride	Chlormethiazole
	Aminoglutethimide	Colistin
	Antimuscarinics	Cyclosporin
	Apomorphine	Dantrolene
	Atropine	Digoxin
	Baclofen	Ergotamine
	Barbiturates	Flucytosine
	Benzodiazepines	Ganciclovir
	Bromocriptine	Griseofulvin
	Buspirone	H_2-*receptor antagonists*
	Carbamazepine	Imipenem

Adverse reaction	Drug	

Psychiatric disorders (contd.)

Confusion *(contd.)*

Interferon-alfa	Piperazine	
Interferon-beta	Quinine	
Lamotrigine	*Quinolone antibiotics*	
Lignocaine	Selegiline	
MAOI antidepressants	Sodium valproate	
Mexiletine	Spironolactone	
Moclobemide	*SSRI antidepressants*	
Nabilone	Topiramate	
Nefazodone	Tocainide	
Nefopam	Tramadol	
Omeprazole	*Tricyclic antidepressants*	
Pamidronate	Vigabatrin	
Pergolide	Zolpidem	
Phenytoin	Zopiclone	

Delirium

Chloral hydrate, Clozapine, Digoxin

Dependence

Benzodiazepines, Chlormethiazole, *Corticosteroids*, Dexamphetamine, *Opioids*, Phentermine, Zopiclone

Depression

Alpha blockers, Aminoglutethimide, *Antihistamines*, *Antipsychotic agents*, Baclofen, Carbamazepine, Clomiphene, Clonidine, *Corticosteroids*, Crisantaspase, Cycloserine, Dantrolene, Dexfenfluramine, Diltiazem, Disulfiram, Ethosuximide, Fenfluramine, *Gonadorelin analogues*, Interferon-alfa, Interferon-beta, Lansoprazole, Levodopa, Mefloquine, Mesna, Methyldopa, Metoclopramide, Nabilone, Nifedipine, *Oestrogens*, Omeprazole, Phentermine, Piracetam, *Progestogens*, *Quinolone antibiotics*, Stanozolol, Tacrolimus, Tetrabenazine, Topiramate, Toremifene, Vigabatrin, Zolpidem

Adverse reaction	Drug	
Psychiatric disorders (contd.)		
Euphoria	Apomorphine	*MAOI antidepressants*
	Baclofen	Nabilone
	Clonidine	Phentermine
	Corticosteroids	Stanozolol
	Dexamphetamine	Tacrolimus
	Ethosuximide	
Excitement	*Antimuscarinics*	Chlormethiazole
	Barbiturates	Dexamphetamine
	Bromocriptine	Pizotifen
	Buspirone	Thyroxine
	Chloral hydrate	Vigabatrin
Hallucinations	Aciclovir	Nabilone
	Amantadine	Nefopam
	Apomorphine	Omeprazole
	Baclofen	*Opioids*
	Bromocriptine	Pamidronate
	Digoxin	Pergolide
	Flucytosine	Phentermine
	Lysuride	*Quinolone antibiotics*
	MAOI antidepressants	Tocainide
	Mefloquine	Zopiclone
Mania	Disulfiram	*SSRI antidepressants*
	Levodopa	*Tricyclic antidepressants*
	MAOI antidepressants	Vigabatrin
Mood disturbances	*ACE inhibitors*	*Gonadorelin analogues*
	Carvedilol	*Opioids*
	Chorionic gonadotrophin	*Progestogens*
		Topiramate
	Ganciclovir	Zopiclone
Nervousness	Amantadine	*Gonadorelin analogues*
	Antimuscarinics	*MAOI antidepressants*
	Buspirone	Methylphenidate
	Cephalosporins	Naltrexone
	Danazol	Nefopam
	Dantrolene	Phentermine
	Dexamphetamine	Phenytoin
	Dexfenfluramine	Piracetam
	Fenfluramine	*SSRI antidepressants*
	Gabapentin	Venlafaxine
	Ganciclovir	Vigabatrin
	Gestrinone	

Adverse reaction	Drug	

Psychiatric disorders (contd.)

Psychosis	Aciclovir	Isoniazid
	Carbamazepine	Levodopa
	Chloroquine	Lysuride
	Colistin	*MAOI antidepressants*
	Corticosteroids	Mefloquine
	Cycloserine	Nabilone
	Dexamphetamine	Nalidixic acid
	Dexfenfluramine	Ofloxacin
	Disopyramide	Phentermine
	Disulfiram	Procainamide
	Ethosuximide	Quinidine
	Fenfluramine	Selegiline
	Ganciclovir	Vigabatrin

Renal and urinary tract disorders

Cystitis	Cyclophosphamide	Tiaprofenic acid
Difficulty in micturition	*Antipsychotic agents*	*Opioids*
	Labetalol	Oxybutynin
	MAOI antidepressants	*Tricyclic antidepressants*
Haematuria	Amsacrine	*NSAIDs*
	Chloramphenicol	Pamidronate
	Ganciclovir	Penicillamine
	Mycophenolate	Sulphasalazine
Interstitial nephritis	*Cephalosporins*	Mesalazine
	Cimetidine	*NSAIDs*
	Ciprofloxacin	Omeprazole
	Co-amoxiclav	Vancomycin
Nephrotic syndrome	Penicillamine	Sulphasalazine
	Probenecid	
Proteinuria	Carbamazepine	Sodium aurothiomalate
	Penicillamine	Sulphasalazine
Renal impairment or failure	*ACE inhibitors*	Cyclosporin
	Aciclovir	Enoximone
	Aminoglutethimide	Ethosuximide
	Aminoglycosides	Foscarnet
	Amphotericin	Ganciclovir
	Capreomycin	Gemcitabine
	Carbamazepine	Imipenem
	Carboplatin	Indapamide
	Cisplatin	Mitomycin
	Colistin	Mycophenolate

Adverse reaction	Drug	

Renal and urinary tract disorders (contd.)

Renal impairment or failure (contd.)	*NSAIDs* Pamidronate Pentamidine Quinine	*Quinolone antibiotics* Rifampicin Sulphinpyrazone Vancomycin
Urinary frequency or urgency	*Alpha blockers* Cisapride Dexfenfluramine Fenfluramine Ganciclovir	Lithium Nicardipine Nifedipine Phentermine Probenecid
Urinary retention	*Antihistamines* *Antimuscarinics* *Benzodiazepines* Disopyramide Enoximone	Ipratropium Nefopam Oxitropium Oxybutynin
Urine discolouration	Danthron Imipenem Levodopa Metronidazole Nefopam Phenindione	Phenolphthalein Rifabutin Rifampicin Sulphasalazine Tinidazole

Reproductive system disorders

Breast pain or tenderness	Bicalutamide Clomiphene Ganciclovir	*Gonadorelin analogues* *Oestrogens* *Progestogens*
Fertility impaired	*Alkylating cytotoxics* *Anabolic steroids* Carbamazepine *Flutamide*	Ganciclovir Nitrofurantoin Sulphasalazine
Galactorrhoea	*Antipsychotic agents* Carbamazepine Cyproterone	Domperidone Flutamide *Tricyclic antidepressants*
Gynaecomastia	*Antipsychotic agents* Bicalutamide Carbamazepine *Chorionic gonadotrophin* Cyproterone Domperidone Flutamide *Gonadorelin analogues*	H_2-receptor antagonists* Isoniazid Omeprazole Sodium valproate Spironolactone *Tricyclic antidepressants* Verapamil

Adverse reaction	Drug	
Reproductive system disorders (contd.)		
Impotence	*ACE inhibitors*	*Fibrate antilipaemics*
	Antipsychotic agents	Finasteride
	Bicalutamide	Indapamide
	Carbamazepine	Naltrexone
	Cimetidine	Omeprazole
	Clonidine	*Opioids*
	Dexfenfluramine	Spironolactone
	Fenfluramine	*Thiazide diuretics*
Libido altered	Acamprosate	Fenfluramine
	Benzodiazepines	Finasteride
	Bicalutamide	Flutamide
	Dexfenfluramine	*Gonadorelin analogues*
	Disulfiram	*Opioids*
	Domperidone	*Progestogens*
Menstruation disorders	*Anabolic steroids*	Itraconazole
	Antipsychotic agents	Misoprostol
	Clomiphene	Nicotine
	Corticosteroids	*Progestogens*
	Cyclosporin	Rifampicin
	Danazol	Sodium valproate
	Gestrinone	Spironolactone
	Gonadorelin analogues	Tamoxifen
	Interferon-beta	
Priapism	Alprostadil	Testosterone
	Clozapine	Trazodone
	Mesterolone	
Sexual dysfunction	*Adrenergic neurone blockers*	Naltrexone
	Indoramin	*SSRI antidepressants*
	MAOI antidepressants	Thioridazine
	Methyldopa	*Tricyclic antidepressants*
		Venlafaxine
Vaginal bleeding	Ethosuximide	Tamoxifen
	Formestane	Tibolone
	Misoprostol	Toremifene
Respiratory disorders		
Alveolitis	Aminoglutethimide	*NSAIDs*
	Amiodarone	Sulphasalazine
	Mesalazine	Tocainide

Adverse reaction	Drug	

Respiratory disorders (contd.)

Bronchospasm	Adenosine	*NSAIDs*
	Amiodarone	Omeprazole
	Antihistamines	Piperazine
	Aspirin	Rifabutin
	Beta-2 agonists	Sodium cromoglycate
	Beta-blockers	Teicoplanin
	Interferon-beta	Vancomycin
	Nedocromil	
Cough	*ACE inhibitors*	Nedocromil
	Fludarabine	Nitrofurantoin
	Gabapentin	Sodium cromoglycate
	Mycophenolate	
Dyspnoea	Adenosine	Nitrofurantoin
	Bicalutamide	Pergolide
	Carbamazepine	Protamine sulphate
	Fludarabine	Rifampicin
	Fluoxetine	Tacrolimus
	Ganciclovir	Toremifene
	Moracizine	Vancomycin
	Mycophenolate	
Nasal congestion	*Adrenergic neurone blockers*	Doxazosin
		Hydrazine
	Butyrophenones	Indoramin
	Carvedilol	Methyldopa
	Chlormethiazole	*Phenothiazines*
	Co-dergocrine	Quinagolide
Pleural effusion	Bromocriptine	Tacrolimus
Pneumonitis	Azathioprine	*Thiazide diuretics*
	Carbamazepine	Tocainide
	Methotrexate	
Pulmonary fibrosis	Amiodarone	Fluoxetine
	Bleomycin	Mitomycin
	Busulphan	Sodium aurothiomalate
	Carmustine	Tocainide
Respiratory depression	*Barbiturates*	*Opioids*
	Butyrophenones	*Phenothiazines*
	Lignocaine	
Rhinitis	Gabapentin	Risperidone
	Pergolide	

Adverse reaction	Drug	

Skin and subcutaneous tissue disorders

Acne	*Anabolic steroids*	*Gonadorelin analogues*
	Corticosteroids	Mycophenolate
	Danazol	Phenytoin
	Ganciclovir	*Progestogens*
	Gestrinone	
Angioedema	*ACE inhibitors*	Nitrofurantoin
	Antihistamines	*NSAIDs*
	Beta-2 agonists	Ofloxacin
	Etidronate	Omeprazole
	Fluconazole	*Penicillins*
	Fluoxetine	Phentermine
	Gemfibrozil	Piperazine
	H$_2$-receptor antagonists	Probucol
	Heparin	Procainamide
	Itraconazole	Quinidine
	Lamotrigine	Quinine
	Mebendazole	*Statins*
	Metronidazole	Tinidazole
Bullous eruptions	Acamprosate	Fluconazole
	Chlormethiazole	Omeprazole
	Ciprofloxaxin	
Epidermal necrolysis	*ACE inhibitors*	Griseofulvin
	Carbamazepine	Imipenem
	Cephalosporins	Indapamide
	Chlorambucil	Lamotrigine
	Ciprofloxacin	Norfloxacin
	Co-amoxiclav	Phenytoin
	Co-trimoxazole	Terbinafine
	Dapsone	Trimethoprim
Erythema multiforme/Stevens Johnson syndrome	*ACE inhibitors*	Diltiazem
	Aminoglutethimide	Ethosuximide
	Amlodipine	Fluconazole
	Carbamazepine	Griseofulvin
	Cephalosporins	Indapamide
	Chlorambucil	Isoniazid
	Chloramphenicol	Itraconazole
	Cinoxacin	Lamotrigine
	Ciprofloxacin	Mefloquine
	Clarithromycin	Methylphenidate
	Co-amoxiclav	Nifedipine
	Co-trimoxazole	Nitrofurantoin
	Dapsone	Norfloxacin

Adverse reaction	Drug	

Skin and subcutaneous tissue disorders (contd.)

Erythema multiforme/Stevens Johnson syndrome *(contd.)*	Nystatin	Ranitidine
	Ofloxacin	Sulphasalazine
	Omeprazole	*Sulphonylureas*
	Penicillamine	Terbinafine
	Pentamidine	Tocainide
	Phenytoin	Trimethoprim
	Piperazine	Vancomycin
Exfoliative dermatitis	Aminoglutethimide	Nitrofurantoin
	Amiodarone	*Sulphonylureas*
	Co-amoxiclav	Tocainide
	Methylphenidate	Vancomycin
Flushing	*ACE inhibitors*	Ondansetron
	Adenosine	*Opioids*
	Anastrozole	*Oxerutins*
	Atropine	Oxpentifylline
	Bicalutamide	Oxybutynin
	Cabergoline	Pentamidine
	Calcitonin	Probenecid
	Calcium channel blockers	Protamine sulphate
	Clomiphene	Quinagolide
	Co-dergocrine	Quinine
	Danazol	Rifampicin
	Epoprostenol	Salcatonin
	Formestane	Sumatriptan
	Gestrinone	Tamoxifen
	Gonadorelin analogues	Thymoxamine
	Levodopa	Thyroxine
	Nicorandil	Toremifene
	Nicotinic acid derivatives	Vancomycin
	Nitrates	
Hair growth	Aminoglutethimide	Formestane
	Anabolic steroids	Gestrinone
	Corticosteroids	Minoxidil
	Cyclosporin	Phenytoin
	Danazol	*Progestogens*
	Finasteride	Tibolone
Hair loss	*ACE inhibitors*	Bicalutamide
	Allopurinol	Carbamazepine
	Amiodarone	Carbimazole
	Anastrozole	Chloroquine
	Antihistamines	Clomiphene
	Azathioprine	Colchicine

Adverse reaction	Drug

Skin and subcutaneous tissue disorders (contd.)

Hair loss *(contd.)*	*Cytotoxic agents*	Omeprazole
	Danazol	Phenindione
	Fibrate antilipaemics	*Progestogens*
	Fluoxetine	Proguanil
	Formestane	Propylthiouracil
	Ganciclovir	Sodium aurothiomalate
	Heparin	Sodium valproate
	Itraconazole	Stanozolol
	Mefloquine	Tamoxifen
	Methylphenidate	Toremifene
	Methysergide	Vigabatrin
	Nicoumalone	Warfarin
Photosensitivity	Amiodarone	*NSAIDs*
	Antihistamines	Omeprazole
	Antipsychotic agents	*Quinolone antibiotics*
	Carbamazepine	Sulphasalazine
	Chlorpropamide	Terbinafine
	Flecainide	*Tetracyclines*
	Griseofulvin	*Thiazide diuretics*
	Indapamide	Triamterene
	Lamotrigine	*Tricyclic antidepressants*
	Loop diuretics	
Pruritus	Acamprosate	Itraconazole
	Alverine citrate	Lacidipine
	Aminoglutethimide	Mefloquine
	Betahistine	Meropenem
	Bicalutamide	Miconazole
	Carbimazole	Nitrofurantoin
	Cephalsporins	*Opioids*
	Chenodeoxycholic acid	Pamidronate
	Chloroquine	Propylthiouracil
	Didanosine	*Proton pump inhibitors*
	Etidronate	*Quinolone antibiotics*
	Felodipine	Sucralfate
	Fibrate antilipaemics	Tibolone
	Fluoxetine	Toremifene
	Flutamide	Trimethoprim
	Formestane	Vancomycin
	Ganciclovir	Verapamil
	Gonadorelin analogues	Zalcitabine
	Imipenem	
Purpura	Co-trimoxazole	*MAOI antidepressants*
	Isoniazid	*Tricyclic antidepressants*

Adverse reaction	Drug	

Skin and subcutaneous tissue disorders (contd.)

Skin discolouration	Amiodarone	*Phenothiazines*
	Bleomycin	Toremifene
	Busulphan	Zidovudine
	Minocycline	
Skin necrosis	Heparin	Phenindione
	Nicoumalone	Warfarin
Sweating	*Antihistamines*	Omeprazole
	Bicalutamide	*Opioids*
	Dexamphetamine	Sodium nitroprusside
	Epoprostenol	*SSRI antidepressants*
	Ganciclovir	Thyroxine
	Gonadorelin analogues	Toremifene
	Levodopa	*Tricyclic antidepressants*
	MAOI antidepressants	Venlafaxine
	Naltrexone	Vitamin D
	Nefopam	Zalcitabine
	Nizatidine	
Urticaria	*ACE inhibitors*	*Macrolide antibiotics*
	Aminoglutethimide	Mebendazole
	Aztreonam	Mefloquine
	Beta-2 agonists	Meropenem
	Capreomycin	Methylphenidate
	Cephalosporins	Metronidazole
	Chlormethiazole	Nitrofurantoin
	Ciprofloxacin	Nystatin
	Dornase alfa	Omeprazole
	Etidronate	*Opioids*
	Fibrate antilipaemics	*Penicillins*
	Fluoxetine	Piperazine
	Ganciclovir	*Progestogens*
	Gonadorelin analogues	Rifampicin
	H_2-receptor antagonists	Spectinomycin
	Heparin	Terbinafine
	Imipenem	Tinadazole
	Interferon-beta	*Tricyclic antidepressants*
	Itraconazole	Vancomycin
	Lansoprazole	Vigabatrin
	Loperamide	Zopiclone

Miscellaneous disorders

Back pain	Alprostadil	*Thrombolytics*
	Captopril	Toremifene
	Danazol	Vancomycin
	Gonadorelin analogues	

Adverse reaction	Drug

Miscellaneous disorders (contd.)

Chest pain

Adenosine
Bicalutamide
Buspirone
Flutamide
Ganciclovir
Lacidipine
Macrolide antibiotics
Milrinone
Moracizine
Mycophenolate
Naltrexone
Nicotine
Ondansetron
Sumatriptan
Toremifene
Zalcitabine

Fatigue

ACE inhibitors
Aciclovir
Amiodarone
Beta-blockers
Buspirone
Calcium channel blockers
Chorionic
    gonadotrophin
Cyproterone
Digoxin
Disulfiram
Doxazosin
Fibrate antilipaemics
Flutamide
Foscarnet
Gabapentin
Gonadorelin analogues
Griseofulvin
H$_2$-receptor antagonists
Indapamide
Lamotrigine
Lansoprazole
MAOI antidepressants
Mefloquine
Mesna
Moracizine
Moxonidine
Propafenone
Risperidone
Statins
Sumatriptan
Topiramate
Toremifene
Tropisetron
Vigabatrin
Zalcitabine

Fever

Aminoglutethimide
Amphotericin
Atovaquone
Atropine
Azathioprine
Carbamazepine
Cephalosporins
Clozapine
Didanosine
Ganciclovir
Hydralazine
Imipenem
Isoniazid
Lamotrigine
Mefloquine
Methylphenidate
Nefazodone
Omeprazole
Pamidronate
Penicillins
Phenindione
Phenytoin
Procainamide
Pyrazinamide
Quinidine
Quinolone antibiotics
Rifabutin
Spectinomycin
SSRI antidepressants
Sulphasalazine
Sulphonylureas
Teicoplanin
Tocainide
Tricyclic antidepressants
Vancomycin
Zalcitabine
Zidovudine

Adverse reaction	Drug	
Miscellaneous disorders (contd.)		
Insomnia	Amantadine	Moclobemide
	Aminoglutethimide	Mycophenolate
	Aminophylline	Nefopam
	Antipsychotic agents	Nicardipine
	Atovaquone	Nicotine
	Bicalutamide	Omeprazole
	Clomiphene	Pamidronate
	Corticosteroids	Pergolide
	Dexamphetamine	Phentermine
	Dexfenfluramine	Phenytoin
	Didanosine	Piracetam
	Enoximone	*Progestogens*
	Ephedrine	Quinagolide
	Fenfluramine	*SSRI antidepressants*
	Flutamide	*Statins*
	Lamotrigine	Theophylline
	Levodopa	Thyroxine
	MAOI antidepressants	Torimefene
	Mefloquine	Venlafaxine
	Methylphenidate	Zidovudine
	Methysergide	

Glossary

Adverse drug reaction (ADR)   A response to a drug which is noxious and unintended and which occurs at doses normally used in man for the prophylaxis, diagnosis or therapy of disease or for the modification of a physiological function.

Black triangle ▼   The symbol used to denote that there is limited experience of the use of the product. All suspected adverse reactions should be reported to the Committee on Safety of Medicines (CSM).

Clearance   The volume of plasma from which a drug is eliminated in unit time. Clearance is the sum of elimination processes by renal, hepatic and other mechanisms.

Committee on Safety of Medicines (CSM)   The CSM is a Government appointed committee that advises on safety, quality and efficacy of new medicines and monitors adverse reactions to medicines already on the market.

Conjugation   Conjugation is a means by which the biological activity of certain chemical substances is altered and the substances made ready for excretion.

Controlled drug (CD)   A CD is a substance controlled by the Misuse of Drugs Act 1971.

Data sheet   A data sheet is a manufacturer's document containing information on the presentation, uses, dosage, administration, side effects, contra-indications and precautions related to a medicine.

General Sale List (GSL) medicine   A GSL medicine is a substance described in a General Sale List Order made under the Medicines Act 1968. It can be bought in non-pharmacy outlets.

Medicines Act 1968   The Medicines Act is the legislative framework that controls the licensing of medicines. It provides the structure for the marketing and use of medicines.

Pharmacokinetics   Pharmacokinetics is the study of the process and time course of drug absorption, distribution, metabolism and elimination.

Pharmacy medicine (P)   A Pharmacy medicine is a substance which is not subject to the prescription only requirements of the Medicines (Prescription Only) Order and which is not included in a General Sale List Order. It can be bought from pharmacies.

Placebo   A placebo is a pharmacologically inactive substance.

Post-marketing surveillance   Post-marketing surveillance is the systematic process that monitors the safety of marketed medicines.

Prescription only medicine (POM)   A POM is a substance in the Medicines (Prescription Only) Order. It may be supplied to the public only on a practitioner's prescription.

Steady state   A point following multiple dosing when the rate of drug elimination is equal to the rate at which a drug enters the body. Steady state is commonly accepted to occur after four or five half-lives. With repeated dosing at steady state, the concentration will rise and fall by an equal amount.

Summary of Product Characteristics (SPC)   A Summary of Product Characteristics is a manufacturer's document containing information on the presentation, uses, dosage, administration, side effects, contra-indications and precautions related to a medicine. From January 1998 all new drugs introduced to the market have a SPC rather than a data sheet.

Therapeutic window   Above a certain concentration, the drug may induce dose related adverse effects: below a certain concentration, the drug may have little or no effect. Between these two concentrations lies the therapeutic window.

Yellow card   A yellow card is the reporting scheme for adverse reactions to drugs. Pads of yellow cards are found in the *British National Formulary* and the *Compendium of Data Sheets and Summaries of Product Characteristics*. Reports are sent to the Committee on Safety of Medicines.

Subject Index

Medicines, Drugs and Chemicals Index

Page numbers of the contents of Appendices 1 and 2 are not included